THE SCHOOL OF PHARMACY UNIVERSITY OF LONDON

MEDICINES, SCIENCE AND SOCIETY, 1842–2012

BRIONY HUDSON
IN COLLABORATION WITH MAUREEN BOYLAN

For Elsevier
Commissioning Editor: Kristine Jones
Development Editor: Andy Albrecht
Project Manager: Julia Haynes
Designer: Mark Rogers

THE SCHOOL OF PHARMACY UNIVERSITY OF LONDON

MEDICINES, SCIENCE AND SOCIETY, 1842–2012

BRIONY HUDSON
IN COLLABORATION WITH MAUREEN BOYLAN

ELSEVIER

AMSTERDAM • BOSTON • HEIDELBERG • LONDON • NEW YORK • OXFORD • PARIS • SAN DIEGO
SAN FRANCISCO • SINGAPORE • SYDNEY • TOKYO

Academic Press is an imprint of Elsevier

Academic Press is an imprint of Elsevier
32 Jamestown Road, London NW1 7BY, UK
225 Wyman Street, Waltham, MA 02451, USA
525 B Street, Suite 1800, San Diego, CA 92101-4495, USA

British Library Cataloguing-in-Publication Data
A catalogue record for this book is available from the British Library

Library of Congress Cataloging-in-Publication Data
A catalog record for this book is available from the Library of Congress

ISBN : 978-0-12-407665-5

For information on all Academic Press publications visit our website at www.store.elsevier.com

Typeset by MPS Limited, Chennai, India
www.adi-mps.com

Printed and bound in China

13 14 15 16 17 10 9 8 7 6 5 4 3 2 1

CONTENTS

ACKNOWLEDGEMENTS

Like so many "big ideas", this one was hatched over a good meal (the last of the Charter dinners), in convivial company and at just the right time … and then it took on a life of its own. I first envisaged this book as a memento for the School's alumni to mark an ending, and in a way to say farewell to the old School of Pharmacy. It very quickly grew beyond that and turned into a plan to create something which, while telling the School's own history, would put it firmly in its social and historical context – 170 years of transformational changes in public health, the creation of a modern primary care medical profession, within an educational sector changed beyond recognition. It also became clear that this wasn't just a retrospective, but "the story so far" as the School enters its new life within UCL.

At each stage, there were key people who saw the potential and provided practical support and excellent ideas: Paul Ayris (Director of UCL Libraries), who introduced me to Suzanne BeDell, Managing Director of Science and Technology Books at Elsevier (and who also lent me a book on the history of UCL that I really will return one day!); Elsevier staff in the US and UK, most especially Kristine Jones and Andy Albrecht; the many colleagues who told me that Briony Hudson was the only possible choice of author because she knew everything and everybody, and would "totally get it"; and most of all, Briony Hudson, who totally got it, and who expertly turned a dinner table conversation into a real history.

Maureen Boylan

"Picture some student, up at the Square in 2013, fingering a copy of the 'Square Chronicle', yellow with age, and learning how Mr Jinks won the Pereira Medal in 1913, or how a year later the 'Square' regained the 'Cup'. One must think of posterity."

Square Chronicle, November 1913

Although Jacob Bell and Theophilus Redwood provided the history of the School and its foundation in their *Historical Sketch of the Progress of Pharmacy in Great Britain*, published in 1880, there was nothing dedicated to its history until more than 120 years after its establishment. In *The Pharmaceutical Journal* of September 1896, there was a call for a history of the School to be written, with past students urged to send their experiences to the *Journal's* editor to be compiled. According to a tribute to Professor Greenish in *The Pharmaceutical Journal* in August 1933, the professor had intended to write a history of the School alongside pharmaceutical education and training in his retirement, but had not had the time. It was T.E. Wallis who took up the challenge with his *History of the School of Pharmacy*, published in 1964. As both student and long-serving staff member, Wallis was perfectly placed to provide a detailed account of the institution and its buildings, illustrated with his own photographs. It has not left my side during the process of writing this book. Three decades later, S.W.F. Holloway's publications, particularly *Royal Pharmaceutical*

Society of Great Britain 1841–1991: A Political and Social History, but also his articles on the School and the Pharmaceutical Society, have been invaluable in providing detail and context.

Many people have been involved in the production of this publication from initial ideas to practical assistance. Maureen Boylan has been a fantastically supportive and enthusiastic collaborator, and the originator of the concept to commemorate the School's latest milestone by putting it into its historical context. Ainley Wade, as a past student, current Fellow and publications maestro, has been the epitome of a reviewer. Anthony Smith has also shared his thoughts and experiences to ensure the accuracy of the narrative.

Michelle Wake and her staff at the School's library, particularly Cherry Trott, who looks after the historical collections, have been extremely good hosts. John Betts and Peter Homan at the RPS Museum, and Martha Krumbach at the RPS Library have made my visits easy and enjoyable. The staff at the Wellcome Library have also been a great help. Morgan Williams, David Phillipson, Tony Moffatt and Eric Robbins have all provided useful contributions. Charles Harmer, Diane and Martin Hudson, and Amy Matthews have all given practical and emotional help that has meant that the project was possible. My final thanks go to Lucy for retaining her afternoon nap.

Our aim in producing this publication has been to commemorate the School's history within its pharmaceutical context. In doing so, we hope not to have missed major milestones, but would be pleased to have our attention drawn to any errors or inaccuracies. Our wish is that the book will prompt past and current students, and pharmacy and educational historians, to explore further the history of the School.

Briony Hudson

ACKNOWLEDGEMENTS

Unsurprisingly, the majority of images in the book come from the collections at the UCL School of Pharmacy and the Royal Pharmaceutical Society Museum. However, many other people and institutions have provided help and illustrations. Our thanks go to:

- Picture Library staff at the National Portrait Gallery, Wellcome Images and the Museum of London
- Olivia Timbs and Stuart Thomas at *The Pharmaceutical Journal*
- Jennifer Richardson at *Chemist + Druggist*
- Emm Johnstone, Gail Nevin, Jayne Grant and Laura MacCulloch at Royal Holloway, University of London
- Alison Hawkins at Hastings Museum and Art Gallery
- Victor Patterson
- Jo Hopkins at The Royal Society
- Professor K.D.Rainsford and Dr. Hans Detlef Klüber, *Inflammopharmacology*
- Sarah Hunt at the University of Sunderland
- Professor Gary Baxter at the Welsh School of Pharmacy
- David Hale at mapco.net
- Mandy Wise at UCL Special Collections
- Professor Peter Houghton and Richard Harper, Pharmacy Department, King's College London

FOREWORD

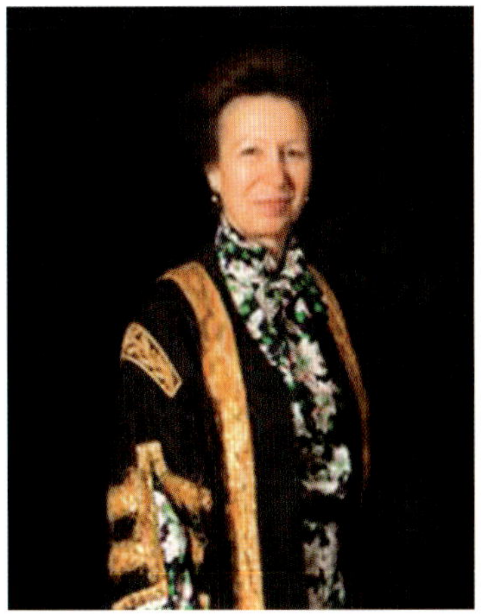

BUCKINGHAM PALACE

As Chancellor of the University of London, I am pleased to introduce this publication marking the 170th anniversary of the School of Pharmacy, and the start of its new incarnation within University College London.

My family's relationship with the School dates back to its very earliest days, when Queen Victoria granted a Royal Charter to the School's parent body, the Royal Pharmaceutical Society, in 1843. This was just two years after the Society's foundation, and one year after the School's. My great-grandfather, King George VI, granted his Patronage to the Society in 1937, and The Queen continues in this role today.

The School 's own Royal Charter was granted by Her Majesty in May 1952, only three months after her accession, and in 1960 my grandmother, the late Queen Mother, then Chancellor of the University of London, officially opened the School's present premises in Brunswick Square. At the opening ceremony she remarked that, as its construction had started as early as 1938, before being badly delayed by the War and post-war shortages, the School was going to inhabit 'the oldest new building in London'.

My own relationship with the School goes back to March 1985 when I attended its Foundation Day event. In 1992, I was delighted to join in the celebrations for the School's 150th anniversary, and it was a great pleasure to visit again in 2008 to open the School's new molecular pharmacy wing.

On my first visit to the School I commented that I was 'aware of the sense of pride which rightly exists among staff and students and the influence which The School of Pharmacy continues to exert, not only inside the profession which founded it and the University which adopted it but also outside, in the wider national and international circles where its activities impinge and influence is felt. Long may it be so.'

I was echoing the sentiments of H.J.Waring, the Vice Chancellor who brought the School into the University of London in 1926, and who promised the University's enduring support for its newest member 'provided that whatever is done is for the progress of science, the good of the nation, and the improvement of the vocation of pharmaceutical chemists and pharmacists'.

At this latest milestone in its long history, I would like to wish the School continued success in the future.

Anne

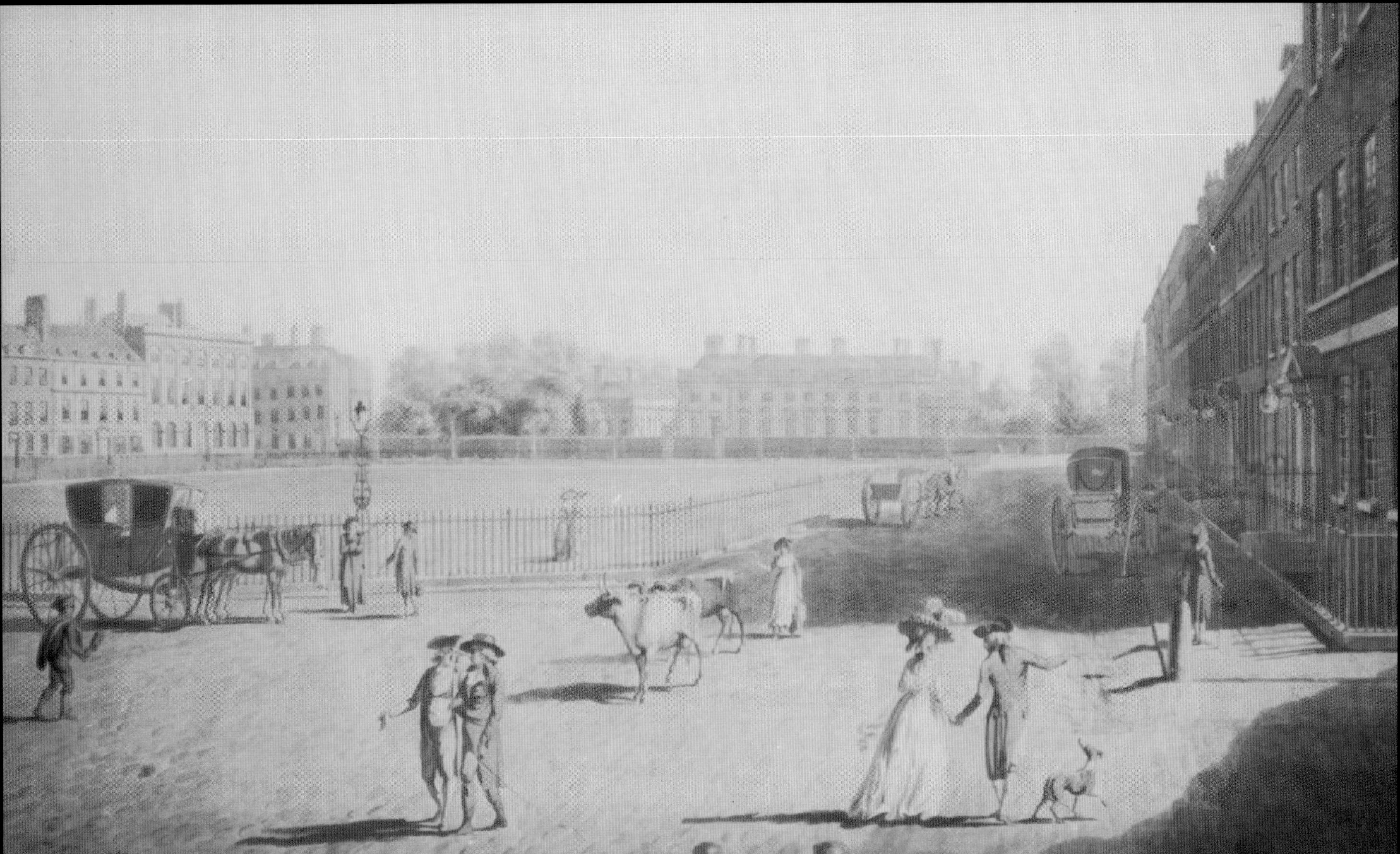

Edward Dayes (1763–1804) created this atmospheric view of Bloomsbury Square, published as an engraving in 1787. Bedford House is shown dominating the north side of the square, while number 17 is clearly shown on the left side with its new neo-classical facade.

MILESTONES

Popular Culture

1843	first Christmas cards sent in Britain
1848	*The Communist Manifesto*, by Karl Marx and Friedrich Engels, published
1849	safety pin patented
1856	first synthetic aniline dye, named mauve, discovered
1859	Charles Darwin's *On the Origin of Species* published

London Life

1841	Kew Gardens given to the nation
1842	*The Illustrated London News*, the first ever illustrated newspaper, launched
1843	Thames Tunnel, designed by Brunel, opened
1843	Nelson's statue publicly displayed before placement on its column in Trafalgar Square
1847	London Zoo first opened to paying visitors
1848	electric lighting publicly demonstrated on the steps of the National Gallery
1851	Great Exhibition
1851	150 horse bus routes operated in London
1853	first free-standing letter box London
1854	very cold winter allowed skating on the Serpentine lake in Hyde Park
1858	Great Stink
1859	Vauxhall Pleasure Gardens closed

National News

1842	Queen Victoria and Prince Albert took their first train journey from Windsor (Slough) to Paddington
1842	Mines and Collieries Act prohibited women, girls, and boys under 10 years old from working underground in mines
1848	Chartist demonstrations in London, Manchester, and Bingley in Yorkshire
1854	John Snow traced cholera to a pump in Broad Street, London
1858	Great Ormond Street Hospital, the first children's hospital in Britain, opened
1858	Medical Act introduced regulated medical practice and education in Britain
1860	Florence Nightingale opened a School of Nursing at St Thomas' Hospital, London

The Wider World

1844	first use of the telegraph, by Samuel Morse
1845–1851	Irish Potato Famine
1846	US/Canadian border defined
1848	California gold rush
1852	submarine patented
1854–1856	Crimean War
1856–1860	Second Opium War in China
1857–1858	Indian Mutiny
1858	first telegraph cable laid under the Atlantic

Drug Developments/Pharmacy Milestones

1842	American William E. Clarke extracted a tooth using ether as an anaesthetic
1844	William Brockeden patented his "compressed pill" (tablet)
1846	Robert Liston, a London surgeon, amputated a patient's thigh using ether
1847	James Young Simpson in Edinburgh first used chloroform anaesthesia
1851	Arsenic Act
1852	Pharmacy Act
1853	Queen Victoria given chloroform for labour pain
1859	*Chemist and Druggist* journal founded

On Wednesday 16th February 1842, Dr Anthony Todd Thomson gave a lecture on materia medica, the raw materials of medicines, at 17 Bloomsbury Square, an eighteenth century house in a fashionable part of London. His audience was a group of chemists, druggists and apprentices brought together by a newly formed professional organisation, the Pharmaceutical Society of Great Britain. For most of them, it was a very different experience from anything that they had encountered before.

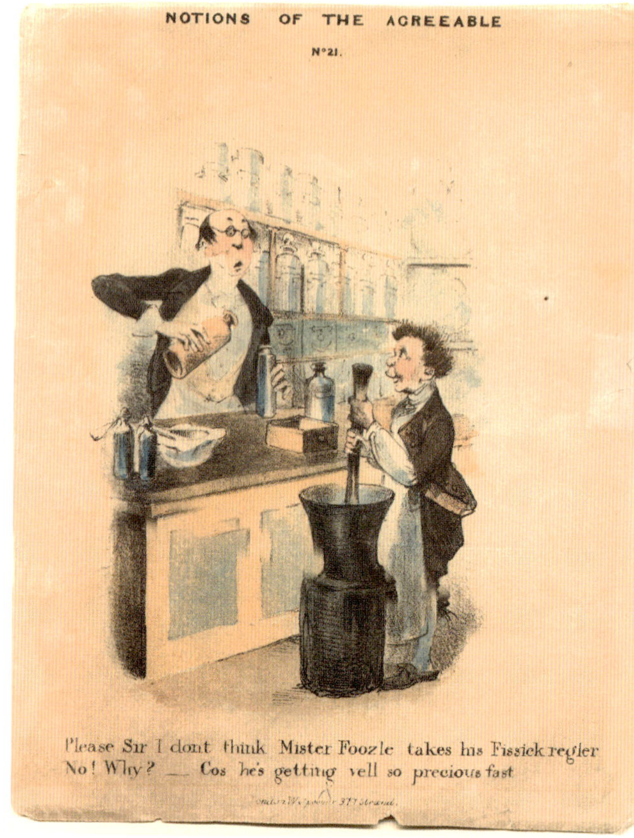
NOTIONS OF THE AGREEABLE
N°21.
Please Sir I dont think Mister Foozle takes his Fissick regler
No! Why? __ Cos he's getting vell so precious fast

Published in the 1830s, this cartoon gives an idea of what the inside of a pharmacy might have looked like in this decade, as well as making the viewer laugh at the apprentice's ignorance and outspokenness.

Royal Pharmaceutical Society Museum

There was no such thing as an average pharmacist in the mid-nineteenth century and, in fact, the term pharmacist was not one that the majority would have recognised. However, there were some common features to the work of someone who made and sold medicines. A pharmacy premises would have contained some kind of laboratory where pills could be rolled, powders mixed and suppositories made. Pharmacy was a craft with manual skills passed from master to apprentice and father to son. The shop itself would probably have had shelves filled with jars, bottles and packets, some bought in from the manufacturer such as Beecham's Pills, Dalby's Carminative and Daffy's Elixir, and others made on the premises. Most customers would come in to buy a preparation for an everyday ailment such as a cough or a boil, or to ask for a family recipe to be made up for them, or in exceptional circumstances, to have a prescription dispensed from a private physician. In some instances, the customer might be an artist wanting to buy some pigments, a farmer wanting a medicine for a horse, or a scientist sourcing a particular chemical. In a world with limited transport, a pharmacy shop would build up a group of local regulars, and the local regulars would come to trust the pharmacist to advise them on their health.

LONDON LIFE

Arguably, the need for medical advice and the production of medicines had never been greater. London in the mid-nineteenth century was crowded, dirty and very unhealthy. In 1801, 20% of people in Britain lived in cities, by 1850 it was approximately 50% and by 1901 it had grown to around 80%. One of the major results of the increasing number of people all living together was a growth in infectious diseases. London's streets were filled with horse manure, night soil men took away as much human detritus as they could, and there was no sewerage system until after the Great Stink of 1858, when the smell of open sewers and cesspits through a very hot summer finally focused the minds of members of parliament (MPs) on the urgent need for a solution to London's sewage problems. The levels of pollution and smog were a catalyst for respiratory diseases, and the high incidence of rickets in cities was partly due to poor diet, but also because access to sunlight was cut by smogs. Average life expectancy in London in 1841 was 37 years (although a shocking 26 years in Liverpool). The average age of death for servants and labourers was only 16 years, according to the Registrar General.

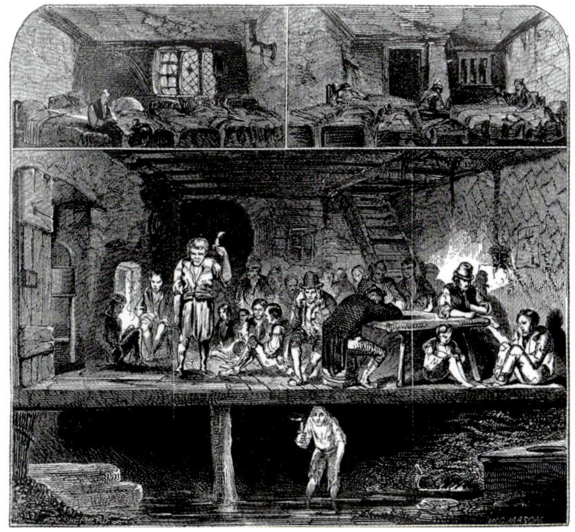

A crowded lodging house in Bethnal Green, east London, shown in Hector Gavin's *Sanitary Ramblings* (1848).

Wellcome Library, London

The close proximity of neighbours and the slum conditions rife across the capital also made epidemics a common occurrence. Between 1831 and 1833 there were two influenza epidemics, followed in the years around 1840 by epidemics of 'flu, typhus, typhoid and cholera. Between 1838 and 1840 in England and Wales, 50,000 people were killed by measles and whooping cough, and in 1840, scarlet fever was responsible for 20,000 deaths in one year. Between 1837 and 1840, a smallpox epidemic killed 6,400 people in London, and in 1854, 10,738 people in London died during a cholera outbreak. Tuberculosis has been estimated to account for 20 million deaths over the nineteenth century. It was, unsurprisingly, the poor, the young and the elderly who were most vulnerable. At the end of the nineteenth century, 20% of infants still died before their first birthday and it has been calculated that children up to the age of five counted for one-third of all deaths in Victorian Britain.

Clearly, chemists & druggists and their medicines and advice could not alleviate the overcrowding or improve the sanitation. It was governmental intervention that was required, and major projects such as Joseph Balzagette's sewerage system. In 1853, an Act of Parliament introduced compulsory smallpox vaccination, the first time that the Government had tried to enforce a medical treatment across the whole population. There were many objectors: an average 2,000 people a year were prosecuted for resistance. Meanwhile, the chemist & druggist offered an option for those who could not afford to see a doctor, and who had enough money to buy some kind of treatment for their symptoms.

They were not without their critics. John Murray, in *Blackwood's Magazine* of July 1841, described "swarms of chemists, who, without education, qualification, or experience, impudently take upon themselves to prescribe for all manner of ailments." In 1844, the Select Committee on Medical Poor Relief saw the chemist & druggist as an unethical pedlar of unreliable potions:

> the easy access to the druggist's shop, vying with the gin palace in its tempting decorations, attracts those who prefer spending a few pence to encountering the formalities and delay attendant on an application to a qualified practitioner. Then the speedy apprehension of the case by the druggist's shopman, a glance being sufficient to satisfy him both as to its nature and treatment, and his ready selection of some drug as a certain cure for the malady of the customer, all this tells wonderfully on the ignorant of all classes.

For those who could not afford the doctor, there were few other options. The only free medical care came from charitable hospitals, such as the Royal Free Hospital, founded in 1828 to provide free hospital care to those who could not afford treatment. The title "Royal" was granted by Queen Victoria in 1837 in recognition of the hospital's work with cholera victims. Friendly societies provided a solution for those who could find a small regular sum, with people making regular contributions in order to draw on them at times of need. There were more than 30,000 societies in operation by the end of the nineteenth century.

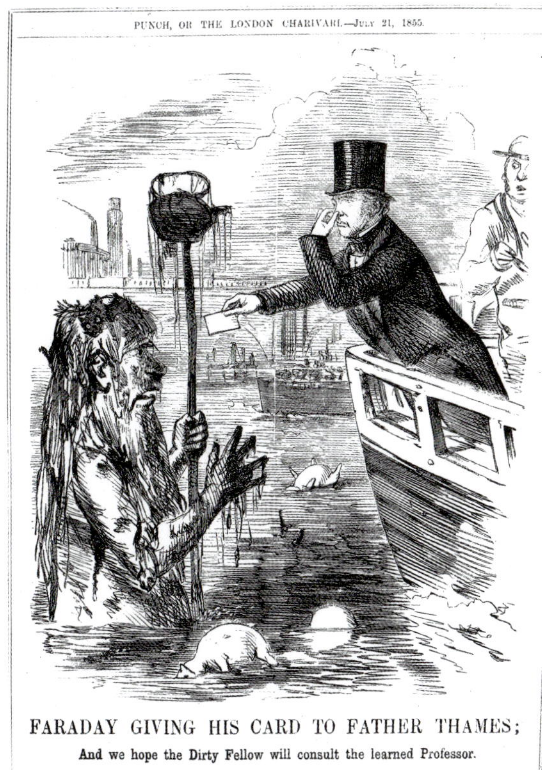
PUNCH, OR THE LONDON CHARIVARI.—JULY 21, 1855.
FARADAY GIVING HIS CARD TO FATHER THAMES;
And we hope the Dirty Fellow will consult the learned Professor.

The condition of the River Thames was the subject of many cartoons including this one from *Punch* in 1855. Pioneering scientist Michael Faraday had carried out a number of experiments to assess the quality of Thames water, and subsequently campaigned for it to be improved.

Wellcome Library, London

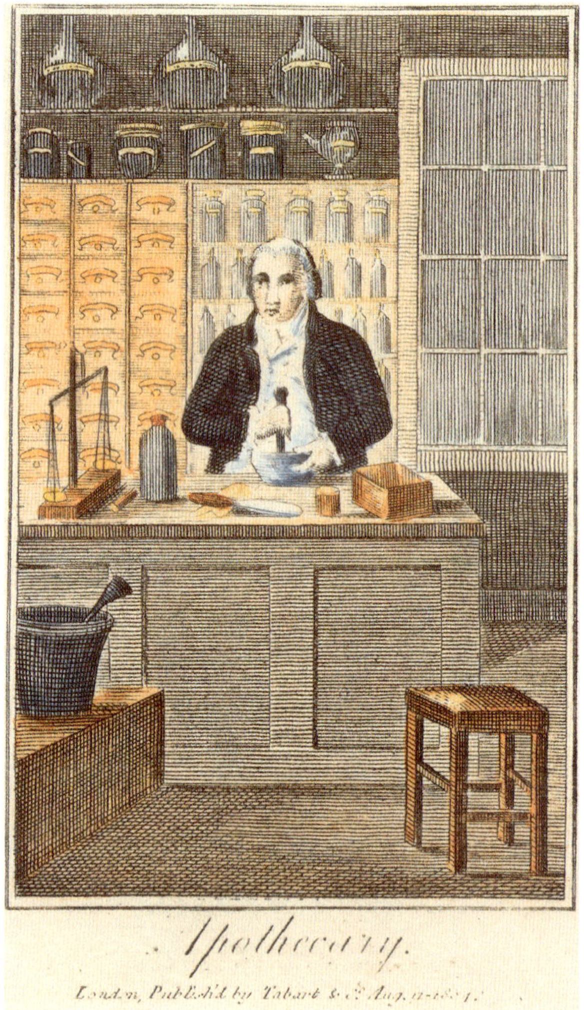

Royal Pharmaceutical Society Museum

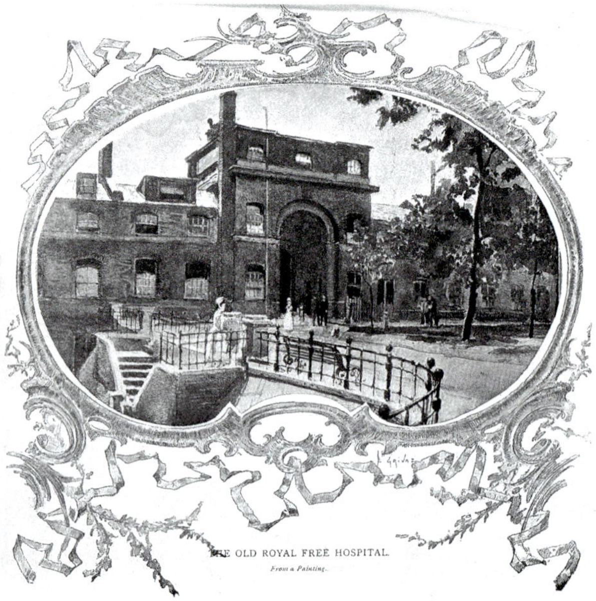

Following its foundation in 1828, the Royal Free Hospital moved to larger premises on Gray's Inn Road in 1844.

Wellcome Library, London

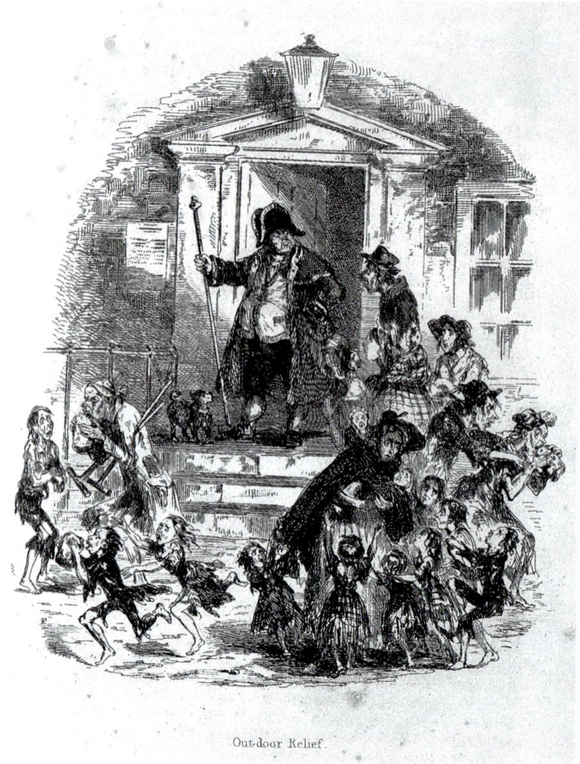

One of the *Sketches in London* published in 1838, showing poor people seeking food at the workhouse door. The Poor Law Act of 1834 had threatened to abolish this form of "outdoor relief" to be replaced by help only if a person entered the workhouse. It is believed that this drawing is by Phiz (Hablot Knight Browne) who illustrated many of Charles Dickens' books.

Wellcome Library, London

BECOMING A PHARMACIST

Before the establishment of the Pharmaceutical Society in 1841, if you made, sold or dispensed medicinal products, you did not have to belong to a particular organisation, work within any legal framework in the way we understand it today, or have any particular qualifications. Most chemists, druggists and pharmacists learnt their trade through an apprenticeship with an established professional before going into partnership or setting up on their own. This was obviously the best way to teach a trainee pharmacist if no university or college courses existed: it was how they developed an understanding of the job and it was a thorough training in most instances. However, there was clearly an issue around quality and consistency of training. Anyone could call themselves a pharmacist and clearly there was no way that the reputation of the profession could rest on such a patchy system.

Before the Pharmaceutical Society, there was another option – to become an apothecary – and there were qualifications that you had to take in order to call yourself an apothecary and work in London. The Worshipful Society of Apothecaries, established in 1617, set up a system of apprenticeship typically lasting for seven years. Although cheaper than training to be a physician, it still cost around 500 guineas (£28,000 in today's money) to set up an apprenticeship in the first half of the nineteenth century. Oral exams were conducted by members of the Society, which included the recognition of ingredients and preparing medicines. Once the exam was passed, the successful new apothecary was entitled to own their own shop.

Between 1815 and 1834, 6,000 new apothecaries' licences were issued, half to surgeons who could hold the dual role of surgeon apothecary. But most apothecaries by the nineteenth century acted as general medical practitioners rather than as experts in the medicines themselves, so the route that most chemists & druggists took was to become an apprentice to an existing pharmacist.

What was it like? William Gelder undertook an apprenticeship with a chemist in Edinburgh and wrote to his father in West Yorkshire in March 1834: "I believe that 6 out of 10 who have served an apprenticeship to a chemist & druggist do not like it on account of the tedious hours … requiring very great mental and bodily attention."

Jacob Bell and Theophilus Redwood were apprentices alongside each other in Jacob's father's John Bell's business in the 1820s. In the Oxford Street shop, the senior assistant with two juniors started at 8am and worked until 11pm, although the shutters were put up at 9pm. Other assistants were on half-duty in the evening in case they were needed. None was allowed to leave the building in the evening without special permission. If off duty, they could go out before breakfast. In the evening, if they were off duty, they were either in the counting house or in the bedrooms. In addition, they were not allowed to talk during breakfast and teatime as they were expected to read, not necessarily pharmacy books, but no light reading material was allowed.

William Tilden was apprenticed, aged 15, for five years from September 1857. Work began at 7.30am, when he had to dust all the bottles in the shop before breakfast. The shop opened until 9pm on weekdays and 10pm on Saturdays, and there were no half-day holidays. Very occasionally, an apprentice was allowed to leave the shop to run errands.

“The indiscriminate sale of drugs by unqualified persons would produce much less injury to the credit and interests of the regular Druggists, if the public had the means of forming a correct estimate of the value of the articles they purchase, and of the qualifications of the parties concerned. But unfortunately in most country towns not only is every Grocer and Oilman a Druggist, but almost every Druggist is a Grocer and Oilman. The Druggist has no badge or credentials to designate his superior qualification; in fact, he is not of necessity more qualified than the Grocer. The blue and red bottles in the windows are common to all; and this is the criterion understood by the public as indicating what is called ‘a doctor's shop’.”

The Pharmaceutical Journal, 1843

By the 1840s, when a Bill was before Parliament for the registration of medical practitioners, a Society of Apothecaries Committee recommended the abolition of the apprenticeship system to be replaced by a two-year course of instruction in pharmacy, and strongly urged that "all chemists and druggists ought to be compelled to undergo an examination in the Latin Pharmacopoeia, pharmaceutical chemistry and materia medica."

Medical students already had materia medica teaching as part of their training. Anthony Todd Thomson gave the fifth ever lecture at University College London Medical School on Monday 6th October 1828, and then lectured daily in materia medica and pharmacy. In 1832, Jonathan Pereira became professor of materia medica at the New Medical School in Aldersgate Street. Aldersgate Dispensary was founded in 1770 by John Lettsom, a Quaker physician, at 36 Aldersgate Street. Lettsom's aim was for it to be a school as well as serve the poor around the area. When Dr Henry Clutterbuck joined in 1807, he started a

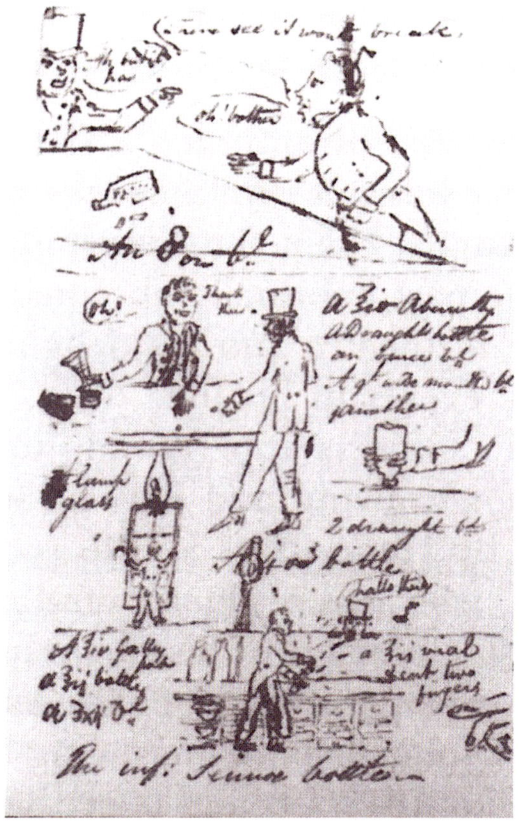

Jacob Bell kept a diary of his apprenticeship in his father's business in the form of illustrations titled "A list of fractures made during the apprenticeship of Jacob Bell. (Motto) 'Save the Pieces!'" It records a series of accidents that he seems to have had as he learnt pharmacy skills.

Royal Pharmaceutical Society Museum

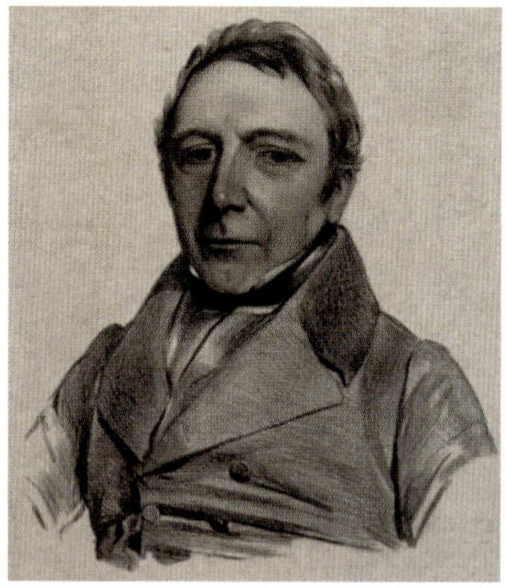

ANTHONY TODD THOMSON (1778–1849)

Wellcome Library, London

ANTHONY TODD THOMSON (1778–1849)

Dr Thomson was professor of botany from 1842 until his death during the session of 1849. Originally from Edinburgh, he qualified as a doctor before moving to London, where he qualified as a surgeon at the College of Surgeons. Although he practised medicine, he also shared his passion for medical botany, initially through a course of lectures in 1810. When the medical department was established at University College Hospital, London in 1828, he was appointed their professor of materia medica and therapeutics.

In 1842, Thomson gave the first ever lecture at the School of Pharmacy, and was appointed professor of botany and materia medica at the age of 64. When Jonathan Pereira joined the staff, Thomson focused purely on botany. One of his key achievements for the School was arranging for students to use the Royal Botanical Gardens in Regents Park.

He was renowned for his long working days. He walked to Regents Park to give his lectures at 7am, and then saw patients until lunchtime. He then worked at the hospital until he gave a 3pm lecture on medical jurisprudence each day. He made house calls on patients into the evening, and then prepared his lectures or wrote publications after dinner. His books included eight editions of *The London Dispensatory* (1811–1844), *Lectures on the Elements of Botany* (1822) and *Elements of Materia Medica and Therapeutics* (1832–1833).

However, he continued teaching at the School until his death aged 71, from pneumonia and pleurisy. On his death, Robert Bentley, past student and prize-winner at the School, then lecturer in botany at the London Hospital, was asked to complete the course, and was subsequently appointed professor of botany.

series of lectures for students, on subjects including materia medica and chemistry. The catalyst for these developments was the Apothecaries Act in 1815, which required that aspiring apothecaries be examined in medical subjects. By the time Pereira was on the staff, his lectures were so popular that he paid for a new lecture theatre himself to accommodate his audiences, apparently costing £700 out of his annual income of £1,000. Pereira was appointed examiner in materia medica at London University in 1839. Medical students could also receive training in what might be viewed as pharmaceutical subjects at Edinburgh Royal Dispensary, and at Apothecaries' Hall in London, but there were no separate schools of pharmacy.

However, if you were not a medical student, there were not many options available. A wave of Mechanics Institutes founded in the 1820s was really the only means of further education for apprentices, but by the 1840s, their courses were more literary and philosophical than scientific. There was no laboratory in the country for practical instruction in chemistry, which meant that some aspiring chemists found the means to study in Paris, Berlin, Göttingen or Giessen.

THE PHARMACEUTICAL SOCIETY OF GREAT BRITAIN

On 15th April 1841, a group of chemists & druggists met at The Crown and Anchor Tavern on The Strand in London to formalise a plan. This meeting had been convened by a smaller committee who had been meeting on a regular basis in recent months in order to fend off perceived attacks from the rest of the medical profession, particularly the apothecaries. In February 1841, Benjamin Hawes, the MP for Lambeth, had introduced a Bill to reform medical practice in Britain. It proposed that the control of the practice of medicine, defined broadly to include pharmacy, would be placed under a body on which pharmacists had no representatives. The result of the April meeting of chemists & druggists was the foundation of the Pharmaceutical Society of Great Britain (PSGB), with the primary aim of raising the standing of the pharmacy profession. They planned to achieve this through education, or as the General Committee of this proto-Society put it in their resolutions, "To benefit the public, and elevate the profession of Pharmacy, furnishing the means of proper instruction." The way they intended to achieve this elevation was through the establishment of a School of Pharmacy.

Speaking at the Introductory Pharmaceutical Meeting of the Society, less than a month later, Jacob Bell explained:

> in order to afford ample means of acquiring the requisite qualifications, and in order to ensure the greatest possible uniformity in the system of education, the chemists and druggists consider it expedient to establish a School of Pharmacy, as a prominent feature in their Society. They propose to institute a regular course of study for the Members of their Society, and more particularly for those who will in future enter into the business of a chemist and druggist. The details of the plan are not yet decided on, but the Laws and Regulations are under consideration, and no exertions will be wanting to bring them into a state of completion as soon as possible.

The Society's founding aims were to unite the profession into one body, to protect its members' interests and to advance scientific knowledge. The Royal Charter of Incorporation, granted swiftly to the new Society in

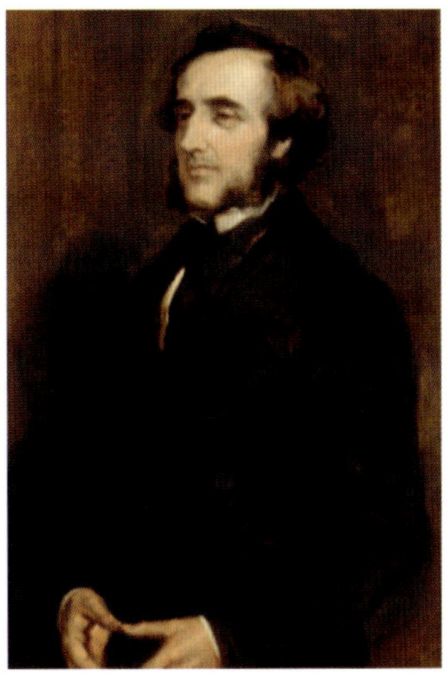

JACOB BELL (1810–1859)

Royal Pharmaceutical Society Museum

JACOB BELL (1810–1859)

Jacob Bell was the leading figure behind the establishment of the Pharmaceutical Society and its early development. As the son of successful Quaker pharmacist John Bell, he started his apprenticeship in his father's retail pharmacy business on Oxford Street. By 1841, he was a partner in the business. The success of the pharmacy meant that he had time and contacts that he could use to benefit the pharmacy profession. He hosted meetings at his house in Langham Place in order to discuss plans to form a pharmacy organisation. He communicated the aims of the early Society through the establishment of *The Pharmaceutical Journal* in 1841, his editorship of it until his death, and his role on the Council, which culminated in his serving as president from 1856 until 1859. He became MP for St Albans in 1850 in order to advance the case for pharmacy legislation. He was also a highly influential patron of the arts, acting as business manager for his friend Sir Edwin Landseer, and with a large circle of artist friends. His death in 1859, aged just 49, left the Pharmaceutical Society without its principal advocate.

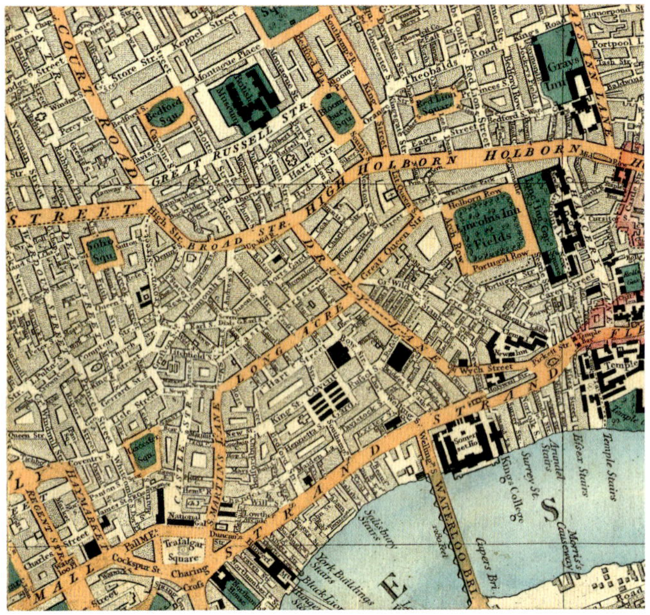

In this detail from *Cary's New Plan of London and Its Vicinity*, published in 1837, you can clearly see that the statue had been erected in Bloomsbury Square, and also appreciate its proximity to both the British Museum and Lincoln's Inn Fields.

MAPCO: Map And Plan Collection Online – mapco.net

February 1843, gave the purpose of "advancing chemistry and pharmacy and promoting a uniform system of education" precedence over "the protection of those who carry on the business of chemists and druggists." Chartered organisations were an elite group. The only other organisations gaining Royal Charters in the same year were the Royal Grammar School in Worcester, Queen Elizabeth's Almshouses, also in Worcester, and Queen's College, Birmingham.

In September 1841, the Society took a yearly lease from the Bedford Estate on a house at 17 Bloomsbury Square. By 1st January 1842, it published a list of its founder members in its monthly *Pharmaceutical Journal*, owned and edited by Jacob Bell. There were 23 honorary members, 665 full members and 263 non-voting associate members (assistants and apprentices). Thirty per cent of members and 40% of associates were based in London. Despite an initial surge and the establishment of 29 local associations, further recruitment of members was slow.

The core group who had met at The Crown and Anchor worked hard to communicate their mission to the wider pharmacy community, who they needed to persuade of the importance of their plans, not least to encourage individuals to subscribe to the fledgling organisation. Their founding aims were three-fold: to establish an organisation that would bring together pharmacy as a profession in the eyes of its practitioners and those outside its boundaries; to establish the profession through a set educational standard; and to protect pharmacists at times of need through setting up a benevolent fund. At a meeting on 25th May 1841, a report was agreed that included the following aim: "the institution of a School of Pharmacy – the development of scientific acquirements, and the exhibition of existing talent will tend to confirm the confidence of the public, and remove our apparent deficiency as pharmacopolists, when compared with other nations." The whole report was printed and 2,000 copies were sent out to prospective members.

These pharmacy education pioneers were well aware that they were working within complicated and contested territories, and decided to meet any possible opposition head-on. On 18th November 1841, a party went to meet with the Royal College of Physicians to explain their educational plans. The College confirmed that they supported the proposals but also that they did not feel that they needed to have any involvement in their execution. To be sure, the Society invited a representative from the College, and from the University of London to sit on a committee formed to set up the first pharmacy examinations. Neither institution sent a representative, and so the Society continued its plans alone. Whether they felt snubbed, or relieved that neither organisation wanted to breathe down their necks, no evidence seems to survive.

What were they trying to achieve? On a practical basis, the Society's founders did not want to set the initial qualifying bar too high, but on the other hand, their underlying aim was to bring credit to the profession by providing it with an academic underpinning to counter the perennial accusations of being merely a trade. As such, they advertised that "the course of education proposed embraces only such subjects as should be known by every person presuming to dispense prescriptions; and though at the outset it would not be stringently enforced, it will be the duty of the Council to extend the examination as circumstances may require." Writing later, having served as a professor at the School, Theophilus Redwood also expressed a by-product of the relatively modest educational standards established by the Society:

> The establishment of an examination in the classics for all future Apprentices, will ensure the possession of that preliminary education which is essentially necessary for the creditable performance of their duties, and their ultimate success as pharmaceutists; and the increased importance and respectability which will be conferred upon Pharmacy by means of this Society will induce many of the more wealthy classes to devote themselves to its pursuit.

The issue of status for the pharmacy profession was inevitably bound up with education. Without any qualifications, those making, dispensing and selling medicines could not escape being grouped with purveyors of dubious quack medicines or grocers with no medical expertise. However, the means of building this pharmacy qualification rested on constructing a recognised body of pharmacy science, as distinct from other medical fields, and this in turn rested on providing the resources for an institution that could encourage and promote these activities, and teach them to the next generation. As Redwood put it, "pharmacy is deserving of a separate and distinct place in the arrangement of the medical profession, and that it is not likely to advance as a science, and to keep pace with other sciences, unless it be followed by a class of persons who devote themselves exclusively to it."

> **"Professional character *prima facie* is supposed to result from liberal and scientific education."**
>
> *The Pharmaceutical Journal, 1849*

In his address at the Council meeting on 12th January 1842, the Society's president, William Allen, referred to the establishment of a school of pharmacy, the establishment and regulation of exams and the appointment of examiners as "among the most important of the means by which the objects of the association were to be attained." He went on to announce an introductory programme of lectures.

Writing in *The Pharmaceutical Journal* of 1st August 1842, Jacob Bell used a fictional generic pharmacy apprentice to explain how the proposed education and examination system would work. The prospective pharmacist must be "examined in his classical attainments", either at the Society's new headquarters at 17 Bloomsbury Square if he lived within 10 miles of London, or by a classical tutor or qualified person acceptable to the examiners if he lived further afield. Bell explained that although some members had suggested that basic achievements in French and Arithmetic, or even Greek or Algebra, should be assessed, the initial test would be based on Latin. Once an apprentice could satisfy an examiner as to their proficiency in Latin, they were able to take the next step, the Minor exam. When the PSGB secretary had received a certificate of qualification, the apprentice's indentures would be agreed and they would be registered with the Society. For an annual fee of one guinea, he could make use of the Society's proposed facilities. Bell suggested that it would then take four or five years to become a qualified assistant.

A prospective candidate for the Minor exam had to show documentary evidence of having been apprenticed or regularly educated by a vendor of drugs or dispenser of medicines. The exam consisted of questions based on the *London Pharmacopoeia* on chemistry, materia medica, botany and pharmacy, a translation of medical prescriptions, a practical pharmacy test, and questions on antidotes for common poisons. If successful, he could join the Society as an Associate. In order to achieve this, the fictional apprentice should "pursue his studies with increased diligence" and attend lectures. If he could not get to lectures, he "should endeavour to supply the deficiency by reading, collecting and studying plants, making chemical experiments on a small scale, and endeavouring to apply the knowledge obtained from books, to the practical operations of the dispensing counter or the laboratory." If successful in this Minor exam, the Associate would be able to progress to the Major exam, a higher qualification available only to proprietors of businesses. Successful Major candidates would become full voting Members of the Society.

Bell knew only too well that there was a balance to be achieved between setting an educational standard that was attainable by a significant proportion of the aspiring profession such that they supported the new Society both morally and financially, and ensuring that the qualification was rigorous enough to provoke the professional respect that the founders were aiming for. He did not rule out raising the standards at a later date: "we are justified in stating that the early examinations will not be unreasonably strict." Equally important was that the educational standard was attainable without having to make the expensive move to London to take part in the School's activities, to avoid criticism from potential regional members that the Society was too London-centric, but also to make sure that there was enough support for a school in London to make it a feasible proposition. He wrote in August 1841 with the financial concerns of potential members in mind: "The School of Pharmacy is not likely, *in the first instance*, to be supported entirely out of the general fund; and during its growth to maturity, those who enjoy its immediate advantages, may be called upon to pay small fees to make up the deficiency."

Enquiry—How can we who reside at a distance from London, derive any benefit from the School of Pharmacy?

Answer.—You will have the privilege of sending your Apprentices to London to complete their education on reasonable terms. It is your duty to afford them every opportunity of learning their business, and it is your interest to possess such facilities as shall induce parents to place their sons under your care. You will also enjoy the gratification of advancing your profession by contributing to a national institution. You must recollect that a very limited number even of the London Members can be within a convenient distance of the establishment, and the necessity of constant attention to business will prevent their deriving much direct personal benefit from the scientific proceedings. But the existence of the School of Pharmacy for the education of the rising generation will confer a degree of credit and character upon every individual connected with it.

From 'Enquiries and Objections Answered', *The Pharmaceutical Journal*, 1 September 1841.

The Pharmaceutical Journal

In the first volume of *The Pharmaceutical Journal* (initially called *The Transactions of the Pharmaceutical Meetings*), Bell reproduced a paper, "On the Constitution of the Pharmaceutical Society of Great Britain", which he had read out at the Introductory Pharmaceutical Meeting on 11th May 1841. He started by stressing how deficient Britain was in pharmaceutical chemistry in comparison with other countries such as France, Germany and America. Although it was possible to obtain a pharmacy education either from the Society of Apothecaries or via the medical schools, neither had pharmaceutical chemistry as their focus, and neither had the aim to raise the standing of the pharmacy profession as a result of their educational activities. Bell had concluded that there was only one way for the profession to achieve this aim:

> Chemists and druggists have been assailed with accusations of ignorance and inefficiency … In assembling together to defend themselves and assert their just rights, they have discovered that a desire for improvement prevails among them as a body, which, in their hitherto disunited condition, has lain dormant, or failed to produce any tangible result. They have also arrived at a conviction that, in their present position, they will be always exposed to attacks … on the ground of their undergoing no regular and uniform course of education, and passing no ordeal as a test of their competence.

However, Bell also stressed that the underlying reason for raising standards was for public benefit, and that chemists & druggists:

> consider that their own interest, as well as the safety and welfare of the public, demand that no person shall become an apprentice in their business who has not had the advantage of an adequate fundamental education; and that no person shall dispense medicines who has not undergone an examination as a test of his competence to perform that important office.

This was a difficult balancing act: to insist that specific pharmacy education was necessary, without offending existing chemists & druggists regarding their own standards, but Bell managed it skilfully:

> In the absence of any uniform system of pharmaceutical education, or any restrictions whatever on those who compound Medicines … it cannot be expected that all dispensing chemists can be equally competent; and, without casting any unjust imputation upon them as a body, we must admit that, among some of their number, a reformation is required.
>
> In every profession and in every trade there must always be a variety of grades, both in respect of moral and mental qualification; but by affording facilities for gaining knowledge, and excluding the incompetent, we must inevitably raise the standard of proficiency.

Bell could demonstrate that the uneven standards across the country had been recognised from outside the Society as well. The second edition of *The Chemist*, a journal aimed at manufacturers, analysts and pharmacists, which first appeared in 1840, stated:

> The retail chemist ought, therefore, to be compelled to undergo a strict examination as to his knowledge of the nature of drugs and their medical properties, so as to enable him to detect any error in prescription and insure his committing no mistake through ignorance.

The fact that the core of founding and early members of the Society included pharmacists from many long-standing pharmacy firms was evidence that Bell's ambitions were shared by other established pharmacy practitioners, who were not offended by the Society's public declaration of the inadequacy of many of their fellow pharmacists. Writing later, Redwood praised this group: "All honour to the worthy band of distinguished pharmacists who laid the foundation for an educational system which, bringing the required knowledge equally within the reach of all, was calculated to undermine the pre-eminence of the great historic houses." The "great historic houses" could clearly see the benefits to be gained through the establishment of a society based soundly on education.

Bell was also treading a fine line with regard to the other medical professions, and the long history of turf wars over diagnosis, supply of medicines and dispensing expertise. Part of his strategy was flattery, and he continued to stress how important it would be for the new Society to work with the medical profession to achieve the highest standards

"In the establishment of an institution for the promulgation of knowledge, the aid of enlightened and experienced men is essential to the complete attainment of success, and the acquirement of that solid foundation on which a permanent and efficient superstructure can be raised."

Jacob Bell, May 1842.

in order to produce pharmacists who could support the physicians and apothecaries to do their job well. He also continued to emphasise that his aim was to establish a separate area of pharmaceutical chemistry which would complement rather than compete with the apothecaries' work. The fact that high-profile physicians, Anthony Todd Thomson and Jonathan Pereira, were willing to accept posts in the fledgling school was valuable bridge-building for the Society. Dr Pereira finished his introductory lecture on materia medica given on 30th March 1842 by saying:

> ... allow me to congratulate the chemists and druggists of this country on the establishment of an institution so well calculated to prove serviceable to them, by improving the education of the rising members, facilitating the acquirement of scientific knowledge, and diffusing important and valuable information among pharmaceutists ... I ascribe the low state of pharmacy in this country to the want of a scientific education by the practical Pharmaceutist. It is one, and I should say the grand, object of this Society to remove this glaring evil.

“ I ascribe the low state of pharmacy in this country to the want of a scientific education by the practical Pharmaceutist. It is one, and I should say the grand, object of this Society to remove this glaring evil. ”

Dr Pereira, 30th March 1842

For seven months of the first year of publication of *The Pharmaceutical Journal*, Bell continued to emphasise the importance of pharmacy education, and how the British situation lagged behind other countries. He started in September 1841 with the reprint of an article from an American journal, "The necessity of colleges of pharmacy in civilized countries" by T.H. Buckler, and for the following six months an article in each publication described the profession in other countries, France, Russia, Norway, the United States, Ireland and Germany. When the Pharmaceutical Society was founded, there were already six schools for education of pharmacists founded in France, the first in 1803, and schools of pharmacy in various German states; in Bavaria, study at a university became compulsory in order to practise as a pharmacist from 1808. In the United States, a College of Pharmacy opened in Philadelphia in 1821, Boston in 1823, New York in 1829, New Orleans in 1838 and Baltimore in 1840.

Bell also continued to explain how the existing teaching available for aspiring pharmacists was insufficient. For example, he reprinted in the September edition of *The Pharmaceutical Journal* a report from the *Medical Gazette* of 30th July 1841 which told of how unsuccessful medical candidates at the University of London were rejected because of "imperfect acquaintance" with chemistry, botany and materia medica. Bell provided this as evidence that medical students were trying to cover too much ground, and the pharmacy-related subjects were treated as being of "secondary importance". He backed this up by printing the full examination papers for chemistry, and materia medica and pharmacy from the University of London in the March 1842 edition. However, the proximity of Bloomsbury Square to the University of London suggests the academic nature of Bell's ambitions, and in practical terms meant that it might be possible to draw on College lecturers as contributors to pharmacy education.

The School of Pharmacy formed the core of a group of measures designed to raise the educational standards of the profession, including the foundation of the Society's library and museum, the establishment of *The Pharmaceutical Journal* in order to share scientific papers and developments with the wider pharmacy community, and a programme of scientific meetings and conversazione held at the Society's headquarters. It is no accident that all of these elements were also components of a learned society's badge of professional and academic honour in the mid-nineteenth century. However, the Pharmaceutical Society did not have many other examples of professional bodies to emulate. The Institution of Civil Engineers, founded in 1818, the Law Society (1825) and the Institute of British Architects (1834) existed, but none had qualifying exams in the 1840s or a compulsory system of education.

The Society presented a report on examinations and education, including arrangements for the Board of Examiners, registering apprentices and relevant fees, at the Annual Meeting held on 17th May 1842, and reported in the June edition of *The Pharmaceutical Journal*. Mindful of the need to demonstrate their credentials to other medical professionals, the Board of Examiners would invite one physician and one public professor in a medical science department to attend each monthly meeting as a visitor. There would be no fees for examinations beyond the existing subscription to the Society.

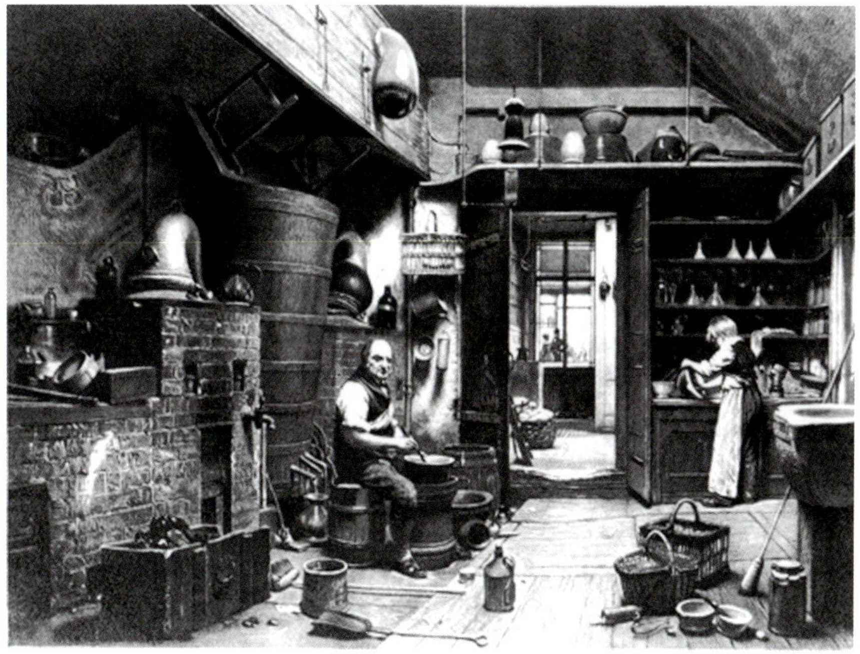

John Bell & Co's business on Oxford Street, London, was typical for a pharmacy of this period in having a laboratory where medicines were made. Bell's laboratory was larger and more productive than most, servicing a busy West End shop. The man in charge was John Simmonds who had worked there since the business opened in 1798.

Royal Pharmaceutical Society Museum

Bell made it very clear that "the foundation of education in our school is chemistry." His ambition was to establish a separate branch of pharmaceutical chemistry that would underpin the practice of pharmacy and, importantly, not overlap with medical teaching. *The Pharmaceutical Journal*, edited by Bell, included both original papers and reprints of recent European developments, and aimed to establish a community of pharmaceutical chemists. In the mid-nineteenth century, before the establishment of a significant pharmacy industry, and with virtually every chemist creating preparations in their own laboratories and back rooms, it was perfectly possible to play a part in the development of pharmaceutical science as part of your everyday work or by following a hunch in your spare time. However, chemistry also played a key part in pharmacy practice. Charles James Payne, writing in *The Pharmaceutical Journal* in 1841, stressed that:

> without some knowledge of chemistry, a man is working in the dark, he can know nothing correctly of the results of, or the reasons for the operations he constantly performs – he can never properly judge the accuracy and quality of his preparation, he can neither detect any error that may occur nor rectify any untoward circumstance that may arise – he has no established data to reason upon – no fixed principles to guide him; but is like a mariner without a compass, exposed to endless confusion and mishap.

The Society had rivals in its chemistry teaching and research with the establishment of the Royal College of Chemistry in 1845 and the Chemical Society in 1841. Bell argued that the Society was aiming to provide a more specific education, but he met criticism from both pharmacists and chemists who did not agree with the idea of creating an independent pharmaceutical science. The most extreme opponents criticised the objective as a vanity project for Bell. There were also critics within pharmacy who

> **"the foundation of the education in our school is chemistry."**
>
> *Jacob Bell, 1842*

wanted the organisation to focus on those who were practising pharmacy rather than the establishment of a scientific society. Bell believed that the two objectives were compatible, and in fact were interdependent. As Redwood expressed it in his introductory lecture on Practical Pharmacy, given on 28th December 1842:

> In establishing a school of Pharmacy, … it is necessary not only to teach those sciences which shall comprise the requisite information for a practical Pharmaceutist, but at the same time to point out the particular connexion which exists between the science taught, and the art to which this knowledge is applied; in fact, to teach the *art*, by illustrating in its practice the principles of the sciences upon which it is founded.

The Society's founders were, of course, well aware that their educational ambitions depended on support from other pharmacists, not least in practical terms. A year after the Society's foundation, they used the May 1842 edition of *The Pharmaceutical Journal* to express their concerns to the membership:

> The prosperity of the Society will be, to a certain extent, influenced by the amount of support enjoyed by the School of Pharmacy. We therefore trust, that those members who reside within a convenient distance, will afford to their assistants and apprentices such opportunities as may be found practicable, of attending the lectures. We presume that it will not be found inconvenient to liberate an associate once or twice a week; and since it is not necessary that every individual should attend lectures on all the subjects during the same season, it will be easy to divide the privilege according to the circumstances. It is very desirable that our school should open with good classes.

Members' support was seen to depend on their buy-in to the approach taken to teaching at the School, and it was continually stressed how practical the lectures would be, even before they started. The Annual Report on exams and education given on 17th May 1842 explained that "It is the Council's intention that the subjects of the lectures shall be of the most practical kind, and be treated with especial reference to the daily pursuits of the chemist and druggist."

However, a proposal made at the Annual Meeting in 1845 for chemists to shorten their apprentices' hours and allow apprentices and assistants time for study suggests the challenges for potential students. Redwood recalled that:

> there was much indifference manifested, both by employers and employed, in acknowledging the necessity for, or even the benefits of, the education that was being provided at so much expense … [this presented] difficulties that had to be contended with in introducing and maintaining an efficient system of sound practical and scientific training for students in pharmacy.

In addition to accusations of indifference by the membership, there was the point that "A feeling also appeared to prevail … that the instruction the Pharmaceutical Society was providing for its students was in excess of what was required." This led to further criticism from members that those students who had attended the school emerged with a conceited and arrogant attitude, not attractive traits for employers.

The number of students remained low into the early 1850s. The Annual Report given in 1852 shows that the Council had decided it was time to take stock:

> It was the desire of the founders to make the School a model School of Pharmacy, complete in all the requirements for theoretical and practical instruction … it becomes necessary to consider whether the advantage derived from the School is an equivalent for the pecuniary sacrifice … The Council are of opinion that the experiment undertaken by the Pharmaceutical Society has had a fair trial. It will be the duty of the next Council to consider in what manner retrenchment may be effected under the circumstances above detailed.

THE PHARMACY ACT 1852

Jacob Bell and his co-founders had always planned that they would apply for legislation to codify the qualifications required for pharmacy. However, looking at the University of London for a precedent, they worried that in applying for legislation, they would be denied because they were both an educating and an examining institution. (The University had set up University College London to provide education whilst remaining as the examining body to avoid this perceived conflict in 1836.) A proposal was made that a College of Pharmacy should be set up to be an examining body, whilst the Pharmaceutical Society would remain as the educating institution. By 1848, it seemed that there would be no problems in this area and that they did not need to set up separate institutions.

Bell's objective for a Pharmacy Act was to improve the qualifications of pharmaceutical chemists, and to establish the principle that all dispensers of medicines had undergone a basic education and passed an exam "as a test of their fitness for the performance of their most important and responsible duties." He wanted to make exams compulsory and separate from medical qualifications. However, the turf wars with other medical organisations continued to dominate discussions. Notably, the Society of Apothecaries objected to toxicology as a proposed examined subject for pharmacists, as they thought it was beyond the areas in which a pharmacist needed to have knowledge. As a result, the Council removed it from their proposal in order not to threaten the progress of the Bill. However, they confirmed that toxicology was only included as the chemical nature of poisons, under a general course of chemistry. In order not to tread on any other toes, the proposal (and final Bill) also specified that pharmacy exams would not include medicine, surgery or midwifery.

The Arsenic Act, passed in 1851, highlighted the wide concern over the control of this poison. Following a series of poisonings and suicides with arsenic, the Act represented the first restriction in Britain on the sale and supply of a harmful substance. It established that arsenic should only be available from medical practitioners and from chemists & druggists, and that it should only be sold to male adults who were known personally to the vendor. Alternatively, the purchaser could supply a written signed and dated order that stated the purpose for which they wanted the poison, and the total quantity required. However, because there was no restriction on who could call themselves a chemist & druggist, it was not clear how the restrictions would be enforced.

A Parliamentary Select Committee was convened to discuss the proposed Pharmacy Act. John Savory, interviewed by the Committee in 1852, explained how hard it was to find suitable men to work as assistants, as the majority of applicants could not even answer very basic pharmacy questions. He was currently employing a Frenchman, a Hungarian and an Italian as their skills were better than English applicants.

The resulting Act was a partial success for the Society. It restricted titles such as "pharmaceutical chemist" and "pharmaceutist" to people who had passed the Society's Major exam, and those that were successful had to appear on a register. It also allowed for the setting up of a separate Board of Examiners in Scotland. However, it did not provide a legal definition of "pharmacy", meaning that anyone could practise it. The status of the profession was not safeguarded through controlled education and registration as Bell and his peers had proposed, largely owing to concerns by the Act's opponents about providing an entrance monopoly to the Society.

TEACHING

The Society's Council discussed setting up a School of Pharmacy at their first meeting on 6th January 1842, with further deliberations at the Society's first evening meeting on 12th January 1842. It was decided that preliminary lectures should be arranged while the selection of permanent teaching staff was considered. This lecture series started on 16th February 1842, with an introductory lecture by Dr Anthony Todd Thomson on materia medica. On 2nd March, Dr Andrew Ure gave a lecture on chemistry, and on 16th March, Theophilus Redwood spoke on pharmacy. On 30th March Dr Jonathan Pereira lectured on "Modern discoveries in materia medica", followed on 12th April by George Fownes on organic chemistry. The series was concluded by Todd Thomson on 11th May with a lecture on botany.

THE OPENING OF THE SCHOOL OF PHARMACY.

Dr. A. T. Thomson commenced his course of lectures on Botany, on Tuesday morning, the 17th of May, and we were glad to see a numerous and attentive audience. Upwards of forty tickets have been taken for the course. The interest which appears to exist on the subject, is not confined to the vicinity of Bloomsbury Square, as we have pupils from Kensington, Sloane Square, Bayswater, Brixton, Walworth, Islington, and Clapham, distances varying from two miles to above five. It is a remarkable fact, that those who come from the greatest distance have hitherto been first in the lecture-room. We mention the circumstance to show that when a sincere desire for improvement prevails, the obstacles relating to time and space appear to vanish.

***The Pharmaceutical Journal*, 1 June 1842.**

The Pharmaceutical Journal

Meanwhile, the Council appointed professors for the subjects they considered key: Dr Thomson in botany, Mr Fownes in chemistry and Mr Redwood in pharmacy. They followed this in 1843 with a professorship for Dr Pereira in materia medica.

The formal teaching courses began with botany by Dr Thomson on 17th May 1842. He gave two lectures per week on medical botany from May to July, starting at 8am. Some of the lectures took place at the gardens of the Royal Botanic Society (RBS) in Regent's Park from 7am, and students were allowed to stay until 10am to study plants in the conservatory and grounds. The RBS had first leased the land within the ring or inner circle in 1840 on a site formerly known as Jenkins's nursery. The renowned architect and garden designer Decimus Burton (1800–1881) was commissioned to design the layout and buildings, which included a large conservatory, built in 1845. The central part of this was opened to the public in 1846. The conservatory was a state-of-the-art building which enclosed an area 175 feet long and 75 feet wide. Other buildings on the RBS site were large palm-houses and a water-lily house. Thomson also voluntarily led demonstrations and walks, or "peripatetic lectures" as they were

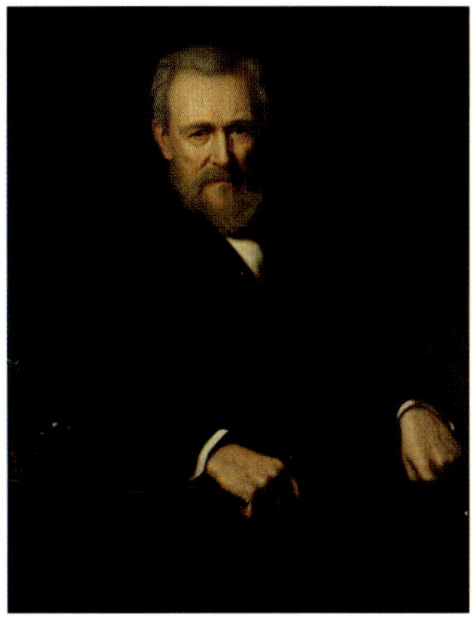

THEOPHILUS REDWOOD (1808–1892)

Royal Pharmaceutical Society Museum

THEOPHILUS REDWOOD (1808–1892)

Theophilus Redwood was born in Boverton, Glamorganshire, and apprenticed to his uncle, an apothecary, in Cardiff. After three years, he moved to London to take up a new apprenticeship in Jacob Bell's pharmacy on Oxford Street and spent seven years there before setting up his own chemical and pharmaceutical factory in Crawford Street. He was appointed professor of pharmacy at the School in 1842 and became director of its first chemistry laboratory on its opening in 1844, but then took over as professor of chemistry and pharmacy when George Fownes had to retire.

Redwood can be credited with the first pharmacy textbook in Britain, *Practical Pharmacy* (1849), an extended and edited translation of a book by the German, Francis Mohr. After Jacob Bell's death in 1859, he shared the editorship of *The Pharmaceutical Journal* with Robert Bentley and John Barnard. He edited the *British Pharmacopoeia* in 1867 and 1885, and was joint author with Bell of the *Historical Sketch of the Progress of Pharmacy* (1880). He was also the Society's first librarian and museum curator. Redwood was president of the British Pharmaceutical Conference in 1876 and 1877.

"Verax", a student in the 1879–80 session, remembered that Redwood, although elderly, was an excellent speaker: "His lectures were models of lucidity, and were remarkable alike for their grasp of principles and a perfect mastery of details. There was no attempt at oratory, but a plain statement of facts conveyed in simple, terse, graphic sentences which any child, versed in its own mother tongue, could have understood."

However, Michael Carteighe, in his President's Jubilee address in October 1892, remembered different qualities: "He was a hard-headed Welshman, and the best point about Redwood was that when you placed him in a difficulty, when you gave him something that it was worth while to fight, or something it was necessary to conquer, or a problem to solve that seemed insolvable, then Redwood was at his best. You had really to get him into a corner."

known, in the RBS's gardens in Regent's Park on the mornings when he was not officially lecturing there. He considered them "a recreation rather than a toil." However, Robert Bentley, later professor of botany, attended Thomson's first lecture course, and was less than complimentary:

> The instruction consisted chiefly in the definition of various words. The professor would write up on the blackboard the words *ovate, obovate, cordate, lanceolate*, etc., and then hold up a specimen by way of illustration – not a very inspiring method. We learned nothing but external forms, and though I had the use of a microscope, I learned nothing of vegetable physiology.

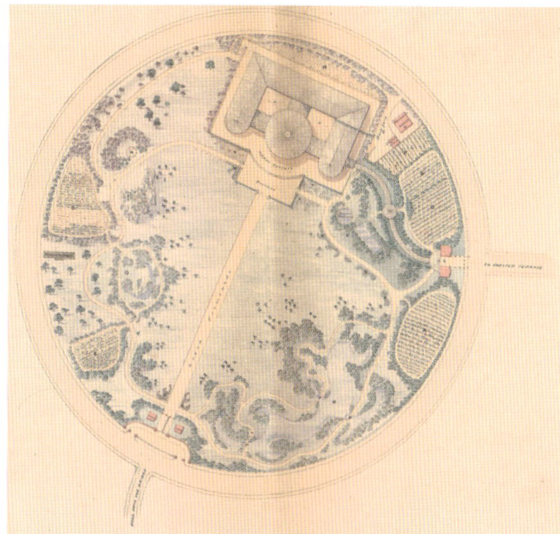

Decimus Burton (1800–1881) designed villas in Regent's Park and the animal houses for London Zoo, before being asked to create the Royal Botanical Society Gardens in the centre of the Park in 1840. Botany students at the School of Pharmacy had lectures in the Gardens, led by Dr Thomson.

Hastings Museum and Art Gallery

The chemistry course started in October 1842, with one lecture per week from October to March starting at 8.30am. Similarly, there was one lecture per week in materia medica and pharmacy from October to March, starting at 8.30am. From evidence presented by G.W. Smith, the Society's secretary, to a Select Committee in 1852, the numbers at the 1842 lectures were 42 students at botany, 71 at chemistry, 78 at materia

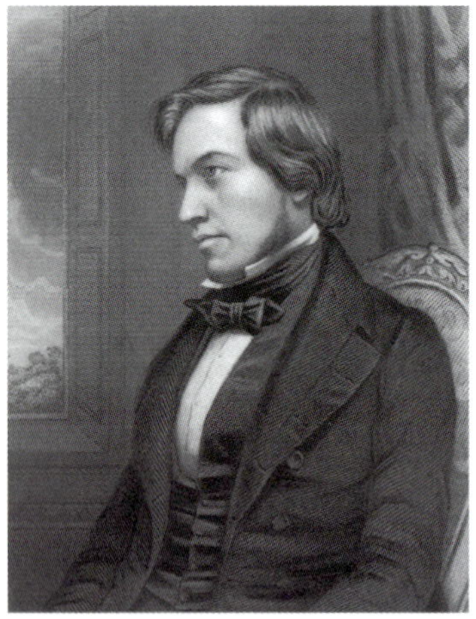

GEORGE FOWNES (1815–1849)

Royal Pharmaceutical Society Museum

GEORGE FOWNES (1815–1849)

Fownes originally followed in his father's footsteps, working with him as a glover near Leicester Square until the age of 22. However, having joined the Western Literary Institute aged 17 or 18, he decided to attempt an academic scientific career. He began work for a Mr Everett, a chemistry lecturer at the Middlesex Hospital, and gained a PhD in Giessen, Germany, after a three-month stay there. On his return, he took an assistant role to Professor Graham at University College, London. In the following year he became a chemistry lecturer at Charing Cross Hospital, and in 1841 he gave an organic chemistry course at the Royal Institution.

He was the first professor of chemistry at the School from 1842. His extensive research resulted in many publications, including a paper on "The artificial formation of a vegeto-alkali", for which he won a Royal Society gold medal. He published the *Manual of Chemistry* in 1844, and became a fellow of the Royal Society in 1845. In the same year he became professor of practical chemistry at University College's Birkbeck Laboratory.

However, he was plagued by ill health. In 1846, he retired from his posts and went to Barbados in the hope of improving his health. Sadly, he died there three years later aged only 34. Joseph Ince was one of his students: "As a lecturer he was remarkable for a singular clearness of explanatory description, given often under distressing circumstances. Some of his experiments, especially in organic chemistry, had to be omitted owing to a difficulty in breathing, painful at times to witness."

medica and 78 at pharmacy. Each student paid 10 shillings and six pence to attend each course.

Although it was planned that the Society's exams were to come into operation in July 1842, there were no candidates until the end of the year. The first associate by exam was admitted on 15th November 1842, and another on 20th December. There were no candidates for the Major exam until February 1844.

According to an article entitled "The School of Pharmacy" in the September 1842 edition of *The Pharmaceutical Journal*, the School opened with a course on botany because they could obtain plant specimens in the summer. Nevertheless, it was without doubt that:

> the foundation of the education in our school is CHEMISTRY … The preparation of drugs which comprehends all pharmaceutical operations, can neither be successfully practised nor clearly understood, without some acquaintance with the ultimate and proximate elements of bodies, their affinities, and the laws relating to combination and decomposition, which constitute the fundamental principles of Chemistry. This science, therefore, which is one of the most interesting, is the most

> **" Lectures are not *absolutely necessary* to the student in Pharmacy … Yet it cannot be denied … that lectures *greatly facilitate* the acquirement of information – that they lessen the labour of the student by directing his researches into the right channel and giving him a methodical plan of study, and consequently this privilege should never be undervalued or neglected by those who have the means of enjoying it. "**
>
> *The Pharmaceutical Journal, 1st August 1842*

> important pursuit to the student in pharmacy, and is calculated to prepare his mind for the reception of other knowledge which he ought to possess.

However, the pharmacy course was also a new and important development for a dedicated school of pharmacy: "This subject is generally treated promiscuously in lectures on Chemistry and Materia Medica, but has not hitherto been taught in this country in a separate course of lectures."

The article was partially a piece of news, but of course also a major advertisement for both the School and the philosophy behind the new pharmacy education. It was stressed that country apprentices were not at a disadvantage to those in the city, especially in relation to materia medica because of the easy availability of plant samples, in comparison with "theoretical study in a large city, where the supply of specimens is of necessity scanty and uncertain." Synopses were provided for all three professors' lecture courses. The standard of education was also emphasised: "It should be our ambition in establishing a School of Pharmacy, to ensure the most complete and efficient education, and to yield to no existing establishments, either in the quality of our lectures or the eminence of the professors whom we engage."

Other major selling points for the School were the supporting departments of the library and museum. The *Journal* trumpeted that the "Museum of the Pharmaceutical Society will afford an opportunity of exhibiting a great variety of specimens, an advantage which is not possessed to the same extent in other establishments where the science of medicine is taught." The Society's museum was created in 1842, alongside the School, as a reference collection for the students and staff. Bell had written in the first edition of *The Pharmaceutical Journal* that the School should be equipped with a laboratory, a library and a "complete museum of materia medica comprising specimens of good and bad drugs."

Bell described the museum soon after it was set up:

> The museum is a front room on the ground floor, 26 feet by 20, containing not a vestige of furniture. The bare boards are well scoured, the ceiling and walls are in a perfect state of repair, but there is not even a chair or table to invite the student to sit down and contemplate what alterations are likely to take place in the apartment within the next six months. On the floor at one corner is a small heap of brown paper parcels, containing a few donations from two or three members, and on the mantel-shelf are about a dozen glasses and bottles, in which are sundry crystals, roots and other substances. These objects form the nucleus of the Museum of Materia Medica of the Pharmaceutical Society of Great Britain.

According to *The Pharmaceutical Journal* in 1858, "many of the early supporters of the Society vied with each other in presenting the most rare and curious specimens, as well as others varying in quality to make the collections as complete as possible." The museum was principally used as a source of lecture specimens by Professors Redwood and Bentley, and increasingly as a collection of examples that could be used as a comparison with others to assess their purity.

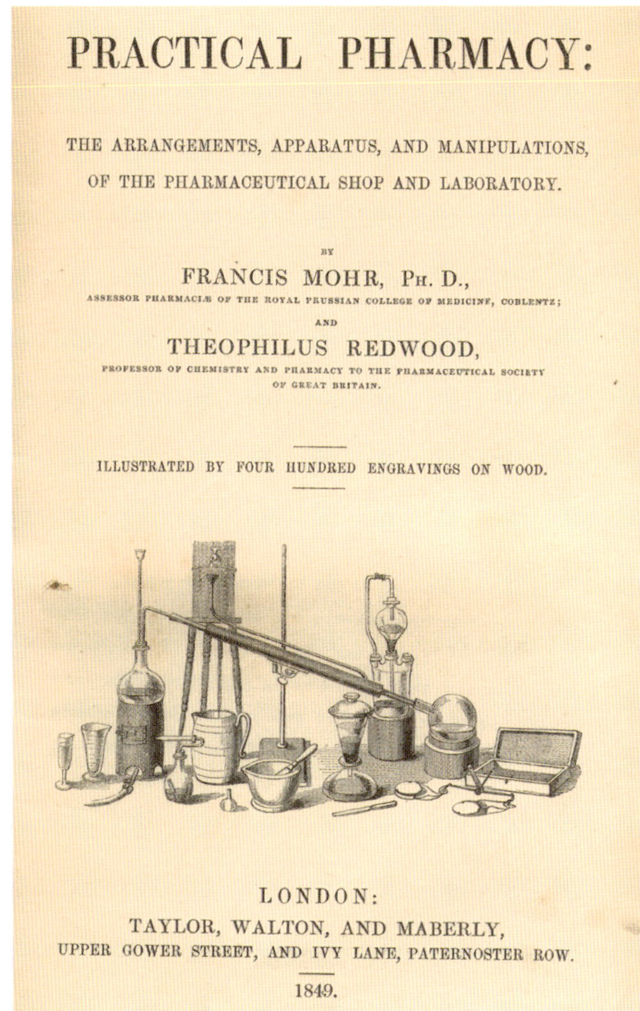

PRACTICAL PHARMACY:

THE ARRANGEMENTS, APPARATUS, AND MANIPULATIONS, OF THE PHARMACEUTICAL SHOP AND LABORATORY.

BY

FRANCIS MOHR, PH. D.,

ASSESSOR PHARMACIÆ OF THE ROYAL PRUSSIAN COLLEGE OF MEDICINE, COBLENTZ;

AND

THEOPHILUS REDWOOD,

PROFESSOR OF CHEMISTRY AND PHARMACY TO THE PHARMACEUTICAL SOCIETY OF GREAT BRITAIN.

ILLUSTRATED BY FOUR HUNDRED ENGRAVINGS ON WOOD.

LONDON:
TAYLOR, WALTON, AND MABERLY,
UPPER GOWER STREET, AND IVY LANE, PATERNOSTER ROW.
1849.

Theophilus Redwood adapted and expanded Francis Mohr's original book to create *Practical Pharmacy*, published in 1849. It was beautifully and usefully illustrated throughout and can claim to be the first specifically pharmaceutical textbook in English.

Royal Pharmaceutical Society Library

The library similarly started without any stock, but with significant ambitions for its contribution to pharmacy education. An article on the library and museum in the February 1842 edition of *The Pharmaceutical Journal* claimed:

> Our course is clear – the first step has been taken, which is the union of ourselves into an ostensible and recognised body; the next step is to prove ourselves worthy of recognition, and capable of self-government. In attaining this end, a variety of measures are indispensable; all of which have reference, directly or indirectly, to education and the promulgation of science. Among these objects, the library and museum are prominent; because, in the first place, they will afford facilities of improvement, which are indispensable to a systematic education; and, secondly, they constitute a tangible and conspicuous feature in our national establishment. The knowledge we possess exists only in the mind, and can only be perceived by its results; but our biblical and pharmaceutical storehouse, which is typical of that knowledge, will be a monument which, while it will afford endless means of instruction, may be considered an heir-loom to be handed down to our successors.

The content of each course was determined first by the ambitions of the Society in creating a distinct programme of pharmacy education, but this also inevitably involved looking over their shoulders to ensure that they were not treading on any other profession's toes. This was particularly true for materia medica. It was stated in *The Pharmaceutical Journal* in September 1842: "Although our lectures on Materia Medica will include an account of the general properties, effects and doses of remedies, they will not comprehend therapeutics and the practice of medicine, and therefore differ from the lectures on this subject in the medical schools." The course did not include pharmacodynamics (effects and uses of medicines) as the medical syllabus did, and had very little toxicology content in order to placate external critics. In his introductory lecture, Pereira again emphasised that he would be sensible to the divisions between pharmacy and medicine. For example, he would stop teaching on the subject of poisoning at the point where the assistance of a surgeon or physician could be obtained. Pereira had to tread very carefully as a physician, teaching in the first British pharmacy school. It has been suggested that his evening lectures in 1842 were deliberately chosen to be uncontroversial, one on food, and one on polarisation of light, rather than on his usual area of materia medica. Politically, pharmaceutical materia medica was destined to be medical botany and pharmacognosy with a little toxicology. The proposed Major exam included the need for knowledge of actions of antidotes and detection of poisons, but initially this was underplayed.

Shellard, the renowned pharmacognosist who graduated from the Square in the late 1930s, argued that Jonathan Pereira could be called the first British pharmacognosist. Pereira's inaugural lecture on 30th March 1842 laid out his approach to the subject, which he divided into three parts: a general study of drugs which he called pharmacognosy and pharmacology, alongside a history of simple drugs which he called pharmacopathia; pharmacy itself; and pharmacodynamics. This lecture appears to be the first reference in Great Britain to classify the study of crude drugs as "pharmacognosy", although it took many decades for this to become the name of the academic course. Pereira's course was lecture–demonstrations, with no practicals. It was assessed with oral exams with practical tests, so that students had to identify crude drugs and detect adulteration. Until the 1890s, materia medica covered the identification of commercial crude

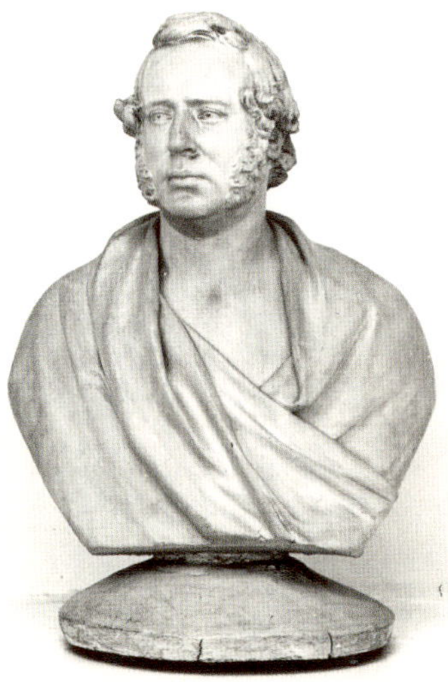

JONATHAN PEREIRA (1804–1853)

Royal Pharmaceutical Society Museum

JONATHAN PEREIRA (1804–1853)

Jonathan Pereira started work with an apothecary and naval surgeon aged 15, and went on to study materia medica and chemistry at the Aldersgate General Dispensary. Aged 19, he became a Licentiate of the Society of Apothecaries and took up the post of apothecary at the Aldersgate Dispensary. He taught a small class there, and published a translation of the *London Pharmacopoeia* for them in 1824. In the following year, he became a Member of the Royal College of Surgeons, and took on the role of lecturer in chemistry at Aldersgate. In 1828, he also started to teach materia medica at the Dispensary. When it was replaced by a new medical school, Pereira became its professor of materia medica. He also took on lecturing in chemistry at the London Hospital, and in 1838 he was elected a Fellow of the Royal Society. In 1839, he was appointed examiner in materia medica to the University of London, and wrote *Elements of Materia Medica* (1839–40). In 1841, he was elected assistant physician at the London Hospital, having taken the Royal College of Physician's diploma. He also received an MD from the University of Erlangen during this period.

Pereira was invited to give introductory lectures in 1842 at the School of Pharmacy on materia medica, and on the polarisation of light. In 1843, he was made professor of materia medica. He clearly inspired Joseph Ince, who recalled "his brilliant exposition and his fine delivery, and found the hitherto dry subject lit up with all the attraction which wit and anecdote and enthusiasm would invest pharmacology, we recognised both the genius of the lecturer and the value of his instruction." Redwood was also extremely complimentary about his colleague: "His lectures were unrivalled for the amount of information conveyed, and the brilliance of the style in which they were delivered. His large correspondence, his powers of original research, his constant application of the microscope, and his unusual facility in explanation, invested the subject with the deepest interest. As a referee he was an inexhaustible source of knowledge, and he was always ready to give further information at the close of his lecture to any inquiring student."

Pereira's relationship with the School became troubled in 1851 when some students supplied "garbled" versions of his lectures to be published in a journal without permission. Pereira suspended his lectures and appealed to the Council to protect him against such actions. Although he agreed to start the lectures again, he resigned a little later, but was persuaded to accept the appointment of honorary professor of materia medica. He clearly remained committed to the organisation, and transferred his specimens from the London Hospital to the Society's museum. However, he died as the result of an accident in 1853.

drugs, detection of adulteration and substitution, and an understanding of the botanical and geographical sources of the specimens that were being studied.

As an incentive for the students, prizes were awarded. For the first two years, these were only in Botany. The first winner was Robert Bentley, who went on to be professor of botany at the School from 1849. From 1844 to 1853, prizes of books were awarded in all four subject areas of botany, chemistry, pharmacy and materia

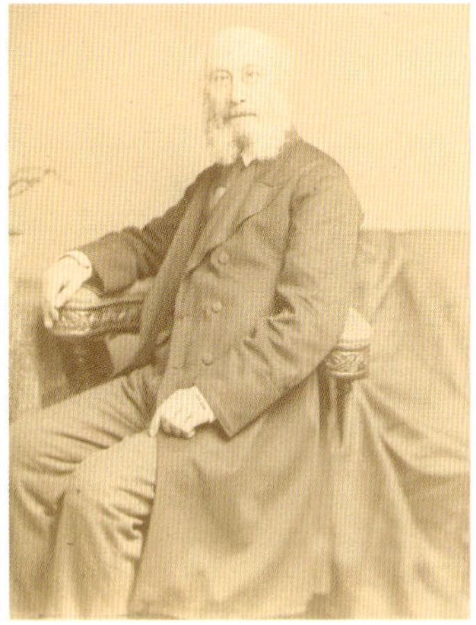

ROBERT BENTLEY (1821–1893)

Royal Pharmaceutical Society Museum

ROBERT BENTLEY (1821–1893)

Robert Bentley served his apprenticeship with a chemist–apothecary in Tunbridge Wells, before joining Jacob Bell's business in Oxford Street as an assistant. He attended Professor Thomson's first course of lectures at the School, and took the first botanical prize awarded. After studying medicine at King's College and becoming a member of the Royal College of Surgeons, he became head of the botany faculty and dean of the Medical School at King's. In 1849, he took over the role of professor of botany at the School of Pharmacy from Thomson. After Pereira's death in 1853, he also held the post of professor of materia medica.

Bentley clearly inspired a great deal of affection in his students. A "former 'Square Man'" reminisced in *The Pharmaceutical Journal* about Bentley's "demonstrations" at the Botanical Gardens: who "can fail to recall every detail of the surroundings, or to retain a trace of the love of his beautiful science which he never failed to impart to his 'boys' … Each felt that the professor was a friend, for he showed a personal interest in each individual. As a teacher too his style was admirable, and his constant revision of the work and cross-examination of students most useful in practising them in the art of concise and lucid reply." A student calling himself "Verax" recalled Bentley in 1879: "In appearance he resembled a country gentleman of the old school, while his well-knit, athletic frame, clear complexion and bright, sparkling eyes, spoke of one whose rambles were taken elsewhere than in the streets of London." He sometimes finished making a complex point by saying "Gentlemen, think this matter well over in your minds until you have both digested and assimilated it and then, in order to fix it indelibly in your memory, take the opportunity of explaining it to the young lady, in whose future you are specially interested, the next time you go for a stroll in the country together."

Bentley was president of the British Pharmaceutical Conference in 1866 and 1867, and chairman of the Garden Committee of the Royal Botanic Gardens in Regent's Park. His publications included *Manual of Botany* (1866), *Textbook of Organic Materia Medica* (1887) and *Medicinal Plants* (1880) written with H. Trimen. He resigned his professorship at the School in 1887, and was appointed emeritus professor.

medica. Bronze medals were introduced from 1854 instead of books, a combined one for chemistry and pharmacy, and a second for botany and materia medica. An additional medal was introduced for practical chemistry in 1863. The prizes were awarded at a special annual meeting, addressed by the professors.

The Council took stock of the School's performance in their report on the second anniversary of the Society on 16th May 1843. The report stated that "the Lecturers have reported their entire satisfaction at the regularity and attention of the Students, many of whom came from long distances." They also reported that they had arranged for 40 lectures on Botany by Dr Thomson over the summer, plus 50 on chemistry, 50 on materia medica and 25 on pharmacy in the autumn and winter. However, the reminder to members to allow apprentices to attend suggested that the number of students did not match the Council's ambitions. The School needed to continue to promote its existence and the value of its teaching to the whole profession. Their main channel was through *The Pharmaceutical Journal*. For example, a report in the *Journal* from the

Pharmaceutical Meeting of 8th October 1845 explained that "No expense was spared in providing the best LECTURERS on the subjects taught in the School, and the courses of lectures were made as extensive as the opportunities for attending them, which the pupils possessed, would admit of."

Of course, the School was not just run by the professors, something that Redwood was certainly mindful of. At the first pharmaceutical school dinner on 17th July 1849, he had sought permission to raise a toast to the past laboratory assistants, Mr Allchin and Mr Edwards, and to the present assistants, Mr Braithwaite and Mr Down.

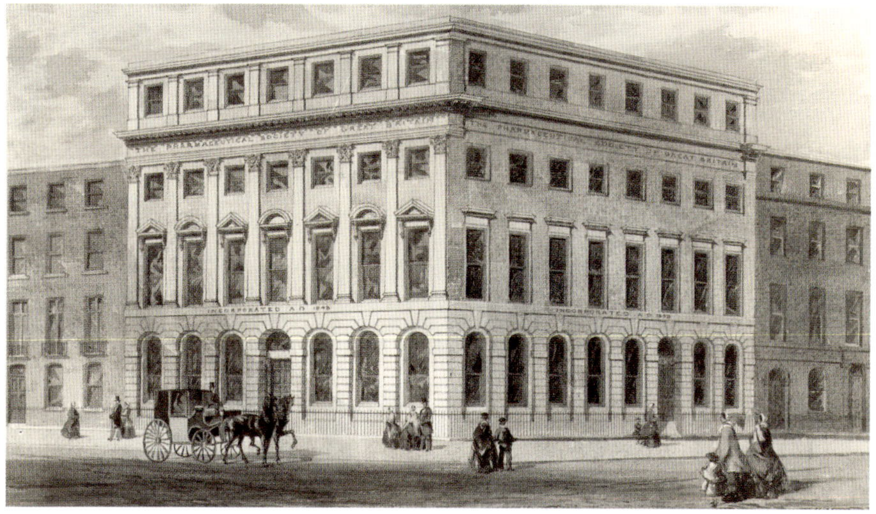

The new third floor, completed in 1860, is clearly shown in this image of 17 Bloomsbury Square by J.C. & G. Lansdown.

Royal Pharmaceutical Society Museum

THE BUILDING

The School was set up in 17 Bloomsbury Square, the house acquired by the Pharmaceutical Society as its headquarters in December 1841. Number 17 was a seventeenth century building, originally built in around 1675 by the Fourth Earl of Southampton for his daughter. It was remodelled by John Nash (1752–1835) into two houses in a neoclassical style as a speculative venture in 1778. Although the Society made many additions and alterations to the building in order to accommodate its needs, it retained the feel of a house, and the ornate ceilings and sweeping staircase remained at odds with laboratory benches and Bunsen burners throughout the Society's occupancy.

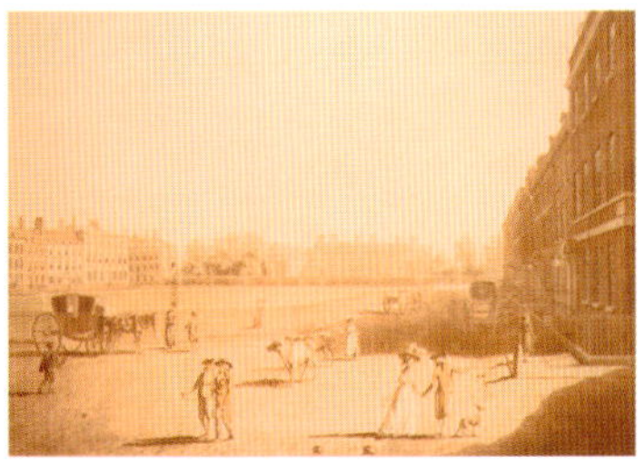

BLOOMSBURY SQUARE

Royal Pharmaceutical Society Museum

BLOOMSBURY SQUARE

First known as Southampton Square after the Earl of Southampton, Bloomsbury Square gained its name in the seventeenth century after the estate passed into the hands of the Duke of Bedford. Originally the site of a cherry orchard with farmland and ponds to the north, the Square itself was a prestige development. The gardens were originally laid out by the leading landscape gardener Humphry Repton (1752–1818). Living in Bloomsbury Square was the height of fashion in the early eighteenth century, and the Duke of Bedford chose to continue to live there as the Earl of Southampton had done, in a large town house which occupied the entire north side of the Square.

Although Bedford House was demolished to be replaced by two terraces of large town houses at the beginning of the nineteenth century, the Square retained its prestigious reputation. For example, the 1806 Bloomsbury Square Act forbade hackney coaches from standing for hire in the square or within 300 feet of it. The residents in the early nineteenth century were of high or professional status: architect James Donaldson, and his son Thomas Leverton Donaldson, who designed University College and University Hall; civil engineer Henry Austin, brother-in-law of Charles Dickens, as a child; George Man Burrows, and his son George (later Sir George) Burrows born here in 1801; the judge Lord Ellenborough; the Disraeli family from 1817 to 1829; Richard Bright, of Bright's disease, from around 1820 to 1831.

In 1816, a statue was erected in the gardens to Charles James Fox, Whig hero of the Duke of Bedford.

In the early years of the Pharmaceutical Society's residence, they had a number of medical and academic neighbours: no. 7 was the home of the Aikin scientific family; Charles (vaccinator who worked with Jenner) and his brother Arthur (geologist and chemist; former Unitarian minister) both died here, in 1847 and 1854, respectively; no. 39 was the site of the Hahnemann Hospital, established in 1850; no. 28 was the office of the secretary of the College of Preceptors, John Parker; no. 5 was from 1853 the office of James Brooks, the Gothic-revival church architect; no. 38 (demolished) was the home of surgeon and editor of the *Literary and Scientific Register*, John W.G. Gutch, who died there in 1862; no. 47 was the home of Thomas Horne, senior assistant librarian in the department of printed books in the British Museum, who died there in 1862; no. 29 was from 1862 to 1864 the home of Herbert Spencer, social philosopher and coiner of the term "survival of the fittest". In 1865, the retired principal librarian of the British Museum, Anthony Panizzi, moved out of the museum and into a house at 31 Bloomsbury Square, which he described as being "in a very unfashionable quarter, though very respectable." Number 23 became the first headquarters of the Metropolitan and National Nursing Association in 1875. In 1870, the Square featured in Charles Dickens's last and unfinished novel *The Mystery of Edwin Drood*: in the novel, a lodging house in Bloomsbury Square is used to provide a temporary haven for a single young lady, away from the threatening behaviour of men.

When G.H. Duckworth walked round this area on 13th July 1898 as part of the project to update Booth's poverty maps, he noted that it remained red, as it had been on the original map; this stood for "middle-class, well-to-do". Number 29 was the family home and office of architect Sir Edwin Lutyens from his marriage to Emily Bulwer-Lytton in 1897 until 1914. In 1902, no. 20 was home to Gertrude Stein, American writer. The Post Office Directory of 1902 lists many institutions here, in addition to the Pharmaceutical Society and the College of Preceptors: the Froebel Society and National Froebel Union at no. 4, the office of the British Asylum for Deaf and Dumb Females at no. 5 and the the Private Schools' Association at the same address, the Royal Institute of Public Health and the Institute of Sanitary Engineers at no. 19, and the Institute of Chemists of Great Britain and Ireland at no. 30.

One of the Society's earliest innovative developments was the establishment of facilities for practical instruction in chemistry. At the Council meeting of May 1843, it had been reported that "The Council have not yet been able to fit up a laboratory, in consequence of the difficulty of doing so at the Society's present house, and it will require much consideration before this essential undertaking is accomplished." However, a back room on the second floor was fitted out for use by eight students, although 10 students were admitted to the first session in October 1844. Practical work was carried out under the direction of Redwood, who admitted later that the whole project was "quite an experiment." However, in terms of educational and professional kudos, it was worth the effort: "The Pharmaceutical Society is entitled to the credit of having been the first institution in which provision was made in this country for carrying out a system of instruction in chemistry and pharmacy by practical operations in which the students were engaged throughout the day under the instruction of a professor."

Demand for the laboratory was great enough for the Society to embark on its first major construction project with the establishment of a teaching laboratory in 1845, which was built in the basement and garden of 17 Bloomsbury Square. A very excited article in the November 1845 edition of *The Pharmaceutical Journal* announced its opening. Those present at the evening Pharmaceutical Meeting on 8th October had been invited to view the new arrangements. Dr Ure had been asked to speak:

> He had seen many Laboratories intended for similar purposes, – he believed he had seen all those in Germany, including the celebrated one at Giessen, and most of those in France, and he was prepared to assert, that the Laboratory of the PHARMACEUTICAL SOCIETY, was, for its size, superior to any of these. It was better provided with conveniences for conducting the various operations of a laboratory, there was a more convenient distribution and arrangement of apparatus, and it was better ventilated and provided with means of getting rid of any injurious or offensive vapours, which often proved detrimental to the health of the students. In all these respects, it certainly was the most compact and commodious Laboratory that he had seen.

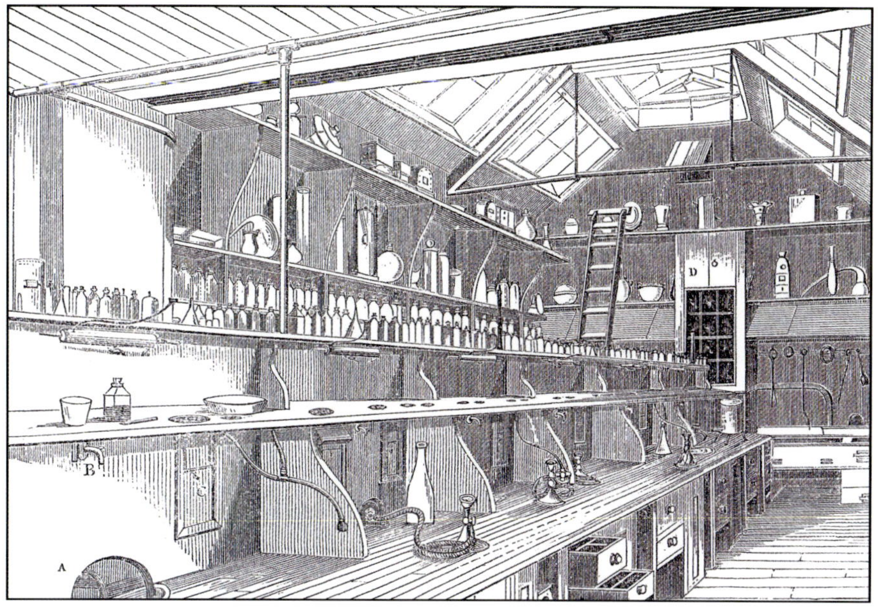

On 1st January 1846, *The Pharmaceutical Journal* published a full guide to the new laboratories including this engraving of the main run of benches with the sand bath and drying closet at the end.

The Pharmaceutical Journal

Instead of the usual evening meeting, a conversazione was held on 12th November 1845 to celebrate the opening of the laboratory. Visitors, members and associates were invited to look around. The laboratory itself had been fitted out to hold 18 students. The Society had planned for up to 400 visitors on the

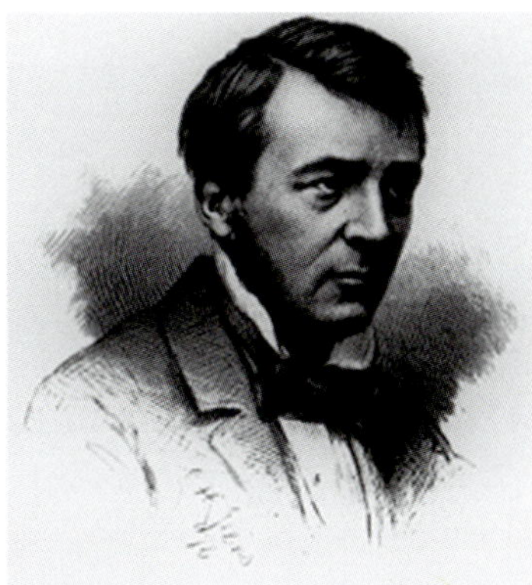

DANIEL HANBURY (1825–1875)

Royal Pharmaceutical Society Museum

DANIEL HANBURY (1825–1875)

Daniel Hanbury was a leading researcher and writer on materia medica. He was the son of Quaker pharmacist Daniel Bell Hanbury, who owned the Plough Court pharmacy with the Society's first president, William Allen, and John Thomas Barry. Daniel served his apprenticeship in his father's business prior to studying in the new practical chemistry laboratory at the Square in 1844. He became a member of the Society in 1857, and continued to work at Plough Court until 1870. He was president of the British Pharmaceutical Conference in 1868 and 1869, and a fellow of the Chemical Society and of the Royal Microscopical Society.

His passion, though, was materia medica, and he travelled widely in both Europe and Asia to find out more about the origins and preparation methods of drugs. After his death, around 200 papers which he had published were brought together by Joseph Ince into one volume, *Science Papers*. His book *Pharmacographia*, written with Professor Flückiger, and published in 1874, remained one of the most valuable references on current and historical materia medica for many decades. His significant collection of books was given to the Society's library and his herbarium of plants from around the world was donated to its museum. He is still commemorated by a medal, awarded by the Society every five years for outstanding research on natural history and the chemistry of drugs.

evening, but double the number attended, which apparently led to some confusion over returning hats and coats. The visitors were given a number of demonstrations during the course of the evening, including the manufacture of sulphuric ether, of alcohol, and of carbonate of ammonia, plus the operation of the furnaces, sand-baths, stills and drying closets.

The previous laboratory, which had been fitted out in 1844 with accommodation for 10 students, was also open, and it was pointed out that the two laboratories could be run together to maximise the teaching space. As the first conversazione that the Society had ever held, they also took the opportunity to exhibit a display of models of crystals in the curator's room, to show off specimens in the library and lecture room, and to invite a supplier of cutting-edge soda-water syphon vases for aerated waters to demonstrate their goods. Although clearly an extremely successful event, it is telling that *The Pharmaceutical Journal* report makes a special note that the tea and coffee supplied was funded by Council members, not Society funds, clearly anticipating some criticism from members.

For those unable to attend, the *Journal* of 1st January 1846 featured a fully illustrated description of the new laboratory, including floor plans, illustrations and labelled diagrams of all the apparatus. Regulations for the laboratory were also given in full.

In 1857, the Society took its next opportunity to enlarge the headquarters when it acquired 72 and 73 Great Russell Street for a period of 90 years. Although it proved expensive, the Society rearranged and extended the majority of the existing rooms: the library, museum, lecture theatre, exam rooms, secretary's offices, and the council and committee rooms.

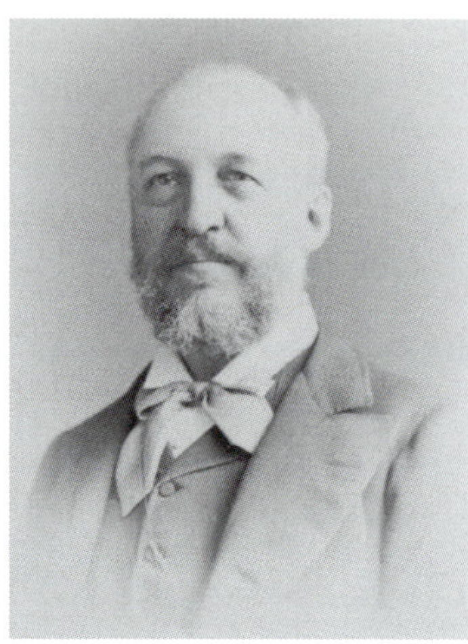

BENJAMIN HORATIO PAUL (1827–1917)

Royal Pharmaceutical Society Museum

BENJAMIN HORATIO PAUL (1827–1917)

Benjamin Paul served an apprenticeship with a chemist & druggist, although he wanted to become a chemist rather than a pharmacist. He came to London in 1844 and started at the School of Pharmacy. He was the Chemistry prize winner in 1845, aged 18, and passed the Major exam in the same year. He then worked briefly as a demonstrator to Professor Redwood, before studying in the laboratory at Giessen under Professor Liebig, graduating with a PhD in 1848. After a short time acting as an assistant chemist in Dublin and Belfast, he returned to London and took on the role of secretary to the Pre-Raphaelite Brotherhood of artists, as he had shared lodgings with Dante Gabriel Rossetti in Bloomsbury. Following this, he managed the business of Professor Thomas Graham, assayer to the Mint and the Bank of England.

However, Paul had started writing on chemical subjects in the 1840s, and worked on a translation of a geology book in the 1850s. He started contributing to *The Pharmaceutical Journal* in 1856 and became editor in 1870, continuing until retirement 32 years later. During much of his time on the *Journal*, he also practised as a consulting and analytical chemist, including taking on the analysis of all of the cinchona bark sold in London, and also significant work on ipecacuanha. Perhaps more surprisingly, recent research has found that Dr Paul spent some time working in the Hebrides devising a way to convert peat into paraffin oil.

Perhaps the biggest change to the building in its history was prompted by a legacy from Jacob Bell. At the Council meeting on 6th July 1859, it was announced that a letter had been received from the executors of Bell's will stating that he had bequeathed £2,000 to the Society. Bell's will stated that the sum was "to be expended in establishing or otherwise increasing the efficiency of a School of Pharmacy, or in promoting pharmaceutical education …" In considering how to spend Bell's legacy, the Council knew that he had wanted to build a laboratory on site. They had been looking for alternative premises for an off-site laboratory without success as the Duke of Bedford did not want a chemical laboratory established on his estate. The Council employed an architect, who confirmed that it would be possible to build the additional floor on top of the entire building. Work must have started in early 1860. Redwood remembered that: "the house of the society was surrounded by scaffold-poles and the arrangements of the establishment were in a state of disorder and reorganization. Students were working at chemical and pharmaceutical operations, not in their accustomed places, but wherever unoccupied space could be found for them, and especially in the room that has since become the library."

"The laboratories, which are nearly finished, are, in extent and with regard to the completeness of the arrangements, unequalled in this country."

The Pharmaceutical Journal, 1860

The opening of the new third floor laboratories also marked the most significant step-change in teaching at the School in the nineteenth century. The new facilities were a source of great pride to the Society: "The laboratories, which are nearly finished, are, in extent and with regard to the completeness of the arrangements, unequalled in this country." An article in *The Pharmaceutical Journal* of 1st September 1860 also explained the impact on the students' progress as they were able to see each other at work: "This is one of the advantages resulting from studying in a public laboratory, where the pupils not only stimulate each other by the emulation which naturally arises, but afford mutual instruction by the inquiries, suggestions, and results, which all contribute in their daily intercourse." Sixty working spaces were provided on the new floor, with each student allocated a working bench with a lock-up cupboard for his belongings. A list of apparatus to be bought by each student was supplied, which included a set of evaporating basins, a retort stand and three rings, two porcelain crucibles and one pair of eight-inch brass crucible tongs, half a pound of small India rubber tubing, and three dozen corks of various sizes.

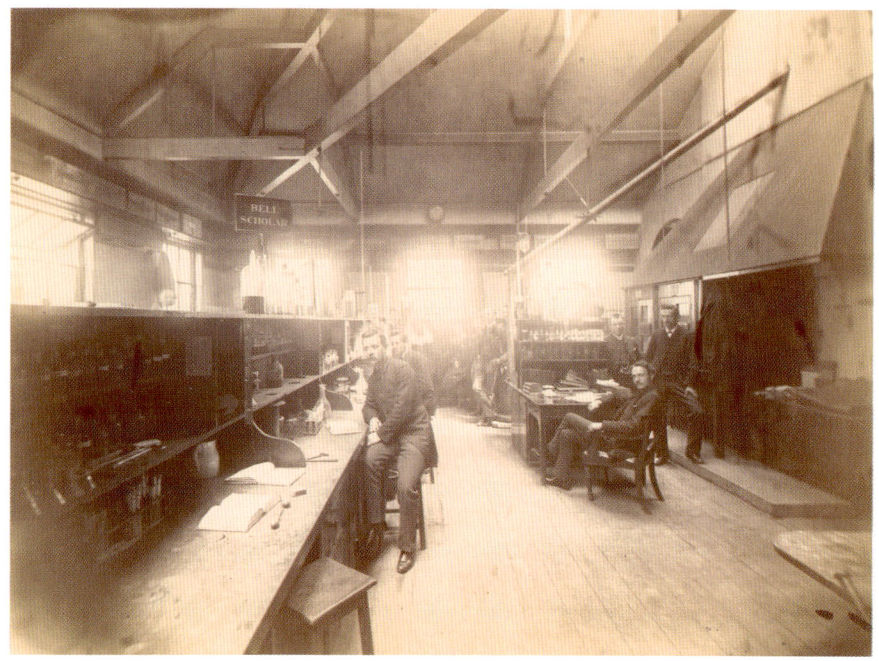

There are no surviving photographs of the new chemistry labs until the early 1880s. This one shows a crowd of students clustered in the background, with the Jacob Bell scholars Fraser McDiarmid and R. Wynn Charles Pierce at their allocated desks. The senior demonstrator is lounging at his desk on the left.

Royal Pharmaceutical Society Museum

A leading article in *The Pharmaceutical Journal* expressed some concerns about the new laboratory. It reported that the Council had admitted that the upkeep of the School's activities cost around £3,000 each year, but there was a very small number of students: "Strange to say, the parties for whom this expensive system was organized appeared to be insensible to the value and importance of the benefits offered to them, or at any rate, they were not prepared at that time to avail themselves of the offer so generally as it was expected they would have done." Bell's legacy had provided the capital sum to allow the Society to build the new laboratory, which was hoped to provide a draw to many new students, but it was recognised that it would not be able to be run as a self-supporting department. The need to significantly increase the numbers of students in order financially to support the educational initiatives was very great.

One strategy which was continued was to promote the membership category of "registered apprentice". Although not compulsory, under the 1852 Pharmacy Act if you passed the classical exam and paid a two-guinea fee, plus a half-guinea annual fee, you received copies of *The Pharmaceutical Journal*, had free admission to the library and museum, were eligible to apply for Jacob Bell Scholarships and were admitted to the Society's lectures for half the normal fees. If you went on to take the Minor exam, you paid a reduced fee of three guineas, rather than five. The Society was clearly attempting to tie apprentices into the educational scheme.

Writing over a decade later, Redwood concluded that the alterations to the building in 1860 led to "a suite of well-lighted and ventilated laboratories, capable of accommodating a large number of students." The changes also had a much-needed impact on teaching and staffing. As Redwood well knew, the current staffing was insufficient for the new set-up:

> It had become the practice for many years past, with a view to economy, to heap many duties on to the shoulders of a few officers, and this was especially the case with regard to the departments alluded to [library and museum], and to the laboratory, lectures, and scientific committees. Formerly the laboratory had been almost always full to overflowing; but now that its accommodation was more than doubled, it was found that in order to keep it in the same satisfactory condition, more undivided attention was required from the professor, and it was therefore decided to appoint a teacher for this special duty.

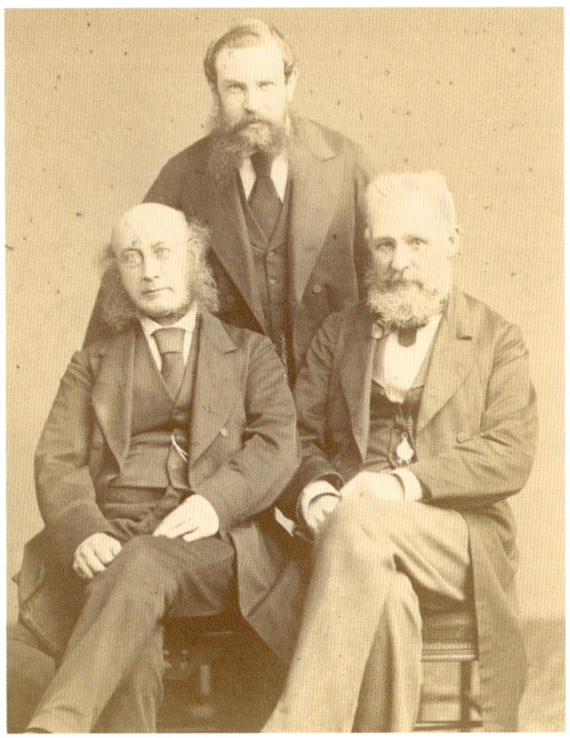

Professors Bentley, Attfield and Redwood were photographed in 1878 by the fashionable photography studio, Elliott and Fry.

Royal Pharmaceutical Society Museum

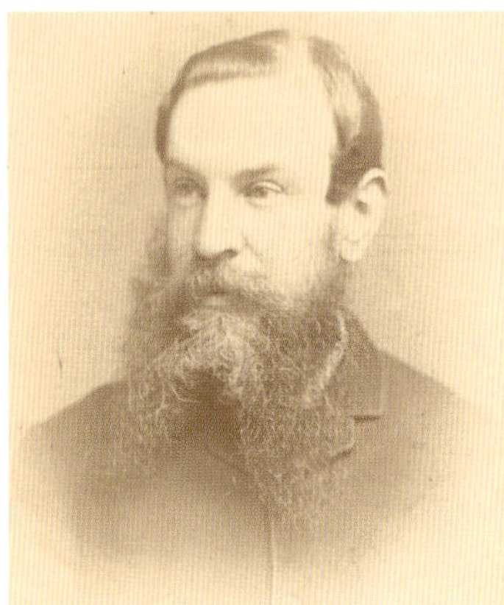

JOHN ATTFIELD (1835–1911)

Royal Pharmaceutical Society Museum

JOHN ATTFIELD (1835–1911)

John Attfield studied at the School after an apprenticeship to a manufacturing chemist. He passed the Major exam in 1854 and became assistant and then demonstrator to the lecturer in chemistry at St Bartholomew's Hospital medical school. In 1862, he gained a PhD from Tübingen, and was appointed director and demonstrator in chemistry and pharmacy at the Square. The post was later changed to professor of practical pharmacy. His *Manual of Chemistry*, first published in 1857, went through 19 editions and was recommended in the School's prospectus until 1900. In 1883, Attfield was awarded a gold medal at the first International Pharmaceutical Exhibition in Vienna for the book, and in 1896 at the Prague International Pharmaceutical Exhibition was awarded the Diploma of Honour, the highest award. Attfield was elected a fellow of the Royal Society in 1880.

Attfield was fiercely opposed to the "crammer" schools that flourished after the 1868 Pharmacy Act, speaking and writing in favour of a meaningful pharmacy education rather than a brief course focused entirely on passing the Minor exam. He was a founder member of the British Pharmaceutical Conference and its president in 1882 and 1883. In the 34 years he spent at the School, it was calculated that he had taught 2,367 students. His retirement party in 1897, attended by over 250 guests, was reported fully in the pharmaceutical press. On the day of his funeral in 1911, the School was closed as a mark of respect.

This teacher was Dr John Attfield, who was appointed to the post of director and demonstrator of chemistry and pharmacy in 1862, as a full-time teacher to concentrate fully on the laboratory. Attfield's appointment was a very satisfying development as he had been a student at the School, and a medallist in chemistry and pharmacy, and in botany and materia medica in 1854.

The new laboratories also provided the impetus for new classes. Mr Braithwaite, one of the principal laboratory assistants, started lessons in pharmaceutical Latin, from 8pm to 10pm. He also provided some tuition in dispensing, in order to make up for deficiencies that had been observed in students in the past. Mr Wood, the other principal laboratory assistant, started a new course on systematic analysis, including detection of adulterations in medicines and food. A move into this area of study clearly showed the School's ambitions for students to attend who wanted to train to be analysts. It was explained that this course was intended to provide support for those who would primarily be studying at home. Both of these courses were made possible with the organisation of "a tolerably good lecture theatre", as Redwood described it, taking over the area where the laboratory had been in the basement. Because it could be divided in two, it was possible to prepare courses in one half of the room while classes were in progress in the other half, thus significantly increasing the School's capacity. The Society's evening meetings were also held in the new lecture theatre, and the old lecture room on the first floor became the examinations room.

Jacob Bell's other major legacy was the scholarships set up in his memory. After his death in June 1859, the Council appointed a committee to form a Capital Fund from which to fund memorial scholarships. The scholarship committee reported back to Council on 20th July that they proposed to set up two scholarships, one for registered apprentices and associates under 21 years old, and one scholarship for associates under 24 years old who had passed the Major exam, "with the view of encouraging the further prosecution of scientific study."

The Council sent out a circular to drum up interest and received nearly £2,000 within a few months, which enabled them to found the proposed two scholarships for £30 each year. The first two scholars were W.A. Tilden and T.W.H. Tolbert, who both received the award in 1861. The report in *The Pharmaceutical Journal* explained that there had been no applications for the senior scholarship, but nine applicants for the junior one. As a result, they had appointed two junior Bell Scholars. As it was the first time that the scholarships were awarded, the Committee wanted to report that the successful competitors had done well in the scholarship exams, but also had "very flattering testimonials" from their teachers, "not only to their diligent cultivation of the science of their profession, but also to the industrious and cheerful manner with which they had performed all the business duties devolving upon them." One of the practical changes made as a result of the scholarships was the establishment of two allotted benches for the Bell Scholars in the practical chemistry laboratory, each marked with a sign.

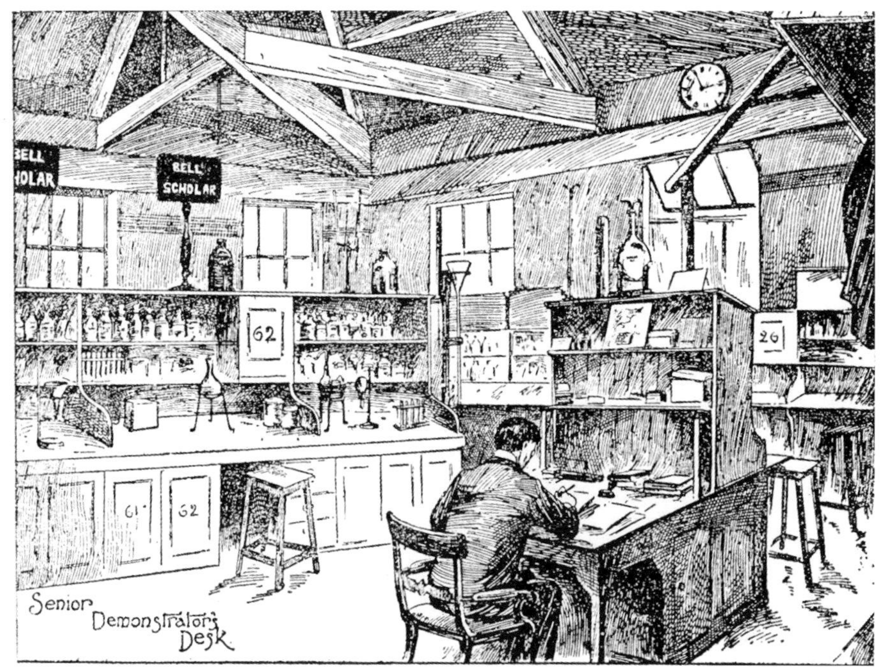

The Bell Scholars were allocated their own desks in the new chemistry laboratory, as shown in this engraving from *The Pharmaceutical Journal* in 1896, with the senior demonstrator's desk in the foreground.

The Pharmaceutical Journal

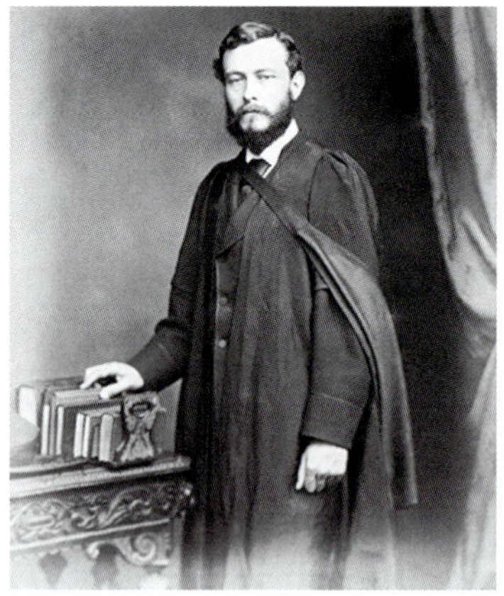

WILLIAM AUGUSTUS TILDEN (1842–1926)

Royal Pharmaceutical Society Museum

WILLIAM AUGUSTUS TILDEN (1842–1926)

W.A. Tilden started his apprenticeship as a pharmacist in 1857, moving from the family home in Bedford to Islington in North London. He became one of the first two Bell Scholars and entered the School in 1861. He passed the Minor exam in 1862, and the Major in 1872. He worked as a demonstrator in the School under Professor Attfield from 1863, gaining his BSc in 1868 and a DSc (London) in 1871. He left London the following year to become senior master at Clifton College in Bristol. In 1880, he became professor of chemistry at Mason College, Birmingham. From 1891 to 1894 he was president of the Institute of Chemistry, and in 1894, he took up the post of professor of chemistry at the Royal College of Science until his retirement in 1909. He was knighted in that year and made emeritus professor of the College. During his retirement he wrote four publications: *The Elements* (1910), *Chemical Discovery and Invention in the Twentieth Century* (1917), *Life of Sir William Ramsay* (1918) and *Famous Chemists* (1921).

His memoirs are rather disparaging about his time at the Square. He wrote about the Bell Scholarship that "I owe nothing whatever in the way of teaching to the scholarship, except the money, for during the session the Professor [Redwood] appeared only twice. The first time he came to receive the fees … The second time he was showing some stranger round the place …" Although he spent 14 years in total at the School, he does not seem to have felt affectionate towards it: "the teaching which existed in 1858 of physics and chemistry was utter rubbish, entirely behind the knowledge and experience of the time." He described Redwood's lectures as "insufferably boring" and went to Hofmann's course at the Royal College of Chemistry instead. He thought that Professor Bentley's teaching in botany was very uninspiring, and also dealt out backhanded compliments to Professor Attfield: "though he cared very little for scientific work, he certainly took good care of the students."

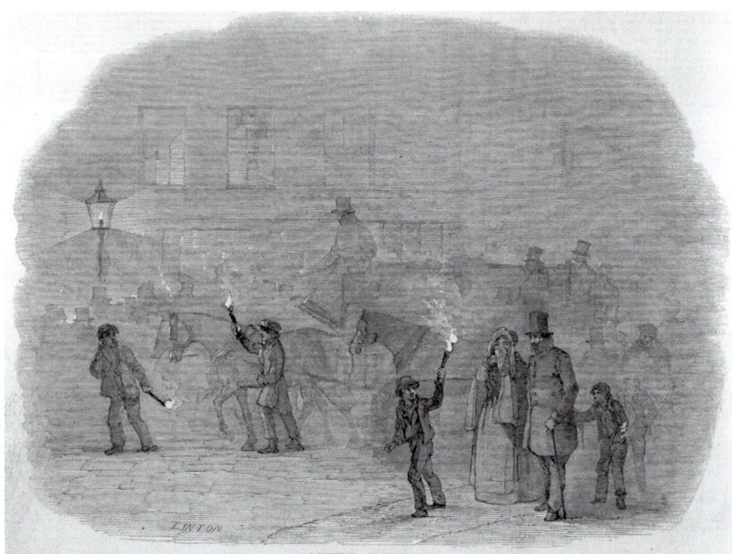

In 1847, *The Illustrated London News* gave an impression of the characteristic dense London smogs.

Wellcome Library, London

THE STUDENT EXPERIENCE

Who were the School's early students, and what were their experiences of pharmacy education? In an article entitled "The Opening of the School of Pharmacy" in *The Pharmaceutical Journal* dated 1st June 1842, it was reported that students at Thomson's first botany lectures numbered more than 40: "we were glad to see a numerous and attentive audience." They came from Kensington, Sloane Square, Bayswater, Brixton, Walworth, Islington and Clapham, two to five miles away from Bloomsbury Square, and were arriving for an 8am start.

The *Journal* took an encouraging tone:

> By rising an hour earlier on lecture mornings, and performing their duties at home with increased diligence, those who enjoy the privilege have the opportunity of proving that the study of the profession is not incompatible with the drudgery of their trade, while it gives a degree of interest and variety to a pursuit, which, when merely followed mechanically, is dull and monotonous.

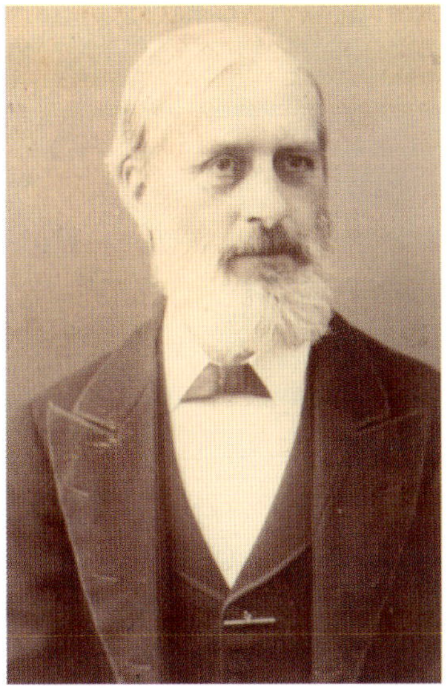

JOSEPH INCE (1826–1907)

Royal Pharmaceutical Society Museum

JOSEPH INCE (1826–1907)

Joseph Ince was born into a pharmaceutical family. His father William became director of Godfrey and Cooke, a business originally founded in about 1660, and became president of the Pharmaceutical Society in 1850. Joseph studied at King's College, and went on to serve as an apprentice to Richard Hotham Pidgeon, first Treasurer of the Pharmaceutical Society. He attended the Schools of Medicine and Pharmacy in Paris for two years after his apprenticeship. On his return in 1847, he entered the School of Pharmacy. He became an assistant at Godfrey and Cooke and stayed on the staff for many years, succeeding his father as director. He passed his Major exam in 1862 and set up his own business for a short while, but gave it up and was lecturer on pharmacy for Dr Muter's School. In 1883, he took on a new role as Dr Redwood's assistant at the Square, and was charged by the Council to set up a department of practical pharmacy.

Ince served on the Society's Council from 1866 to 1869 and was also an examiner for six years. He assisted Jacob Bell with *The Pharmaceutical Journal*, for which he wrote many articles. He was also the author of *Latin Grammar of Pharmacy* and of *Elementary Dispensing Practice*.

However, Joseph Ince, who was a student at the Square in 1847, told a slightly different story: "It did happen in some cases, that an assistant who had far to come had started his long walk without breakfast and over-taxed his strength in the struggle to combine the pursuit of science with business operations."

The *Journal* included an article in February 1843 "in order to give an idea of the course of reading and study which ought to be pursued by candidates for admission as Associates." The piece included a description of the exam, a suggestion of possible books to read, and a reminder to look at plant specimens, advising that it is possible for the general public to go to the Royal Botanic Gardens at Kew, which first opened to the public in 1841. The author refused to be definitive about the time it would take for a student to prepare for the exam, stating that it would vary for each candidate.

Ince remembered a fellow student in the chemistry course in 1847, John Baker Edwards, who worked his way through a printed list of chemicals very rapidly. As the first to prepare chloroform in the class, his peers found it very exciting, "for we had read about but had never seen the famous anaesthetic." Edwards mixed it with alcohol to make chloric ether and handed it round to taste:

> Instantly the compound took effect in a disastrous and unexpected manner; they began to sing and shout and race round the benches. The tumult was at its height when Redwood, startled by the uproar, ventured to appear in time to witness a free fight, and one of the combatants reposing in the sand-bath. Order was soon restored, and a short explanation allayed the professor's fears.

Ince's reminiscences, published in the *Journal* in 1903, contain other vivid memories. He clearly enjoyed Thomson's classes in the RBS gardens in Regents Park: "Well do I remember these matutinal botanical rambles and the hot tea and coffee, cake, and bread-and-butter provided at a stall outside the gardens … Not seldom did Jacob Bell ride up on horseback and sit in the museum lecture-room – a student, like the rest." However, Ince's enthusiasm did not seem to always result in punctuality. He recalled that some lectures were given in the room next to the library, with folding doors creating an antechamber once the lecture had begun: "Late comers had to listen penitentially outside, and make good resolutions for the future."

Another student in 1847 was Richard W. Giles who, having passed the Major exam, joined his father in business in Clifton, Bristol, and went on to form the Bristol Chemists' Association. As a student, he was not quite so diligent: "The approach of these [Society's] examinations could always be predicted from the group of eager students gathered around the drawers. But at other times, and except for the occasional visit of one or two of Dr Pereira's class bent on verifying some point in his morning's lecture, the museum was not much frequented by us."

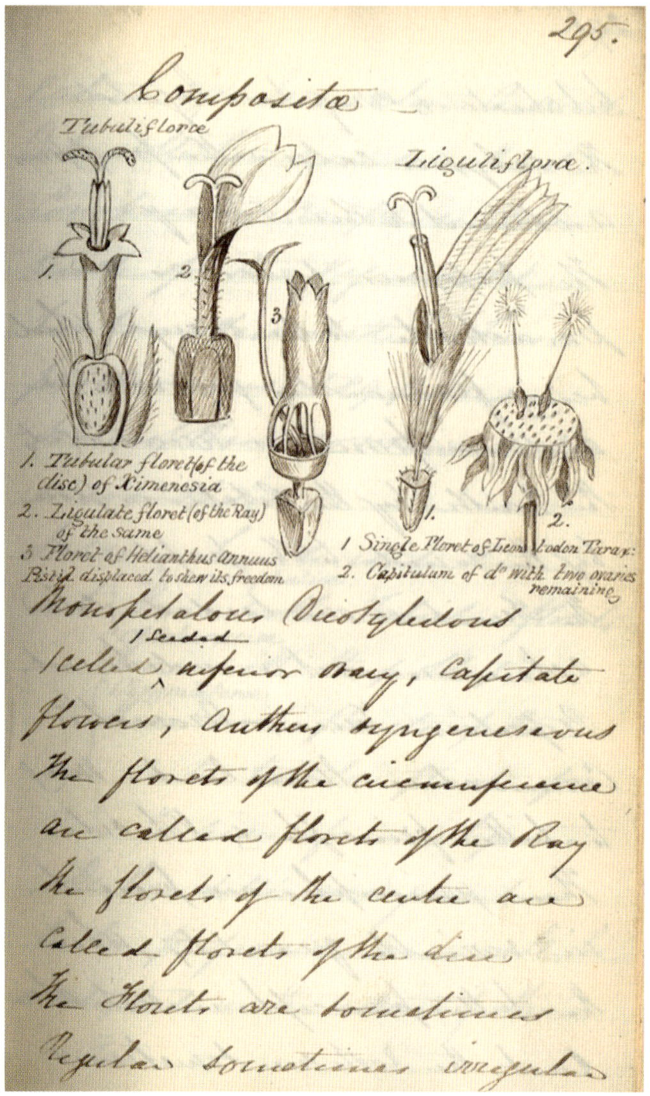
295.
Compositæ
Tubulifloræ
Ligulifloræ.
1. Tubular floret (of the disc) of Ximenesia
2. Ligulate floret (of the Ray) of the same
3 Floret of Helianthus annuus Pistil displaced to shew its freedom
1 Single Floret of Leontodon Tarax:
2. Capitulum of do with two ovaries remaining
Monopetalous Dicotyledons
The florets of the circumference are called florets of the Ray
the florets of the centre are called florets of the disc
The Florets are sometimes regular sometimes irregular

R.W. Giles produced detailed illustrations as part of his lecture notes for the 1847-8 session. These show features for members of the Compositae or daisy family: Ximenesia, Helianthus annuus (sunflower) and Leortodon tarax.

Royal Pharmaceutical Society Museum

In 1848, some students experienced a different role when they were enrolled as special constables to defend the area against Chartist demonstrators in Russell Square. As shops and houses were boarded up, special constables' staffs were provided to workers at the British Museum and students at the Square, headed by Professor Redwood. In the event, the demonstrators dispersed and no damage was done.

William (later Sir William) Tilden went to see the Society's first laboratory in the early days of his apprenticeship, around 1857: "There was an irritating vapour in the place and furnaces from which the fumes proceeded. The teacher had on a black skull-cap, and altogether the scene reminded one of the description of an alchemist's laboratory." Joseph Ince also recalled that the fumes would rise "to the discomfort of the Council whilst holding their deliberations; irate messages from the upper regions were not infrequent." Redwood had no choice but to devise an efficient ventilation system. The laboratory students were clearly keen as, in May 1850, a "Laboratory Class" was formed to meet on Saturday mornings in the Council room. A minute book was kept with a résumé of each meeting. The class continued to meet until 15th March 1856.

In 1853, a phytological club of the Pharmaceutical Society was founded by associates and junior members. Its object was the extension of study and the application of the science of botany, with Robert Bentley as president. The club continued until 1860.

Although the majority of the early students were already based in London, apprentices from the provinces did attend, living in London for a period of months in order to study at the School. However, there was also a small number of overseas students. In 1847, a French student attended from Mauritius, under British control since 1810. A Parliamentary Select Committee called to discuss the proposed Pharmacy Act included a hearing on 22nd April 1852 from C. Baschet, a resident of Mauritius who was studying for a diploma at the School, which was one of the European qualifications needed to set up and run a business in Mauritius. At the Annual Meeting in 1848, it was reported in typically bigoted nineteenth century terms that "It is also gratifying to find that some [students] have come from distant countries, and one of these, an intelligent African, is probably the first native of that soil who will apply a knowledge of chemistry acquired in an English school, with the view of promoting the arts of civilization among his coloured brethren."

The Society's faith in the student body was enhanced in 1849 with their proposal for an annual pharmaceutical school dinner. Having commented on their apathy in the previous edition, an advert for the dinner stated that:

> it is gratifying to observe that a very different spirit animates those who have experienced the benefit of the improved education which it was a leading object of the Society to introduce. As a means of promoting harmony and extending the interest in this important branch of the Institution, a Pharmaceutical School Dinner is proposed … Originating as it does among the Students themselves, the proposition has been warmly seconded by many of the Members of the Society, who are desirous of encouraging this evidence of zeal in the cause of pharmaceutical education among the Junior Members of our body.

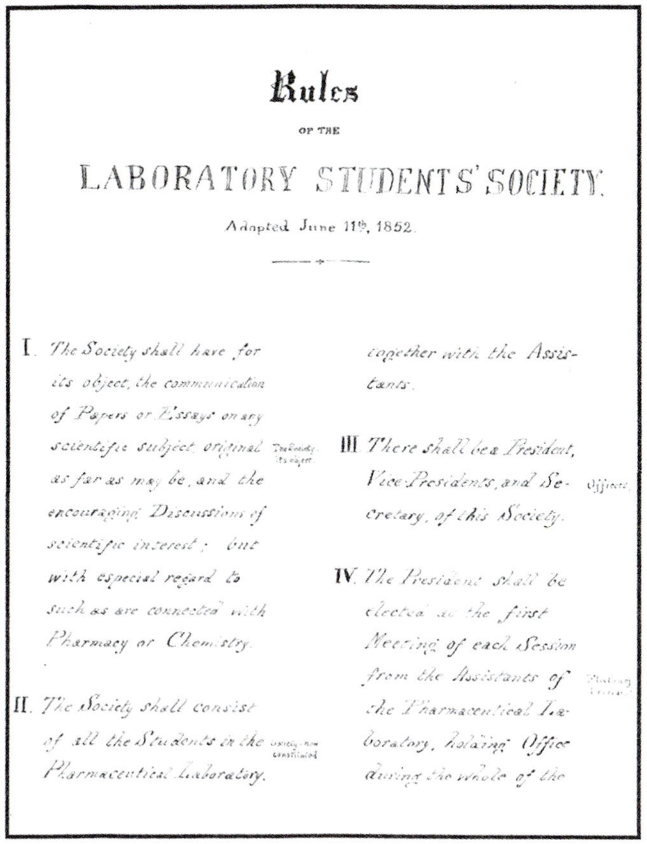
Rules
of the
LABORATORY STUDENTS' SOCIETY.
Adopted June 11th, 1852.

I. The Society shall have for its object, the communication of Papers or Essays on any scientific subject, original as far as may be, and the encouraging Discussions of scientific interest; but with especial regard to such as are connected with Pharmacy or Chemistry.

II. The Society shall consist of all the Students in the Pharmaceutical Laboratory, together with the Assistants.

III. There shall be a President, Vice-Presidents, and Secretary, of this Society.

IV. The President shall be elected at the first Meeting of each Session from the Assistants of the Pharmaceutical Laboratory, holding Office during the whole of the

The minute book of the Laboratory Students' Society, founded in 1852, started with their rules.

Royal Pharmaceutical Society Museum

The inaugural dinner was held at the London Tavern on 17th July 1849. Dr Copland, a leading physician and Fellow of the Royal Society, acted as chair and 134 guests attended. There were a number of toasts and speeches, including one by Mr Rogers of Honiton, who spoke on behalf of the past students:

> He had been accustomed, as an apprentice, to mix various ingredients together, of the nature and composition of which he was almost as ignorant as the pestle with which he stirred them in the mortar … He had to thank the School of the Pharmaceutical Society for unveiling the mysteries of science to his mind, and teaching him the principles upon which alone his business could be safely and satisfactorily conducted.

It was clearly a good-natured event. Pereira responded on behalf of the professors, "it must be remembered that those who attended the school were generally the best men from among the whole body – those who studied Pharmacy from pure love of the subject."

"it must be remembered that those who attended the school were generally the best men from among the whole body – those who studied Pharmacy from pure love of the subject."

Dr Pereira, 17th July 1849

"It may safely be affirmed that a more orderly, industrious, and intelligent class of students does not exist than that which usually assembles in Bloomsbury Square. They have all one ultimate object in view, the completion of their practical and scientific qualifications as pharmaceutical chemists."

The Pharmaceutical Journal, 1860

OTHER SCHOOLS

It has been estimated that there were around 3,000 young men in the pharmacy profession in the 1840s. With fewer than 80 students in lectures and 25 in the laboratory, the School was only reaching a small proportion of the total. Other than continuing with a traditional apprenticeship, what could the majority do to gain formal pharmacy education?

Initially, apprentices and assistants were advised through *The Pharmaceutical Journal* to attend lectures, but if these were not available, to read, study plants, carry out chemical experiments and apply the knowledge they had obtained to the practical operations of the dispensing counter. Of course, although lecture attendance was advised, it was out of the question for the majority of aspiring pharmacists.

Provision of formal pharmacy education outside London was rare. In 1848, Dr G.D. Fripp, physician to Bristol General Hospital, addressed the Bristol Chemists' Association. He suggested that schools of pharmacy should be annexed to existing medical schools as some subjects were common to both. Some pharmacy students did attend lectures at medical schools, but the emphasis provided was not specific to pharmacy and there was not enough practical work to suit the needs of aspiring Society members. Another approach was taken by the Society. The first list of founders of the Society includes members who are indicated to be local officers. These names suggest that there were at least 29 pharmaceutical associations in place in Britain at the end of 1841, and certainly some had established some kind of educational provision, including Bath, Bristol, Colchester, Exeter, Liverpool, Manchester, Newcastle and Norwich.

Various reports in *The Pharmaceutical Journal* described the situation in Manchester. In April 1842, a conversazione was held in Manchester at which a Mr Woolley proposed that regional schools of pharmacy should be established attached to medical schools, as pharmacy subjects were already being taught there. The *Journal*'s editorial voice, presumably Jacob Bell, agreed that provincial schools should be established with branches working with the "parent establishment". He made the point that the Society had to make sure that everyone was working with one system so that it was to everyone's advantage. The momentum in Manchester continued with a meeting of local pharmacists at the Manchester Mechanics Institute in December 1842 to discuss arrangements for the establishment of a school, which led to a series of lectures in pharmaceutical chemistry beginning on 11th January 1843, held in the Royal Medical Institution, Pine Street. This followed the precedent of a course of lectures on pharmaceutical chemistry given at Pine Street Medical School by John Dalton in 1824. The report suggests that the lectures given in 1843 were very general, delivered by John Davies, lecturer in chemistry at the medical school. They followed with a course in Medical botany, which 43 members and associates attended. Interestingly, this meant that the proportion of people attending in relation to total Society membership of the area was higher than in London. The report concludes by saying that similar courses were also being arranged in Bristol, Bath, Liverpool, Newcastle, Norwich and Birmingham.

In 1843, the Society established a scheme for "branch schools". They were to be organised and managed by local members, but the Society would provide an annual grant equivalent to one-quarter of the total annual subscription income for that area. The only stipulations were that lectures had to be given in essential pharmaceutical subjects and that pharmacy lectures had to be given by a teacher with practical knowledge.

An article appeared in the *Journal* on 1st April 1843 providing an update on progress. In Manchester, the lectures on pharmaceutical chemistry given by Mr Davies were reported, alongside a course of lectures given in Bristol. The branch in Bath wanted to arrange some on chemistry and pharmacy, plus enthusiasm had been expressed in Liverpool, Newcastle, Norwich and Birmingham. However, the parent body had to continue to keep its attention on the overall picture: "Our object is to establish an effectual and permanent system of education; in effecting which object, no contingency should be overlooked; and whatever plans are proposed, must be considered, with reference not merely to any particular locality, but to the general interests and requirements of the society at large."

By 1844, Society grants had been given to Manchester, Norwich, Bath and Bristol. However, it was very difficult to set up successful branch schools. As was the case in London, apprentices worked long hours, and at a distance from any institution that could host the lectures, meaning that they would probably have to walk as there was no public transport in most areas. People attending the lectures in Manchester came from Bolton, Bury and Rochdale, and therefore could make use of the new train system, but this was the exception. Masters also had to let their apprentices go. In 1850, pharmacists in Edinburgh agreed that freedom to attend lectures should be written into indentures.

However, the situation was difficult from the start. In 1843, the Society's membership demanded a reduction in subscription, and it was halved in 1844. The members were told that this would affect provincial schools and the Benevolent Fund, and this was really the death knell to the existing branch schools. In London, the Royal College of Chemistry opened in 1845, and based its teaching laboratory on the Society's, opened earlier in the year. The early attendance figures suggest that a small proportion of those taught at the RCC entered the pharmacy profession.

At the opening of the fourth session of the Society's School in 1845, it was described as a national establishment, intended to serve the needs of the whole country. Whilst appreciating that in order to take advantage of it you had to be able to live and study in London, the Society clearly refocused its efforts on the central educational establishment. Ironically, from 1848 to 1852, three-quarters of the students attending the laboratory courses were not Londoners. However, in 1849, following a visit by Jacob Bell, the Liverpool Chemists' Association was founded, which organised lectures, and formed a library and materia medica museum. Although the initial response to the initiative was poor, these beginnings developed into the Liverpool School of Pharmacy, the last of the private schools to be taken over by public authority in the mid-twentieth century. The establishment of similar schools outside London was slow until the impetus provided by the 1868 Pharmacy Act.

However, the Society's foundations allowed for the development of a core of educational pioneers. Its powers to elect honorary members explicitly enabled the Society to achieve its educational objectives.

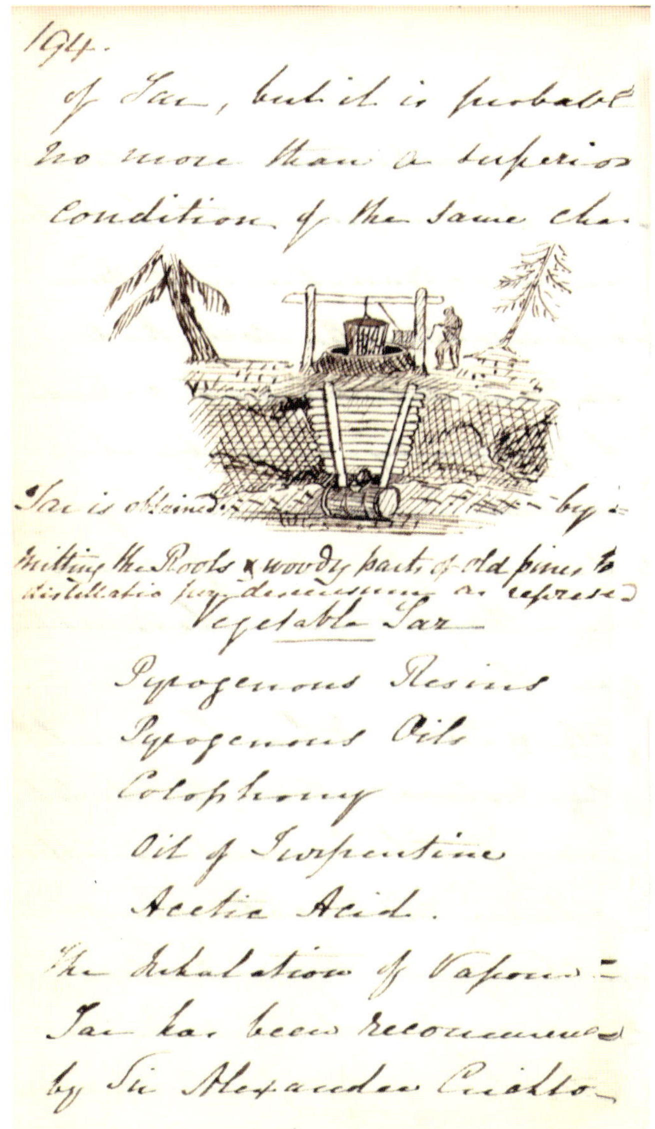

The notes that R.W. Giles, from Bristol, produced for the materia medica lectures given by Jonathan Pereira in the 1847-8 session survive in the Royal Pharmaceutical Society's collection. The book is filled with detailed drawings such as this one from a lecture on making tar.

Royal Pharmaceutical Society Museum

The initial list of honorary members included John Dalton, who had already given lectures in Manchester. And, of course, as the School itself developed, the Society's founders hoped that it would provide teachers both for its own classes in the future and for developments in the provinces.

A letter published in the *Journal* in 1852 proposed a more creative approach. Mr Henry Scholefield of South Shields explained that although many students across the country could read the relevant books and attend public lectures, they were not benefiting from the teaching at Bloomsbury Square. He proposed that a reporter be employed to add a description of experiments to the lecture scripts being used by the Bloomsbury Square lecturers, with a list of apparatus and specimens exhibited. He felt sure that it should be possible to find someone in most towns who was competent to "rehearse and illustrate" the lectures so that people in the country could attend and have lectures that were specially written for pharmacists. He wrote:

> There is no doubt that an attendance at Bloomsbury Square, where there is the finest museum of the kind in the world, and where there is an opportunity for practical study in the Laboratory, would be of infinitely greater value than the system here proposed; but as "half a loaf is better than no bread", so I think to those who are precluded from availing themselves of London attendance, would a recitation of the lectures delivered there be hailed as a considerable boon, and awaken a lively interest in the pursuit of a deeper and more practical insight into what are now to many of them hidden mysteries.

However, Mr Scholefield's suggestion fell on unreceptive ears. Pereira's lectures had been produced unauthorised in the previous year, and so both the lecturers and Council were against the idea.

Professor Attfield, remembering earlier events at the British Pharmaceutical Conference in 1872, recalled the result of the decision by the Council to invest in the School from the mid-1840s:

> Thenceforward the school in the metropolis ceased to be simply a metropolitan school. As a mere London school it probably would, like the other schools, have been closed for want of support, but affording educational occupation for students during the whole of the day, it attracted just a sufficient number of pupils from the whole area of England and Wales to warrant the Council in maintaining it, and from time to time increasing its efficiency. While still the school in London, it ceased to be the London school, but became what it has since continued to be, the School of Pharmacy for the whole of Great Britain.

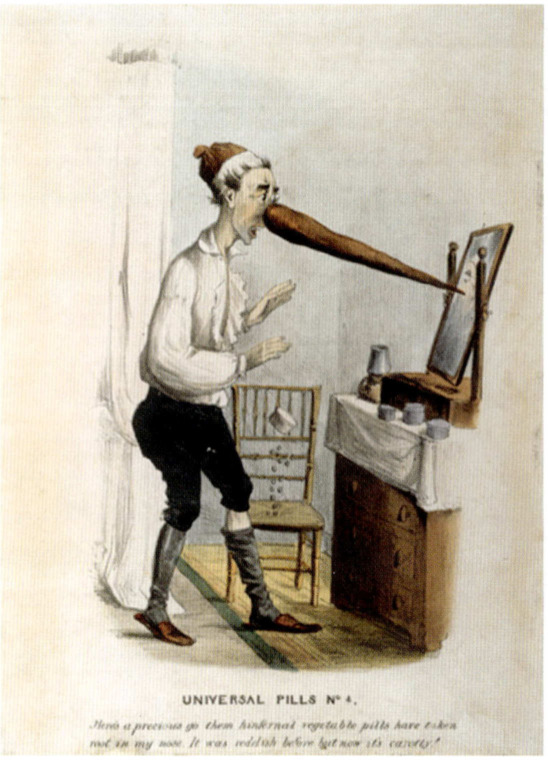

James Morison's Hygeian Vegetable Universal Medicine was spectacularly successful, but as an untrained medicines manufacturer, Morison represented everything that the Pharmaceutical Society was trying to improve. Launched in the 1820s, Morison claimed that his two pills could treat any disease by purifying the blood. As strong laxatives, Morison's recommendation to take them in high quantities led to a number of deaths, and he was strongly opposed by the medical establishment led by *The Lancet*. Even so, at the time of his death in 1840, he was worth about £500,000 and it has been calculated that he sold more than a billion pills.

Royal Pharmaceutical Society Museum

ADVOCACY

The growth of discussions around compulsory pharmacy education which accompanied and followed the 1852 Pharmacy Act appeared to have benefited the School. The likelihood of legislation controlling pharmacy qualifications raised issues and led pharmacy students to further levels of activity. In order to raise awareness and engender an informed debate, in 1856 the Society's Council put out a paper for wide distribution and for insertion into public papers entitled "On the Education of Dispensers of Medicine and the Sale of Poisons". It gave facts about pharmacists' education and examination, the Society's Royal

Charter, the 1852 Pharmacy Act and the history and current efforts of the Society to improve the quality of medicines. It stressed that all of this had been achieved as a voluntary organisation.

Writing in July 1857, Bell said that the School had never been so well attended, with an increase in the number of exam candidates. The number of botany students was particularly impressive, with more than 80 students in the current session. Chemistry sessions were also well attended, although Bell commented that not enough students were attending for long enough periods to gain a competent knowledge of the subject.

"It has been shown that much good has arisen from the establishment of the Pharmaceutical Society, the members of which, being specially educated in the knowledge of drugs, are better able than heretofore to make proper selections and to detect adulterations."

Parliamentary Select Committee, 1856

However, a lack of awareness of the Society's activities to date stretched right to the top of the political establishment. In 1858, Jacob Bell wrote to the Prime Minister, Lord Derby, to oppose the Government's proposal to set up a new Board of Examiners to examine for a "Licensed Druggist" qualification in order to control the sale of poisons. Although the principle of controlling the sale of poisons through educational standards was one that Bell supported, the proposal would have undermined all of the Society's existing work in this area. The proposal was that "Licensed Druggists" would be examined by a board appointed by the Royal College of Physicians, the Society of Apothecaries and the Pharmaceutical Society, rather than allowing the Society to regulate its own profession. Drawing on its national network, the Society was able to force the withdrawal of the Bill under pressure from pharmacists through their MPs from across the country.

The value of the Society's educational standards was also gaining recognition by others outside pharmacy. During the Crimean War, army officials expressed a preference for dispensers with a PSGB certificate, and in 1857, the Director-General of the Army Medical Department refused to engage any candidate to be sent to India who did not have a PSGB certificate.

The death of Jacob Bell in 1859, aged just 49, deprived the Society of its most informed and energetic advocate. As Redwood eulogised:

> [Bell's] short life had been devoted to the one chief object of his ambition, the union of the whole body of chemists and druggists in association, for the establishment of a sound and comprehensive system of pharmaceutical education, for the attainment of parliamentary recognition and support in securing to a body of qualified pharmacists the privileges to which they were entitled, for elevating the professional status of such a body, and for generally advancing the interests of pharmacy.

CHAPTER 2

"THE COMMENCEMENT OF A NEW ERA": 1862–1895

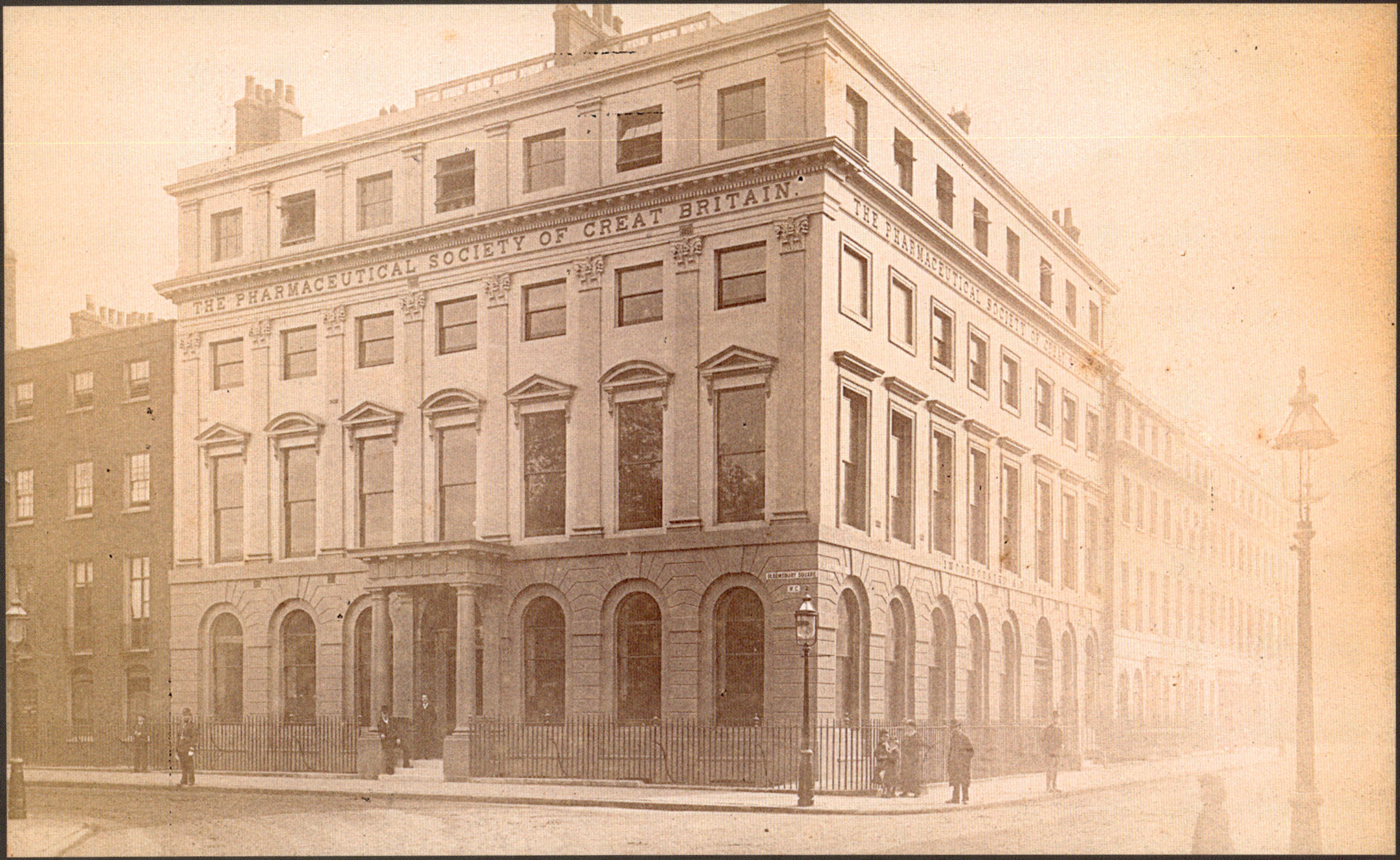

Reproduced with permission from the Royal Pharmaceutical Society Museum

MILESTONES

Popular Culture

1871 William Gilbert and Arthur Sullivan first collaborated on a now-lost opera called *Thespis*
1871 Rugby Football Union formed
1874 safety razor patented
1877 first test match played between England and Australia
1877 first Lawn Tennis Association tournament held at Wimbledon
1882 first electric tram-car
1884 Benz announced the first petrol-driven car
1887 gramophone demonstrated in the USA
1888 Football League founded
1888 Kodak cameras came on the market
1894 first Benz car imported from Germany into Britain

London Life

1861 first trams demonstrated in London
1863 first underground railway in London opened
1865 Jumbo arrived as the first elephant at London Zoo
1868–1870 London struck by "velocipedomania"
1870 first commercial tram route opened between Brixton and Kennington
1870 new Palace of Westminster opened after 30 years of construction
1870 Londoners had their first continuous supply of water, although for many this was via a street pump
1879 first telephone exchange opened in London
1880 Madame Tussaud's grandsons moved her waxwork attraction to its current location on Marylebone Road
1887 Lloyds Bank on Lombard Street was first UK building to have electric lighting inside
1888 Bryant and May match girls marched from Bow Road to Westminster on 24th April in protest at their working conditions; nearly 700 girls went on strike on 5th July
1888 Jack the Ripper murders shocked the city
1889 dockers' strike
1889 Charles Booth's *Life and Labour of the London Poor* published, revealing that 35% of Londoners lived in abject poverty
1889 London County Council established
1890 first electric underground line opened from Bank to Stockwell
1892 work started to build Blackwall Tunnel under the Thames
1894 Tower Bridge opened after 13 years of construction

National News

1861 Prince Albert died of typhoid on 14th December
1867 end of transportation of convicts from Great Britain to Australia
1867 Second Reform Act doubled the British electorate
1868 Trades Union Congress established
1871–1872 more than 50,000 people killed by smallpox in Britain and Ireland
1875 Public Health Act tackled housing, sewerage, drainage, water supply and contagious diseases for the first time
1880 attendance at school made mandatory for children under the age of 10
1892 Keir Hardie elected as the first Labour Member of Parliament

The Wider World

1860–1870 Maori Wars in New Zealand
1861 Italian unification
1861–1865 American Civil War
1863 International Red Cross founded
1869 Suez Canal opened

Life for the vast majority of people in Britain in the later nineteenth century was hard, and in London perhaps harder than anywhere else. Although measures had been introduced to make improvements to public health, disease was still virtually unavoidable. In 1866, 5,596 people were killed in a cholera outbreak in East London, even though John Snow had discovered that the disease was spread through dirty water in 1854, and the capital's sewerage system was nearly completed. Charles Booth's famous survey, *Life and Labour of the People in London*, published in 1889, suggested that around one-third of Londoners lived in terrible poverty. Nevertheless, although perhaps not obvious to the man on the street or the woman in the slums, there were glimmers of hope. In 1870, a continuous supply of water was made available to Londoners for the first time, although for many this was via a street pump. In the same year, an Education Act introduced universal elementary schooling.

The Crimean War (1853–1856) was the first major conflict to be widely reported in the growing number of newspapers, and brought concerns about nursing to public attention. Florence Nightingale became a national figure and her subsequent work to improve conditions in hospitals back in Britain kept this issue at the forefront. The amazing rate of medical scientific advances in this period,

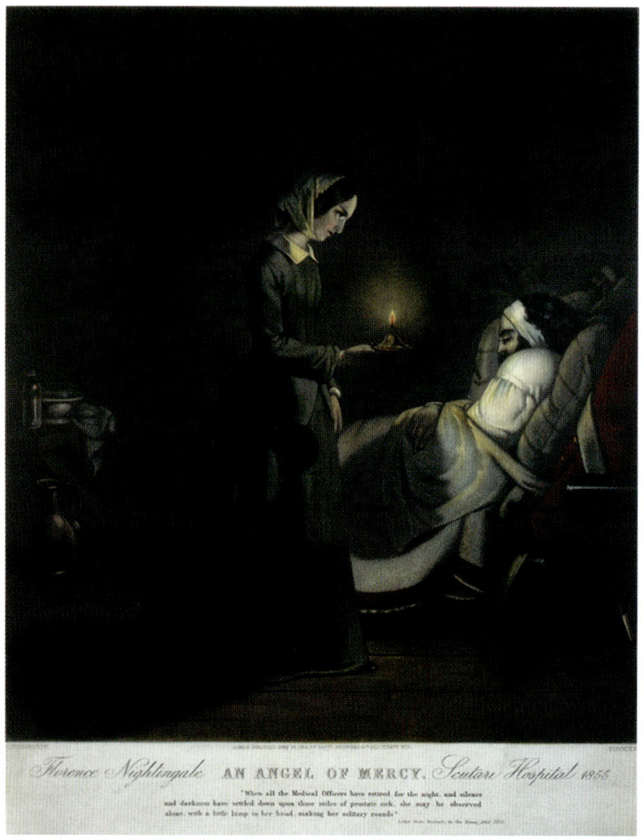

Florence Nightingale, depicted here as the famous "lady with the lamp", led the nurses caring for thousands of soldiers during the Crimean War. On her return, she demanded a Royal Commission to investigate the conditions in military hospitals. Her subsequent campaigning, education initiatives, research and publications established nursing as a respectable profession.

Wellcome Library, London

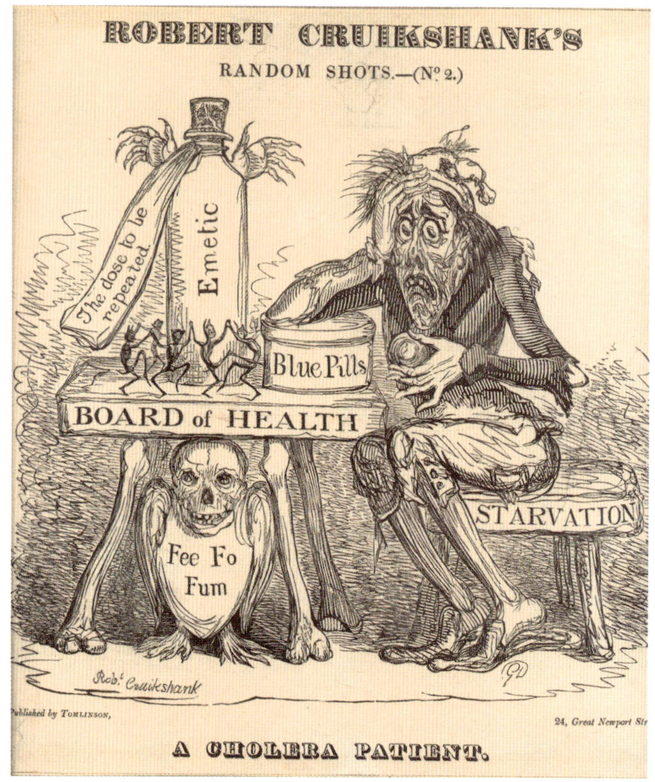

It is not known when this caricature was produced, but the horror and hopelessness of being a cholera patient is only too clear.

Royal Pharmaceutical Society Museum

including anaesthetics and antiseptics, was coupled with public health reforms prompted by continued industrialisation and urbanisation. A Sanitary Act in 1866 was quickly followed by a Factory Act and a Workshop Act, both in 1867, and an Artisans' and Labourers' Dwellings Act in 1868. All of these measures were intended to improve living or working conditions, and provide minimum standards of sanitation, safety and hygiene.

For the pharmacist, there was no shortage of products to sell, if customers could afford them. It was an era of a seemingly limitless number of proprietary medicines, promoted by ubiquitous advertisements. One famous example is Holloway's Pills and Ointment, first produced by Thomas Holloway in the 1830s. By the 1860s, this self-made man had established an international market and was spending over £40,000 each year on advertising. A lasting memorial to his wealth, and to his philanthropy, is Royal Holloway College, opened after his death in 1886. The 1880s also saw the rise of multiple pharmacies, most notably

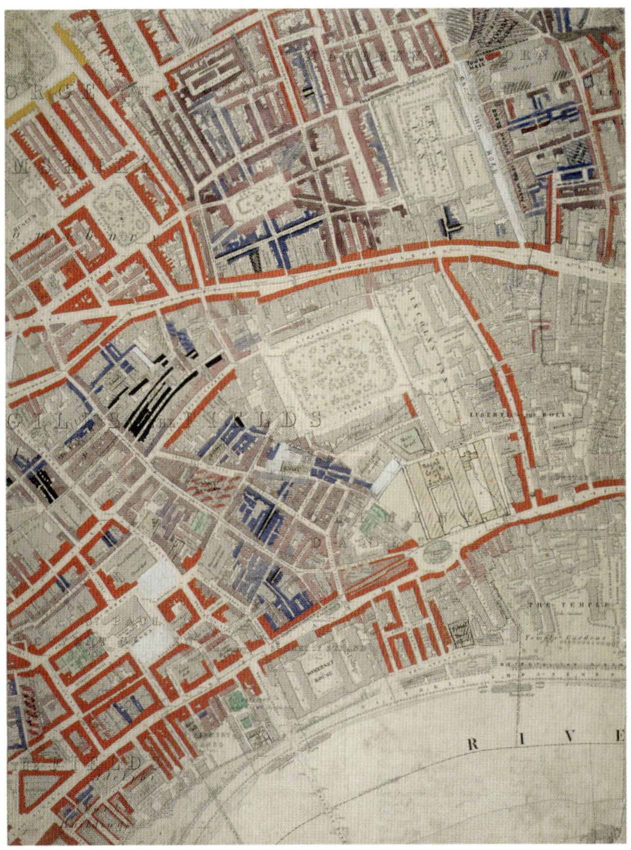

Bloomsbury Square itself was shown in red on Charles Booth's poverty map of 1889, indicating well-off inhabitants. However, as was the case across the whole of London, you did not have to travel far to reach streets coloured black, or "semi-criminal."

© Museum of London

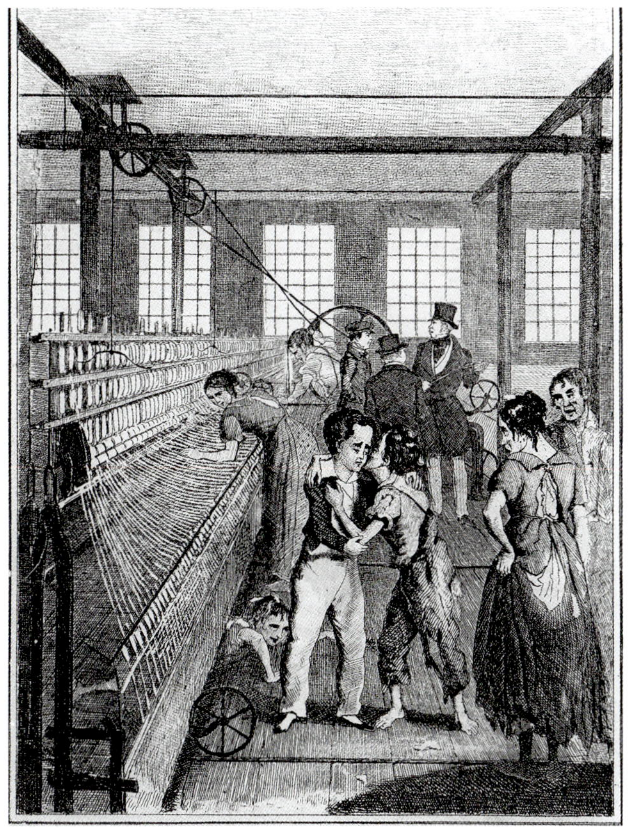

Life and adventures of Michael Armstrong, the factory boy **by Frances Trollope was first published in parts in 1840. She visited factories in Manchester where children were working in order to write a convincing novel, but was criticised for allowing readers to find out about these working conditions.**

Wellcome Library, London

1871	German unification.
1875	onwards European "Scramble for Africa"
1876	Bell patented the telephone
1879	Edison invented the incandescent electric lamp
1885	Indian National Congress formed
1894–1895	Sino-Japanese War

Drug Developments

1863	German chemist Johann Friedrich Wilhelm Adolf von Baeyer discovered the first barbiturate
1865	Joseph Lister successfully used carbolic acid (phenol) to aid the healing of an 11-year-old patient's broken leg
1869	chloral hydrate introduced as a hypnotic
1874	diamorphine (heroin) synthesised from morphine
1875–1884	micro-organisms responsible for amoebic dysentery, gonorrhoea, typhoid, leprosy, malaria, tetanus and pneumonia identified
1879	Burroughs, Wellcome and Co. formed
1879	Louis Pasteur accidentally discovered the principle of vaccination when he found that chickens did not develop cholera when exposed to weakened cholera bacteria, and were then immune to the disease
1881	Louis Pasteur developed a vaccine against anthrax, which he publicly demonstrated on sheep
1882	Robert Koch isolated the tuberculosis bacillus
1883	first edition of *The Extra Pharmacopoeia* published, edited by William Martindale and Dr William Wynn Westcott
1884	Robert Koch isolated the cholera bacillus
1885	Louis Pasteur developed a rabies vaccine
1889	Oskar Minkowski and Joseph von Moring deduced that the pancreas produced a hormone vital to glucose control in the body; this hormone was later isolated and called "insulin"
1890	Emil von Behring announced his development of "serum therapy" to treat tetanus, diphtheria, pneumonia and cholera: an animal's blood was rendered immune to a disease by the injection of the relevant toxin; this extracted serum could then be used to treat another animal or human
1894	Ronald Ross began his work on malaria, leading to the proof that the disease was transmitted by mosquito bites
1895	X-rays discovered by Wilhelm Röntgen

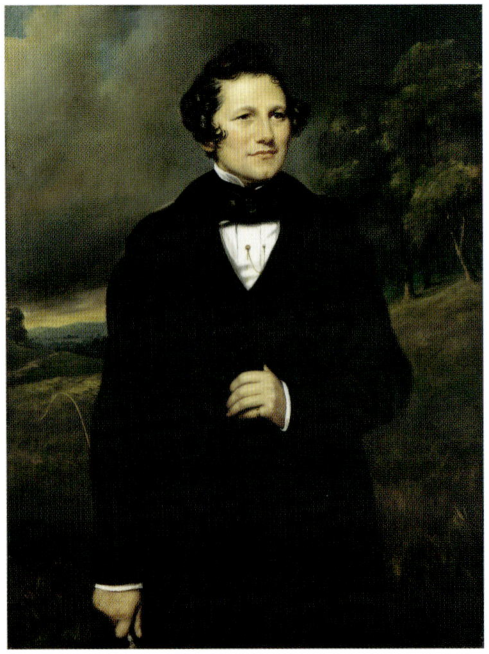

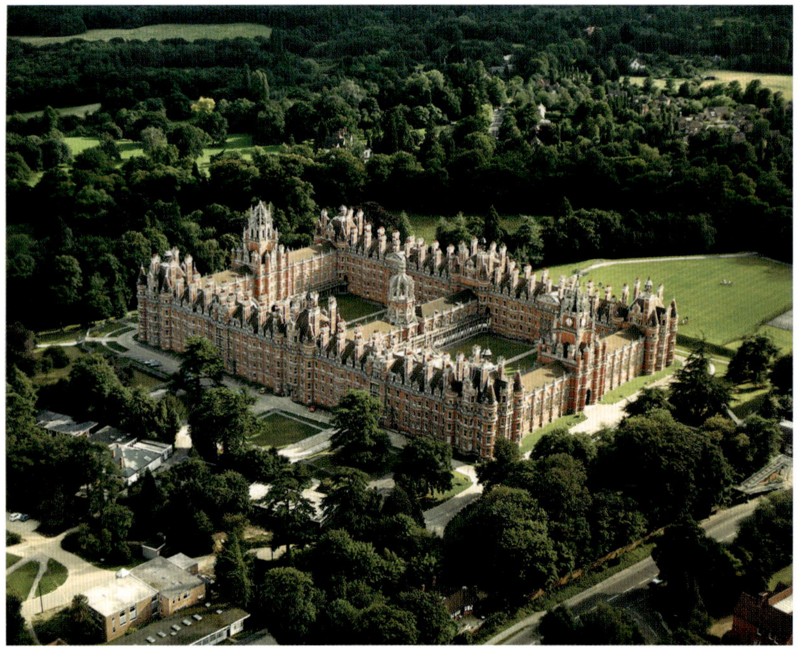

Thomas Holloway made enough profits from selling his pills and ointment in the mid-1800s that he was able to fund a sanatorium and a ladies' college, now Royal Holloway College, University of London. At its height, he was spending £40,000 annually to advertise his products internationally. He claimed that his pills and ointment would treat a wide range of diseases, although once their formula was discovered in the late 1800s, the pills were shown to be simply laxatives.

Thomas Holloway by William Wallace Scott, 1845. Royal Holloway, University of London, Both reproduced by kind permission of Royal Holloway, University of London

Boots, and the beginnings of a scientific pharmaceutical industry. Work as a retail pharmacist was often hard as hours were long. In 1892, the Shop Hours Act finally put some restrictions in place to safeguard retail workers from overwork. As late as 1890, shops could be open from 8.15am to 8pm on weekdays, and to 9.30pm on Fridays, and to 11pm or midnight on Saturdays. Criticism of quackery or profiteering was obviously not without foundation, but many pharmacists took their role in the community and their duty towards public health very seriously.

"The fatal error [of the Pharmaceutical Society] is that they have ignored the fact that the best of all knowledge is gained by experience, open and free to every sincere inquirer, and not packed up in a box, the key to which is only to be found at Bloomsbury Square."

The Chemist and Druggist, 1862

As far as the School of Pharmacy was concerned, *The Pharmaceutical Journal* viewed the early 1860s with an optimistic tone:

> If the efforts thus made to render the school of pharmacy fully efficient should be responded to by pharmaceutical students as they ought to be, and as we trust they will be, the present session may prove the commencement of a new era, in which the provisions for education so liberally made and maintained for many years, will be not only received, but sought after, and not only recognised, but appreciated and duly acknowledged by young men who, in their turn, will become creditable members of the pharmaceutical body, and active promoters of pharmaceutical education.

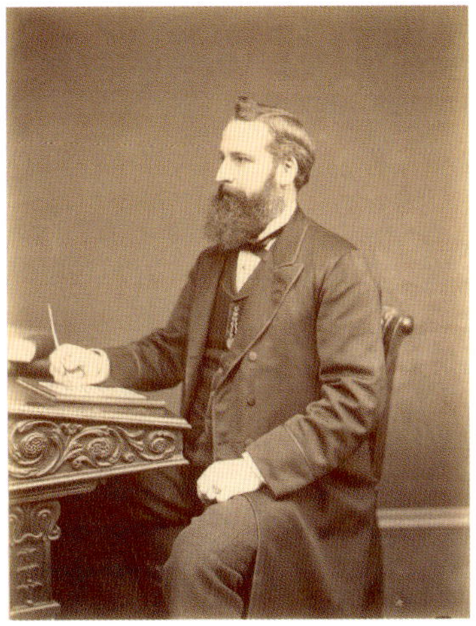

WILLIAM MARTINDALE (1840–1902)

Royal Pharmaceutical Society Museum

WILLIAM MARTINDALE (1840–1902)

William Martindale studied at the School following an apprenticeship with his uncle in his native Carlisle. He passed the Minor exam in 1864 and the Major exam in 1866. He then became an assistant at Morson and Son's pharmacy. In 1868, he joined University College Hospital (UCH) as its first qualified dispenser. He also taught pharmacy at UCH's medical school and became a demonstrator of materia medica at University College. In 1873, he bought the pharmacy of Hopkins and Williams in New Cavendish Street in the West End of London. He served as an examiner for the Society from 1873 to 1882, a member of the Council from 1889, treasurer in 1898 and president in 1899.

However, his name lives on because of the book that he started with co-author Dr William Wynn Westcott. The first edition of *The Extra Pharmacopoeia* was published in 1883, to provide descriptions of drugs not covered by the *British Pharmacopoeia. Martindale: The Complete Drug Reference*, as it is now known, is still published in both hard copy and electronic form by the Pharmaceutical Press, and used by medical professionals all over the world.

William Martindale was a Mayor of Winchelsea and thereby a Warden of the Cinque Ports. In 1899, he suffered a recurrence of a previous illness and his son took over his business. Martindale committed suicide with cyanide in February 1902.

THE PHARMACY ACT 1868

Having invested financially in brand new facilities at the Square, what the Society's Council wanted was the realisation of their ambition for compulsory registration for pharmacists, based on a national standard of pharmaceutical education. In 1864, the recently formed General Medical Council (GMC) threatened to bring pharmacists under their control. In response, a requisition signed by more than 300 members was presented to Council asking them to convene a general meeting to consider application for legislation to make pharmacy qualification compulsory. The members' motivation was that "it is highly desirable for the protection of the public", but of course this move was also inextricably tied to the ongoing issues around the pharmacy profession's status within the medical landscape.

The Pharmacy Act of 1868 was a key milestone for the profession, and in particular for pharmacy education. In fact, its primary purpose was to control the sale of poisons, and it was public fears about increases in cases of poisoning that had contributed to its creation. The Act established a register of people who might "keep open shop for retailing, selling or compounding poisons." But in setting up this safeguard, the qualification for inclusion on the register was based on a person's education. In short, the Act made the Minor exam the test for admission to the register. The Pharmaceutical Society had achieved its founding aim to control entry to the profession via a set educational standard. As the Society had a school and was also the examining body, the Privy Council was given authority to see that exams were properly conducted, by sending inspectors known as Visitors to assess standards and procedures.

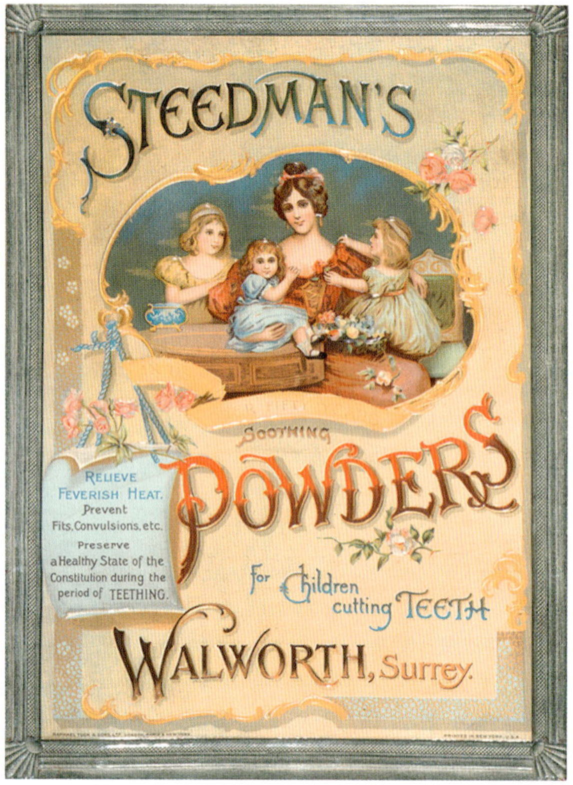

John Steedman first made his soothing powders to relieve infant teething pain in the early 1800s. They continued to be made for more than a century after his death in 1846. Steedman admitted that the powders had once included opium, but when they were analysed in 1909, they were shown to contain mercurous subchloride (calomel). The product still contained mercury until the 1940s.

Royal Pharmaceutical Society Museum

Critics of the Act pointed out that the standard of the Society's exams had been lowered because principal pharmacists now only had to pass the Minor exam, which had originally been set up for assistants. This put the Major exam into a different light as an optional extra for the more academic pharmacist.

Nevertheless, the Act provided a much-needed stimulus for pharmacy education. In the 1868–9 session, there were nearly 60 students at the Square. In the following session, the first after the Act, this increased to 90 students for chemistry lectures, 93 for botany and 96 for the laboratory course. The Act also obviously meant a marked increase in candidates from across the country for the Minor exam. This in itself put pressure on apprenticeships as the primary means for entering the profession, and questions were asked about whether they were "professional" enough with the associations with trade and manual work. Apprenticeships were also criticised because they passed on the conservative practices of the previous generation rather than teaching cutting-edge methods, and of course were of an inconsistent standard. However, they provided a source of cheap and well-motivated labour, and without a network of educational centres across the country, were the best way to feed new entrants into the profession.

However, according to reports from Society members, prospective pharmacy students continued to struggle after the 1868 Act, in that very few business owners took their role as instructors seriously and very few establishments carried out enough dispensing for it to provide adequate experience. Long opening hours also meant little time for private study, and there was a shortage of introductory texts in chemistry, botany and pharmacy for those who could not afford to study at the Square.

Politically, the parliamentary debates leading up to the 1868 Act had done the Society's reputation good at a high level. Many agreed that the Society had done an excellent job up to that point in raising the profession's status and developing a solid foundation of educational initiatives. Lord Elcho, debating the Bill in Parliament, called for support for the Society: "They have done great public service since their incorporation. They have a most excellent school of pharmacy; they have excellent and extensive laboratories; lectures of the highest class are delivered at the institution, and it is a body whose opinions are entitled to respect and consideration."

> **"They [PSGB] have done great public service since their incorporation. They have a most excellent school of pharmacy; they have excellent and extensive laboratories; lectures of the highest class are delivered at the institution, and it is a body whose opinions are entitled to respect and consideration."**
>
> *Lord Elcho, 1868*

PRIVATE SCHOOLS

One of the major results of the 1868 Act was the rapid development of private, and later institutional schools, in London and in the provinces. Private schools provided a variety of full- and part-time courses leading to the Major and Minor exams. Perhaps the best known was the London College of Pharmacy, which was founded in 1899 by Henry Wootton. It had a very good exam record, which probably explained its longevity, as it was the last private pharmacy school in London to close in 1945.

Clearly, the increase in competition had a significant impact on the Society's School. The growth in student numbers experienced immediately after the Act quickly disappeared, and by the 1879–80 session, there were only 29 students for chemistry and pharmacy, 40 for botany and materia medica, and 38 in the laboratory.

There were two proprietary schools in 1870, and five by 1880 (four of which were in London). By 1890, there were five in London; the Manchester College of Chemistry and Pharmacy, owned by W. Spencer Turner, a pharmaceutical chemist; and the Liverpool School of Pharmacy, closely linked to the local association. By 1900, there were 22 private schools: 10 in London (two for women students), three in Scotland, two in Birmingham, two in Manchester and one each in Leeds, Liverpool, Newcastle, Sheffield and Southsea. Not all succeeded: South West London College in King's Road Chelsea and Central School of Pharmacy in Marylebone Road both failed.

The first private school was set up before the 1868 Act in 1861 by J.C. Braithwaite, who had been an instructor in the laboratories at the Square. He started teaching from his home in Kentish Town, and by 1863 had moved to a larger building with a laboratory to hold day and evening classes. In 1870, the increase in students meant that he enlarged the laboratory and laid out a botanic garden. He called his establishment "The North London School of Chemistry and Pharmacy". In 1870, John Muter, a chemical analyst, opened "The South London School of Chemistry and Pharmacy" in Kennington Road.

Probably the most successful private school was Wills' Westminster College of Pharmacy, established by George Sampson Valentine Wills. He started by organising a pharmacy correspondence course, and in 1874 fitted out two rooms at his house in Southwark as laboratories where he taught 10 part-time students. He moved soon afterwards to bigger premises with full-time students, and moved again to Kennington Road and set up two halls as laboratories and a lecture theatre. His success was shown when he bought Trinity Baptist Church in Trinity Square, and converted the galleries into laboratories for 74 students and the nave into a lecture theatre. In 1899, it was estimated that 4,000 chemists & druggists had successfully registered with the Society via Westminster College.

The core issue which explained the popularity of the private schools was that courses at the Society's School continued to be aimed towards the Major exam and average attendance was five months. In contrast, attending a private school meant focusing for a short period specifically on passing the Minor exam, and therefore taking a course tailored to the minimum requirements of the 1868 Act. In 1872, it was reported that students were passing the exam after six weeks spent learning 500 model questions and answers.

The other major contrast between the private schools and the Society's School was financial. Although the School was linked with the Society, which was the examining body, with staff who were authors of the standard textbooks, proprietary schools were better value for money and had very concentrated three-month courses specifically run to pass exams. Their courses were held in the evening, so they were easier to attend, and their fees were much lower. In 1895, the Minor exam course at the Square cost £18 and ran for six months. This would be more than £1,000 in today's money. At Westminster College, the three-month full time course cost eight guineas, or 12 guineas for six months, or 15 guineas for the whole year (around

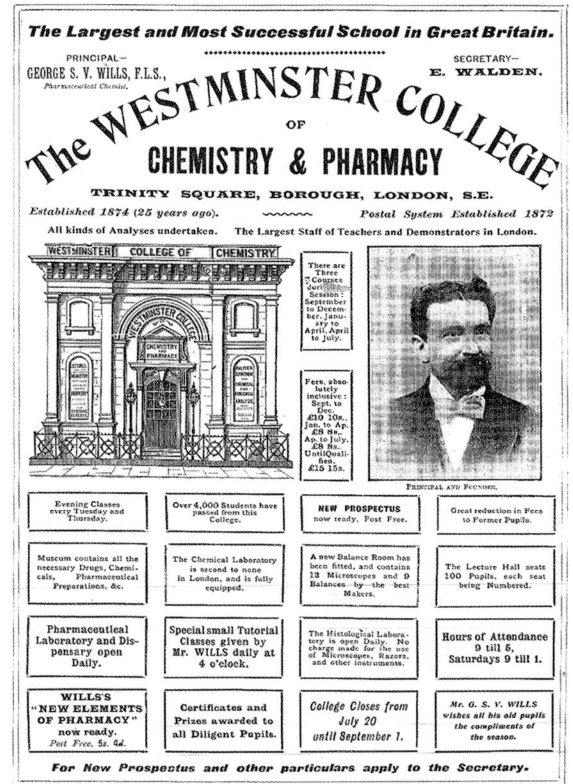

The Chemists' and Druggists' Diary **for 1900 contained 10 adverts for schools of pharmacy. The Westminster College of Chemistry and Pharmacy highlighted its 25 year history, its new Balance Room, and the fact that over 4,000 students had passed the Society's exams from the College. George Wills, a past student at Bloomsbury Square, is pictured as the Principal and founder.**

Chemist + Druggist

£900 in today's money). Evening courses, which ran three times a week on Tuesday, Wednesday and Thursday from 7pm until 9pm, cost one guinea for three months or £2 12s 6d for a full year (around £160 in today's money). As the *Chemist and Druggist* put it in an editorial in 1896, "The School of Pharmacy, owing to its seniority, comprehensive and lengthy curriculum, and comparatively high fees, does not enter into competition with schools which are run at a profit."

Critics of the private schools, most notably led by Professor John Attfield, stressed their negative impact on the pharmacy profession, and blamed the 1868 Pharmacy Act. Students only wanted to study what was needed for the exam, and in as short a time as possible. In the third edition of his textbook, published in 1871, Attfield wanted to credit students with more wisdom than this: "It is unnecessary to advise you to avoid studying merely by way of 'preparation for examination.' You will not so mistake the means for the end. You are studying to fit yourself for your position in the world ..."

"The legislature, with the concurrence of the followers of the calling, have in pharmacy placed a barrier between the public and dangerous incompetence. Surely it is to the interest of *all* parties that this barrier should be as sound and strong as possible?"

Professor Attfield, 1880

Professor Attfield campaigned for 30 years for regulations that would require candidates to produce documentary evidence of having "diligently and deliberately" studied for an appropriate period at a properly supervised and publicly recognised school of pharmacy, in order to get rid of cramming. In a pamphlet written in 1880, he distinguished between two types of knowledge required by pharmacists, and stressed the importance of the gradual and thorough acquisition of "knowledge which relates to a pharmacist's mind rather than a pharmacist's fingers." Not surprisingly, George Wills was a strong opponent of Attfield and did not think it should matter where or how a candidate gained his knowledge as long as he passed.

The high failure rates, as a result of the superficial education provided at these "crammers", caused great concern, and were discussed in detail at the British Pharmaceutical Conference in 1872. An investigation by the Society in 1881 showed that the failure rates in the academic subjects of chemistry, botany and materia medica were twice those in the practical elements of pharmacy, dispensing and prescription reading. The solution that they implemented was to require a certificate of attendance at a recognised course which followed a specified curriculum, and to divide the exam into two parts: science and practice.

PROVINCIAL EDUCATION

The Pharmacy Act in 1868 also provided a new impetus for educational courses in the provinces. The Society encouraged local associations to run classes in order to meet the needs of the Act, first by requesting local associations to report on their needs, and secondly to apply for small grants to assist in delivery of classes. The *Journal* published the results in full tables. They showed that nine out of 26 associations had succeeded in setting up classes to cover all three Minor exam subjects for the 1869–70 session. The Society awarded grants of either £10 or £20 for apparatus or books. For example, it gave £10 to Aberdeen to buy apparatus to teach chemistry, materia medica and botany. The last recorded grant seems to have been

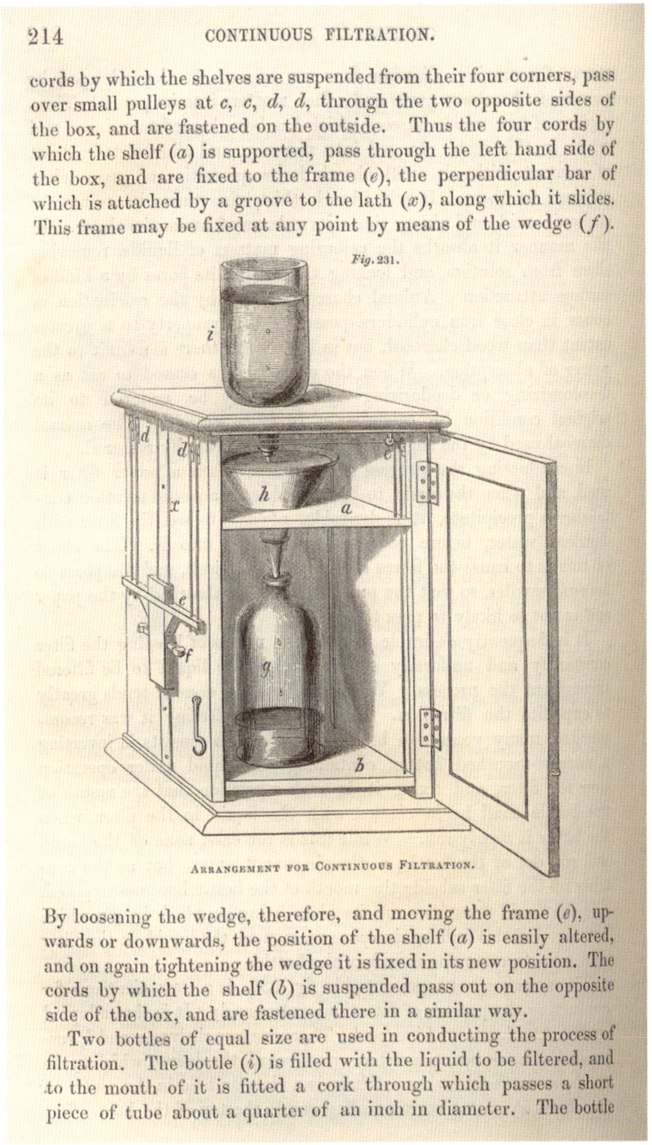
214 CONTINUOUS FILTRATION.

cords by which the shelves are suspended from their four corners, pass over small pulleys at *c*, *c*, *d*, *d*, through the two opposite sides of the box, and are fastened on the outside. Thus the four cords by which the shelf (*a*) is supported, pass through the left hand side of the box, and are fixed to the frame (*e*), the perpendicular bar of which is attached by a groove to the lath (*x*), along which it slides. This frame may be fixed at any point by means of the wedge (*f*).

Fig. 231.

ARRANGEMENT FOR CONTINUOUS FILTRATION.

By loosening the wedge, therefore, and moving the frame (*e*), upwards or downwards, the position of the shelf (*a*) is easily altered, and on again tightening the wedge it is fixed in its new position. The cords by which the shelf (*b*) is suspended pass out on the opposite side of the box, and are fastened there in a similar way.

Two bottles of equal size are used in conducting the process of filtration. The bottle (*i*) is filled with the liquid to be filtered, and to the mouth of it is fitted a cork through which passes a short piece of tube about a quarter of an inch in diameter. The bottle

Mohr's and Redwood's *Practical Pharmacy* (1849) contained over 400 wood engraving illustrations to help the student understand how to set up and use the apparatus needed for the experiments it described. This example shows adjustable apparatus for continuous filtration.

Royal Pharmaceutical Society Library

to Liverpool Pharmaceutical Students' Society in 1896 for £20 to buy a materia medica cabinet and specimens, to be entrusted to Liverpool University College for use in pharmacy classes.

Understandably, the educational provision by local associations varied widely. For example, Bristol had science classes at the School of Mines, Plymouth in the Science School, Manchester at Owen College, and Glasgow in the Mechanics' Institute. In Newcastle, classes were run through the Durham University College of Medicine, where H.B. Proctor was appointed to the chair of practical pharmacy and the university reader in chemistry gave the course in pharmaceutical chemistry. Durham's Medical School Library was made available, and the first session of 1869–70 had 16 pharmacy students. In Leicester, assistants and apprentices formed a co-operative, and researched and read papers for each other. They later organised formal lectures and a library and materia medica cabinet.

Provision of a high standard of pharmaceutical teaching outside London remained a hotly debated topic in the 1870s, led primarily by Society Council member George Schacht. At the request of the Council, the British Pharmaceutical Conference in 1870, held in Liverpool, devoted a great deal of time to the issues. Schacht's paper analysed the current situation. He calculated that an average of 1,693 men entered the profession each year. The Square could never physically accommodate all of these students, and so for those living outside London, he proposed three possible options: local pharmaceutical schools, local medical schools or local science classes run by the local authority. He concluded that most local pharmaceutical associations were not in a position to establish local schools. He confirmed that medical school courses were expensive, and that the key courses for pharmacists, chemistry and botany, were not as important for medics, and so not of a high standard. He had found that of the 232 existing science schools, only 13 taught both chemistry and botany. His conclusion was that the Council should support local associations working with science schools, but should also investigate running short courses supporting students to work through textbooks.

"it would be scarcely an exaggeration to assert that the basis of the Society's existence during its entire history, has been the one fact that it aimed to educate the pharmacists of this country to a higher professional standard; and the content with which its members have seen its large resources lavished upon the school at Bloomsbury Square, may be taken as a proof how fully they have recognized scientific education to be an absolute duty."

George Schacht, 1871

"The laboratories at Bloomsbury Square are overflowing; there is no lack of students now ready to spend money for knowledge which they would have found doubly useful if obtained earlier."

F. Baden Benger, 1870

F. Baden Benger, speaking on "The Apprenticeship and Early Training of Pharmacists", thought that special technical schools should be set up for pharmacy students. He concluded that if a pupil spent a year at a technical school, he would also be more useful as an apprentice. In general discussion, the Conference delegates bemoaned the poor standard of education that children received, and hoped that it would improve as a result of the 1870 Education Act, and a wave of new schools. It was noted that during the Crimean War (1853–1856), dispensers had been dismissed because they could not spell one-syllable words.

At the Society's AGM in the same year, Schacht emphasised that the 1868 Act had given the Society the responsibility for admitting people into the profession. He argued that it was also therefore the Society's responsibility to provide for their education to reach the required standard. As such, this provision should not be wholly centred on London. Resources for education should be distributed generally across the country, rather than concentrated upon one school. It was not that he wanted funding to be withdrawn from the School, simply not fully concentrated on it. The Meeting agreed a resolution that urged on the Council "the desirability of considering some scheme by which the resources available for such purposes may be more generally distributed."

However, by the following year, Schacht had come up with a more drastic proposal, that the Society stopped funding a school at all, and simply acted as an examining body: "I propose that the Society cease to appoint and employ any professional teachers, and cease to maintain any school-buildings or laboratories of instruction, except in the now unavoidable capacity of owners of property." His proposal was that the Society would set and organise an exam once a year to be held across the country. It would be marked centrally, but could be taken anywhere. The idea of "provincial education" would disappear, as pharmacy education would be a national scheme.

Schacht was not leading a vanguard. J. Schweitzer, also writing in *The Pharmaceutical Journal*, felt that a central school was the best way forward. He saw that a scheme of provincial schools would be counterproductive:

> Instead of possessing what we should now have in London, at least, one good effective centre of instruction, provided with the best masters, the largest laboratory, the completest library, and the richest museum, an institution of which all of us can be proud, you would have jealousy everywhere, and a number of elementary schools all good for very little, and all alike contemptible in the amount of knowledge they would diffuse.

He went on to suggest that the Society should spend any money it had for education on its own School, perhaps even opening it for free. If Bloomsbury Square became full to capacity, they should open another school, perhaps in Edinburgh. G.W. Sandford, Society president on three occasions in the 1860s and 1870s, felt that the Square should be left to its own resources, beyond the Society providing accommodation for teaching. He suggested that the School should be self-supporting on students' fees. However, his fellow Council member, Robert Hampson, pointed out that this was currently unfeasible as there were not enough students willing to pay the fees to study at the Square. He put this lack of demand down to limited support from either medics or the general public for "improved, or even passable, pharmacy."

What was certain was that the Society's provincial schools were failing, with very few students, and so the longer term provision of pharmacy education outside the Square would have to be provided elsewhere. At the British Pharmaceutical Conference in 1895, the president, N.H. Martin, saw the future in universities:

> We have only to take the University Colleges throughout the country and we shall find ready to our hands laboratories and eminent professors, with capable assistants and demonstrators, who are prepared to teach physics, chemistry and botany as they ought to be taught, and who can and will teach these subjects in any of their technical applications. We have only to add to each of such colleges a man with a thorough knowledge of pharmacy and materia medica, and who would devote his whole time to teaching, to make our school of pharmacy complete. Many of the Bell scholars who have been trained at Bloomsbury Square, as well as others who have passed the Major examination, and to whom a life of teaching has many other attractions than retail pharmacy, would be available for this post.

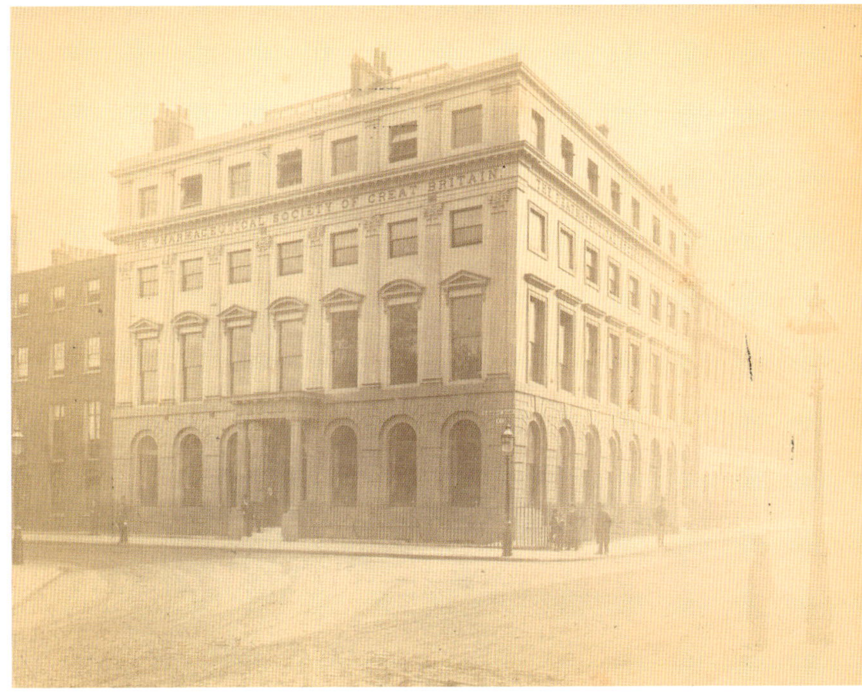

The earliest surviving photograph of 17 Bloomsbury Square dates from around 1883. You can see clearly the new floor added to house the laboratories, and the Pharmaceutical Society's name below the architrave.

Royal Pharmaceutical Society Museum

Martin also added that a library and museum with a pharmacy focus would be required, but otherwise, having pharmacy schools as part of universities would additionally benefit the students, rather than being in a special school with a narrow experience.

EXAMINATIONS

Prior to the compulsory exam established by the 1868 Pharmacy Act, the Society had created a new modified exam, first held on 26th October 1864. It had been recognised that established chemists who wanted to codify their educational standing were currently being deterred by the fact that they had to sit the same exams as their assistants. The Council meeting on 6th June 1864 resolved to set up a new exam for chemists & druggists who had been engaged in business for at least five years, or who were at least 30 years old. Seventeen candidates took the first exams in October, of whom 14 passed. The exam syllabus covered prescriptions, materia medica, pharmacy, chemistry and botany.

The main exams remained as the Minor, now the Qualifying exam for pharmacists to appear on the compulsory register, and the Major exam for those wanting to achieve a higher educational level. The Minor exam was held twice a year in two centres, London and Edinburgh. The exams continued to be oral tests with items laid out on tables for identification and discussion, such as crude drugs, medicinal plants, apparatus, pharmacopoeias and specimen prescriptions.

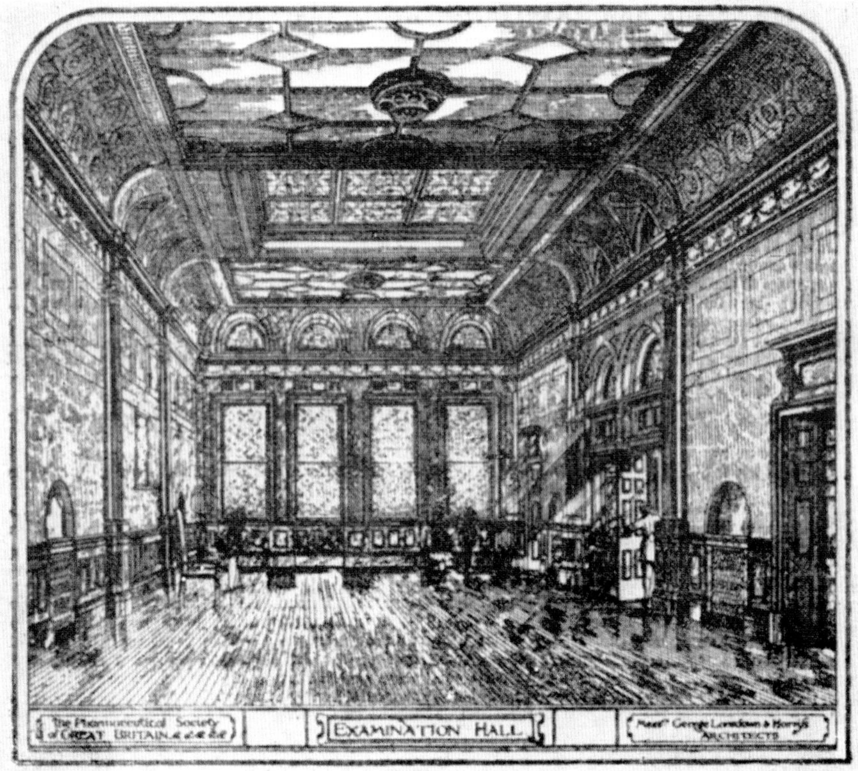

The basement examination hall was created in a new building in 1886. The large room was used for oral exams, with an exam dispensary and an exam laboratory as part of the complex.

The Pharmaceutical Journal

H. Lucas, principal of the South of England College of Pharmacy, published his memories of the exams he took in 1891, in *The Chemist and Druggist* in 1939. The exam extended to two days, with one day of theoretical papers and one day of practical exams. However, the theoretical exam was still purely oral. Lucas remembered that the results were given individually on the second day, and unsuccessful candidates had to leave by the back door into Pied Bull Yard, later Galen Place. Lucas felt that the contrast with his experiences in the 1930s perhaps explained any failures in the earlier decades: "... every public, secondary and grammar school to-day has its physics and chemical laboratory, and many a biology laboratory, so that at school a foundation is obtained in those subjects on which pharmacy is based." In contrast, the Visitor appointed by the Privy Council, Dr Thomas Stevenson, reported in 1891: "It is evident that many young men of defective education still unsuccessfully attempt to enter the business of pharmacy." The Major exam, with its six-hour chemistry practical within a three-day series of exams, was way beyond the capabilities of all but the most gifted and brave students. Its exalted reputation endured for many years. Two decades later, Bernard Gill, who took the Minor in 1913, explained that the general feeling was that there was no advantage in taking the Major unless you wanted to go into teaching, research or hospital pharmacy. He concluded that only the "snob factor" made others take the exam so that they could put PhC (pharmaceutical chemist) after their names. A note in the *Square Chronicle* in February 1913 suggested a similar attitude towards those students who decided to go for the higher qualification: "The Major Session is drawing to a close, as evidenced by the haggard looks and irritable manners of those who inhabit that celestial palace 'The Major Lab'."

In the decades following the Pharmacy Act, the exam failure rates became increasingly alarming. In the late 1870s, about half the candidates failed the Qualifying exam, and by 1896, when the *Journal* published a full analysis, of 793 candidates for the Minor, only 260 passed. For the five-year period to 1899, the failure rate for all candidates in London and Edinburgh averaged 67%. An article in *The Pharmaceutical Journal* by G.S. Taylor in September 1895 laid much of the criticism at the students' feet. He believed that many certificates presented by those wanting to take the Qualifying exam to show that they had been working for three years, were being falsified. The reality was that students could not demonstrate basic skills such as handling scales or spreading a plaster. Taylor also commented that students who had been to a crammer often arrived at the exams mentally and physically exhausted. He also encouraged students to be proactive during their apprenticeships:

> Above all things, don't go about grumbling at your employer's neglect, which may be fancied instead of real, and taking no pains to help yourself . . . We are often met with the statement that the examinations are so much "stiffer" than they were; possibly this is so, but on the other hand, see what facilities the present offers compared with the past! Books, classes, lectures, laboratories, scholarships, and the curtailment of hours of business, all favour the student of the present day, and if he neglects to take full advantage of all these opportunities he only has himself to blame.

Until 1888, the assumption was made that practical pharmacy was taught by doing an apprenticeship, but as it did not seem to be up to standard for all students, a Practical Pharmacy course was introduced in this year, under the direction of Joseph Ince, with a room fitted out for instruction in pharmacy and dispensing.

Another strategy was to increase the amount of written and published support for pharmacy students through the publication of textbooks, mainly written by staff at the Square. The Society's Council was concerned about the lack of textbooks for students, in spite of the range of compendiums and dispensatories that had been published in the early part of the nineteenth century. Professor Redwood recorded later that: "Even books and periodical publications, conveying educational knowledge in the department of pharmacy, were at this time wanting ... The Pharmacopoeia, published in Latin, would have been a sealed book to many who were supposed to use it, if it had not been for an English translation." Redwood contributed in his own subject with the publication of *Practical Pharmacy: The Arrangements, Apparatus, and Manipulations, of the Pharmaceutical Shop and Laboratory*, in 1849. This book was based on a translation of Dr Mohr's *Manual of Pharmaceutical Technology*, published in German. Redwood, in its preface, explains that he made many more additions than he had originally anticipated in order to include "the most practically useful information" for English pharmacists. The book's contents are extremely practical, including suggestions on how to heat, light and ventilate a shop or dispensary, alongside illustrated sections on pharmaceutical apparatus.

Professor John Attfield published his *Manual of Chemistry* in 1867, and helped to cement the position of pharmaceutical chemistry as a separate subject to chemistry and medicine. Most of the existing chemistry textbooks were translations of European works, so Attfield's *Manual* written in English was very popular. He described the book in the preface to the first edition as "essentially a handbook of Practical Chemistry . . . intended as a laboratory guide for medical and pharmaceutical students, and as an aid to the study of pharmaceutical chemistry by the pupils of medical practitioners, and chemists and druggists." It included recent research and chemical theory as well as details of experiments, and was written to appeal to students. Attfield included lists of apparatus that were needed

RULES

TO BE OBSERVED BY

THE STUDENTS IN THE LABORATORIES.

1. The Laboratories are open for Students, from Ten A.M. to Five P.M. daily, except Saturday.

2. The Students are required to observe the above hours, and to conduct themselves in a quiet and orderly manner whilst in the Laboratories or in the house of the Society.

3. Each Student on commencing the Laboratory Course, is provided with a working-bench fitted with lock-up cupboards, etc., and is supplied with certain articles of apparatus; he is held responsible for the safe keeping and restoration of these. Any damage done by a Student must be repaired at his own cost.

4. Each Student is expected to keep his bench and the apparatus supplied to him clean and in working order, and to leave them in that state at the close of the day; to make use of the means provided for carrying off noxious gases and vapours, and to avoid waste in the use of gas and chemicals.

5. Such operations only can be performed as are sanctioned by the Director.

Students' Laboratory Handbook, 1862.

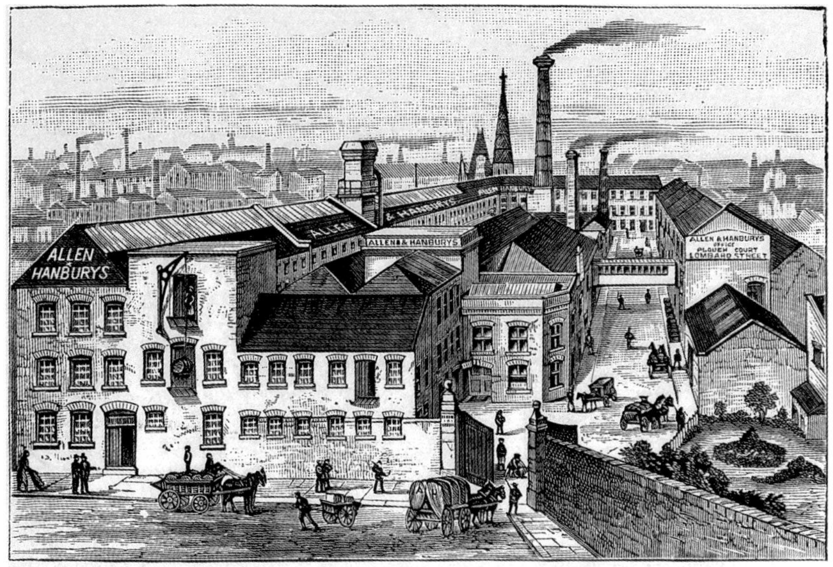

GENERAL VIEW OF THE WORKS AT BETHNAL GREEN.

Shown here in 1892, Allen and Hanburys' extensive factory complex at Bethnal Green was a far cry from the beginnings of the business at Plough Court in the City of London in 1715. In 1957, the company merged with Glaxo.

Wellcome Library, London

"The course of instruction is arranged according to the requirements of the Pupil, chiefly in reference to his previous knowledge and future pursuits. Each Student works independently, he can therefore commence a course of study of any length at any date."

PSGB Calendar, 1870

for different experiments including their prices, and, after the 1868 Pharmacy Act, he also indicated which sections of the book were relevant for which exams. Although the book was tailored to British pharmacy students, based on Attfield's experience at the School, it had nine American editions, alongside its 19 British editions, which demonstrated its usefulness to all pharmacists.

The Pharmaceutical Society also published guidance specifically for students who used its facilities at the School. A series of Laboratory Handbooks, dating from 1862 onwards, survive in the Royal Pharmaceutical Society's collections. In general, they provide rules for use of the laboratories, lists of apparatus provided and required, chemicals used and the syllabus for the courses. By the 1920s, the contents in *Chemical Laboratory Notes* start with instructions for the "General method of procedure for the examination of an unknown substance", illustrating possible results for different groups of elements, and end with tests for organic substances.

TEACHING

One of the major selling points of the Society's School in this period was the quality and reputation of its teachers and facilities.

Materia medica and botany

The Society's museum was its primary resource for materia medica research and teaching. By 1863, the museum had expanded to occupy three rooms of the Society's headquarters. After Professor Redwood's retirement as curator in 1867, the Society agreed to a full-time curator post, at an annual salary of £150. Between 1867 and 1872, there were three museum curators.

James Collins was appointed in 1868 and was clearly very enthusiastic. He wrote papers on various museum specimens and tried to obtain more, but he did not keep the place tidy, which was fundamentally what the Council wanted. Notes from the Society's Library, Museum and Laboratory Committee from May 1868 state that: "the Committee visited the museum and found it very dirty. Mr Collins promised

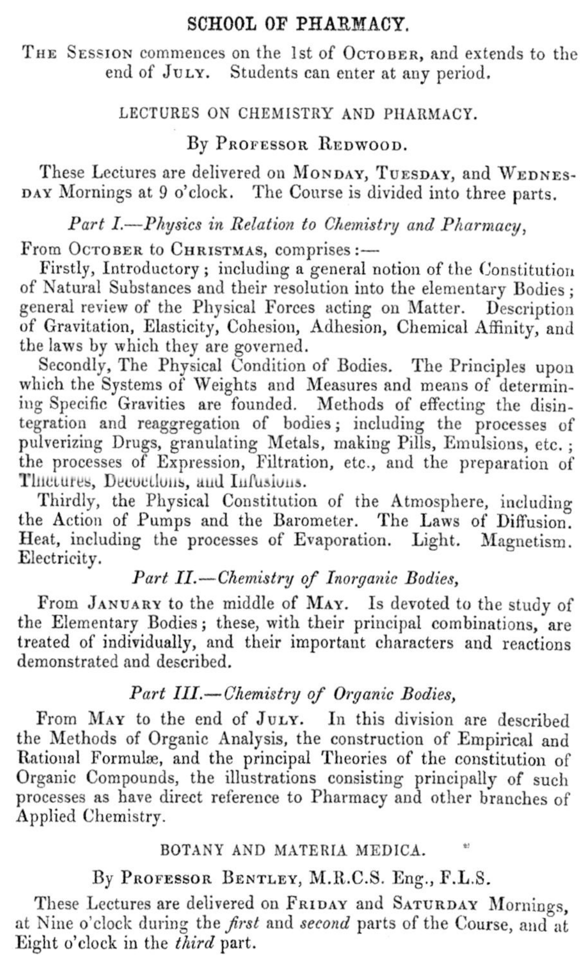

SCHOOL OF PHARMACY.

THE SESSION commences on the 1st of OCTOBER, and extends to the end of JULY. Students can enter at any period.

LECTURES ON CHEMISTRY AND PHARMACY.

By PROFESSOR REDWOOD.

These Lectures are delivered on MONDAY, TUESDAY, and WEDNESDAY Mornings at 9 o'clock. The Course is divided into three parts.

Part I.—Physics in Relation to Chemistry and Pharmacy,

From OCTOBER to CHRISTMAS, comprises:—

Firstly, Introductory; including a general notion of the Constitution of Natural Substances and their resolution into the elementary Bodies; general review of the Physical Forces acting on Matter. Description of Gravitation, Elasticity, Cohesion, Adhesion, Chemical Affinity, and the laws by which they are governed.

Secondly, The Physical Condition of Bodies. The Principles upon which the Systems of Weights and Measures and means of determining Specific Gravities are founded. Methods of effecting the disintegration and reaggregation of bodies; including the processes of pulverizing Drugs, granulating Metals, making Pills, Emulsions, etc.; the processes of Expression, Filtration, etc., and the preparation of Tinctures, Decoctions, and Infusions.

Thirdly, the Physical Constitution of the Atmosphere, including the Action of Pumps and the Barometer. The Laws of Diffusion. Heat, including the processes of Evaporation. Light. Magnetism. Electricity.

Part II.—Chemistry of Inorganic Bodies,

From JANUARY to the middle of MAY. Is devoted to the study of the Elementary Bodies; these, with their principal combinations, are treated of individually, and their important characters and reactions demonstrated and described.

Part III.—Chemistry of Organic Bodies,

From MAY to the end of JULY. In this division are described the Methods of Organic Analysis, the construction of Empirical and Rational Formulæ, and the principal Theories of the constitution of Organic Compounds, the illustrations consisting principally of such processes as have direct reference to Pharmacy and other branches of Applied Chemistry.

BOTANY AND MATERIA MEDICA.

By PROFESSOR BENTLEY, M.R.C.S. Eng., F.L.S.

These Lectures are delivered on FRIDAY and SATURDAY Mornings, at Nine o'clock during the *first* and *second* parts of the Course, and at Eight o'clock in the *third* part.

Pharmaceutical Society *Calendar*, **1870.**

Royal Pharmaceutical Society Library

to have it cleaned by Monday . . . " Collins was dismissed in October 1868. As a result, the Council approved a more detailed job description that included working hours, their expectations regarding care of specimens, and the level of support expected for professors and students.

Edward Morell Holmes was appointed to the post as a result of advertisements in *The Times*, *The Telegraph*, *Athenaeum* and *The Pharmaceutical Journal*. He started at the Square in 1872. By October 1873, his frustration was beginning to show. Holmes reported to the Library, Museum and Laboratory Committee that Professor Bentley was in the habit of taking up to 100 specimens away from the museum and keeping them on the table in the lecture room for up to a week. The Committee approved this practice as acceptable. Holmes responded with a report that explained the damage this was causing to historical specimens, and that it was not necessary because the students could use the specimens in the museum. In addition, "the employment of the museum simply as a specimen cupboard for lecture purposes has deprived the collection of many valuable specimens which would otherwise have been given." As a result of this report from Holmes, the Committee interviewed the professors, and agreed to a separate collection for lecture purposes. Holmes established a separate collection for students in a separate room in 1875 so that they had access at all times.

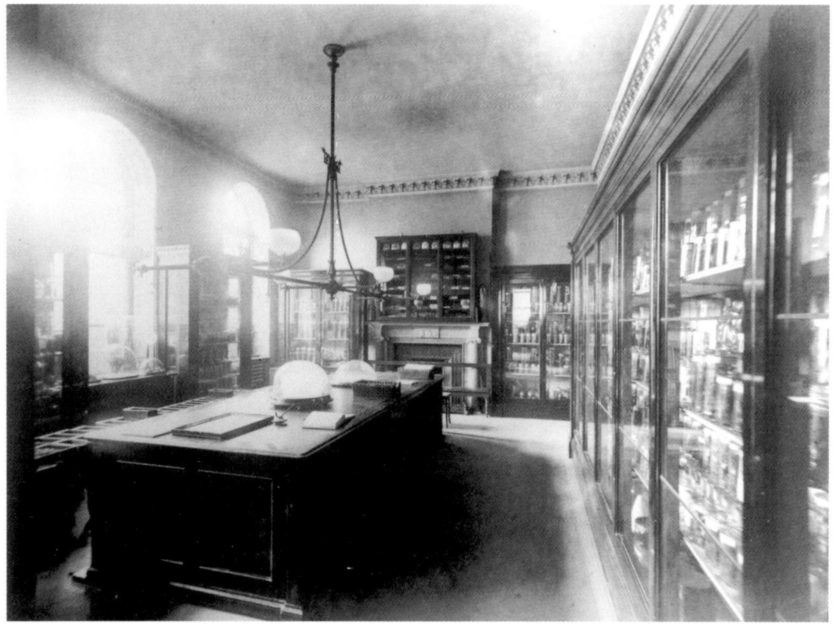

Although the Museum started with no collection, by the time this photograph was taken in the early 1880s, it occupied two large rooms on the first floor and already had significant numbers of specimens.

Royal Pharmaceutical Society Museum

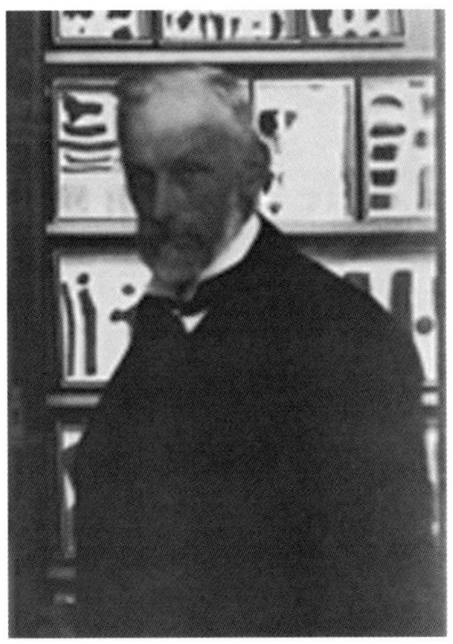

EDWARD MORELL HOLMES (1843–1930)

Royal Pharmaceutical Society Museum

EDWARD MORELL HOLMES (1843–1930)

E.M. Holmes served his apprenticeship in Chelsea and passed the Minor exam in 1860 at the age of 17, the youngest student to achieve this at that point, even though he had apparently only bought one book by Pereira. He worked in Plymouth and London before taking the Major exam in 1864. He returned to Plymouth to work as a pharmacist for six years. He was appointed as curator of the Society's museum in 1872 out of a field of 24 candidates, and remained in the post for 50 years until his retirement in 1922. He also served as the School's lecturer in materia medica from 1887 to 1890 and built up the museum collections to over 20,000 specimens. He collected samples of crude drugs from around the world, established separate teaching collections, published full catalogues and reports, wrote more than 600 articles and notes for *The Pharmaceutical Journal*, and was an active member of the Museums Association.

Holmes served as the botanical referee for the General Medical Council for the 1898 and 1912 editions of the *British Pharmacopoeia.* He wrote all of the entries on drugs from G to V in the *Encyclopaedia Britannica*, 9th edition. In 1897, Holmes received the first memorial Flückiger medal, established to commemorate the co-author of *Pharmacographia* with Daniel Hanbury. He was awarded the Hanbury gold medal in 1895 and was president of the British Pharmaceutical Conference in 1900. His achievements far exceeded the Society's definition of his post: "They reflect the man, not the office, for there is no record that his predecessors did much else than keep the place tidy." His private collections of mosses, lichens, algae and shells were given to many universities and museums.

Holmes continued to apply to the Committee for improvements to the museum's facilities. He made a request for chairs so that lady students could sit down while looking at the specimens. The Committee replied that they should be treated in the same way as men. He also asked for his own microscope as the two in the Society were in constant use by the professors.

Holmes' major project was a complete published catalogue of the full collection. He started work in 1874, and it was published in 1878. The preface explains the collection's use for students and the catalogue's approach to support this, which included references to journal articles, the fact that many specimens in the museum were the actual ones used in the articles, and directing students to works easily available in the library. There were also notes to help students to examine specimens. The catalogue shows that students were using the collections for research. For example, the convolvulin specimen "was prepared from the Museum specimen of Tampico jalap, by a student in the laboratory of the Society . . . " and the samaderin specimen was described as "Examined by Mr Hutchinson, student in the laboratory . . . "

Holmes also solicited a huge number of donated specimens from around the world, including by taking trips himself, such as to Paris in 1878. He also acquired material from exhibitions including the 1886 Colonial and Indian Exhibition in London. In addition, material was provided by students, such as the samples of okra (*Abelmoschus esculentus*) "presented by Mr J. Smith, a native of the Gold Coast, and formerly a pupil in the Laboratory, PSGB." Other samples reflected recent developments, such as pilocarpine phosphate: "These specimens were presented by Mr A.W. Gerrard, who was the first to prepare the alkaloid in this country. See Joun.Chem.Soc. Oct.1876 p.367 P.U.[3] vol.v., p.965." Others were bequests, including the paraffin or marsh gas series left to the museum in his will by William Allen, the Society's first president. Many of the specimens are described as "as met with in commerce" or "commercial specimen", and many of these were donated by manufacturers. The animal collection was less current. Many of the specimens showed native, rather than Western current, usage, and others were historical, suggesting that the collection was more of curiosities than of research material.

Holmes reorganised the museum based on the geographical source of specimens. To improve his own knowledge, he spent one day each week at the Royal Botanic Gardens at Kew to discuss issues with staff there.

Robert Bentley resigned as professor of botany and materia medica in 1887, and was succeeded by Joseph Reynolds Green. As Green was a pure botanist, he was not able to give materia medica lectures, so Holmes was appointed lecturer of materia medica to give them instead. Holmes was not keen to take on this duty, but clearly did what he could to support his teaching, including reorganising the students' museum room to show the common drugs and their adulterants as dealt with in his lectures. In fact, the room stayed this way until the School was evacuated in 1939. Holmes also made up envelopes with sets of the common drugs for students to take away, although this practice was stopped by Council in 1915. Holmes introduced practical classes which involved chemical studies and some use of the microscope for histology. The histology laboratories, provided on the first floor from Green's appointment onward, were used for practical botany from 1887 and practical pharmacognosy from 1920. In 1926, it was refitted with benches supplied with water, gas and electricity, and became a much better facility for both chemical and microscopical work.

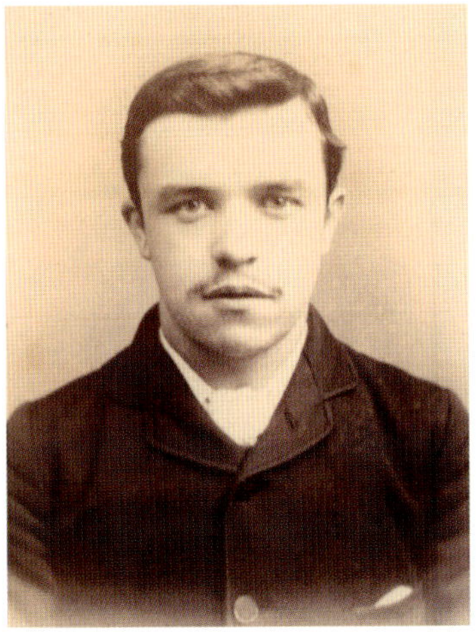

THOMAS ANDERSON HENRY (1873–1958)

Royal Pharmaceutical Society Museum

THOMAS ANDERSON HENRY (1873–1958)

Thomas Henry entered the Society's laboratories in 1893 as a Jacob Bell Scholar, having served his apprenticeship in Barrow-in-Furness. He passed the Major exam in 1894, and spent two years in the research laboratories as the Redwood and Manchester Scholar successively. In 1896, he moved to the scientific staff of the Imperial Institute, and gained a Salters' Research Fellowship and a Doctor of Science degree. He later became superintendent of laboratories at the Institute. Until his retirement in 1943, he was director of the Wellcome Chemical Research Laboratories for 24 years.

He had a large number of scientific papers published, many of the earlier ones with Sir Wyndham Dunstan. He was best known as the author of the standard work *The Plant Alkaloids*, first published in 1913. However, his research interests developed to include tropical medicine and chemotherapy, particularly for tuberculosis. He served on the committees of the British Pharmacopoeia Commission and the *British Pharmaceutical Codex*. He was described in a tribute as "a modest, unassuming man of small stature but of big heart."

In 1890, Henry Greenish was appointed as lecturer in materia medica, and Holmes was no longer required to teach. He was made professor of materia medica in 1893, continuing his role alongside being curator of the museum. After Greenish's appointment, he introduced microscopical studies as a means of identifying powdered drugs, a new development in pharmacy teaching, into practical classes for Major students. However, he met with some criticism as many pharmacists did not own microscopes.

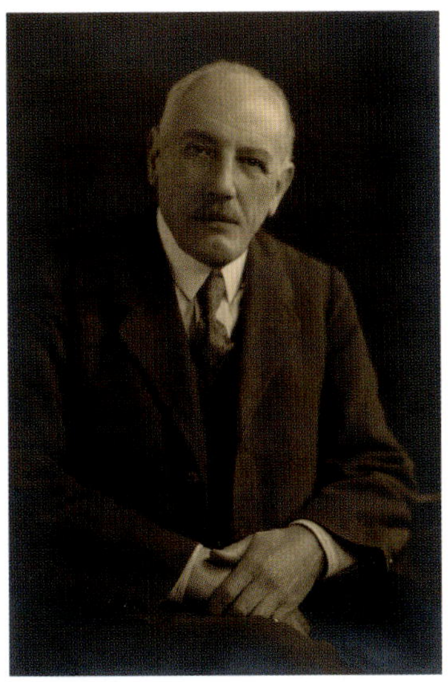

HENRY GEORGE GREENISH (1855–1933)

Royal Pharmaceutical Society Museum

HENRY GEORGE GREENISH (1855–1933)

Henry Greenish was born into a pharmaceutical family. His father, Thomas Greenish, was president of the Pharmaceutical Society from 1880 to 1882, and president of the British Pharmaceutical Conference in 1886. After serving his apprenticeship with his father, he attended the School from 1873, winning a Bell Scholarship in 1875 and passing the Major exam in 1877. He was a distinguished student with silver medals in all available subjects, and became a demonstrator in the chemical laboratory. Having spent two years at the University of Dorpat studying with the leading pharmacognosist, Professor Dragendorff, and a short period at the University of Vienna, he returned to the Square in 1880 as lecturer in materia medica and was made professor in 1893. He became professor of pharmaceutics in 1900. An eminent expert in his subject, he was awarded the Hanbury gold medal in 1915 and an honorary doctorate from the University of Paris in 1919, and was president of the British Pharmaceutical Conference in 1922. He published numerous research papers, but his most well-known publication was the textbook *Materia Medica* (1899), which went through six editions.

Greenish became dean of the School in 1896 and continued his support for students' social events, particularly botanical rambles. He was commemorated by the Greenish Memorial Scholarship, first awarded in 1936, for the first year student who had shown most promise. The award enabled students to continue with their studies either for the pharmaceutical chemist qualifying exam or for the final exam of the Bachelor of pharmacy degree of London University.

Chemistry

Chemistry had been viewed as the bedrock of teaching in the School from its establishment. The museum's collections supported this teaching with a separate chemistry museum from early in its history. The museum catalogue, published in 1878, shows that its specimens included samples of recently discovered elements such as thallium and indium. Chemistry itself was in an exciting period, with the Periodic Table having been published by Mendeleev in 1871.

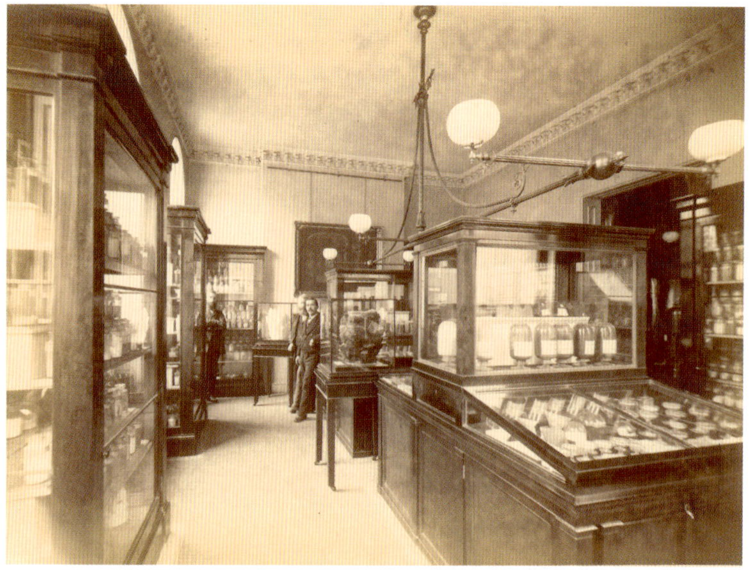

The Chemistry Museum, on the ground floor of the building, provided materials for teaching and private study in tandem with the main collection of materia medica. Taken in about 1883, this photo shows three shadowy figures at the back, presumably staff.

Royal Pharmaceutical Society Museum

The Society's aim was to establish a separate branch of pharmaceutical chemistry. The Adulteration Acts of 1860, 1872 and 1875 also marked a new use of applied chemistry with chemical analysis of water, food and drugs, and the consequent appointment of public analysts. In 1874, Professor Redwood became the first president of the Society of Public Analysts. Professor Attfield and Benjamin Paul were also founding members. Paul was public analyst for Westminster as well as editor of *The Pharmaceutical Journal*. A number of Jacob Bell Scholars also earned their living through public analysis: Thomas Tickle (Bell Scholar, 1892) in Exeter and analyst to the Chemists' Defence Association, John Evans (Bell Scholar, 1897) for Sheffield, and Edward Harrison (Bell Scholar, 1890), who set up the Harrison and Self firm of analysts and was engaged by the *British Medical Journal* to work on

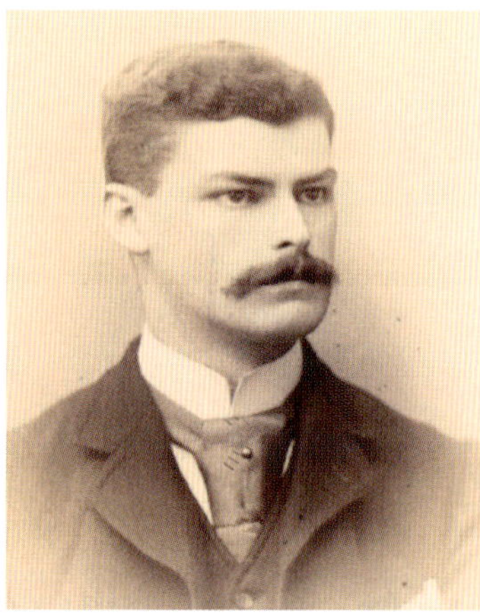

THOMAS TICKLE (1871–1960)

Royal Pharmaceutical Society Museum

THOMAS TICKLE (1871–1960)

"Tommy" Tickle served his apprenticeship in his native Devon before entering the School in 1892 as a Jacob Bell Scholar. Having achieved the Major exam, he was awarded a Salters' Research Fellowship and studied at University College London, gaining his BSc in 1901. He was elected a Fellow of the Institute of Chemistry in 1903.

In 1901, he was appointed public analyst for Exeter, and in the following year, Public analyst for Devon. He was also agricultural analyst for Devon, Exeter and Plymouth. Much of his work outside his official roles arose from the National Health Service drug-testing scheme. He also undertook Food and Drugs Act samples for the Chemists' Defence Association from 1908 onwards. He served on the Society's board of examiners and was a member of the British Pharmacopoeia Commission from 1932 to 1948.

their landmark publication *Secret Remedies*. Professor Redwood himself was a leading figure in the field. Between 1875 and 1892 he held the post of public analyst for the London parishes of St Giles and Holborn, St James and St John, Clerkenwell, the County of Middlesex and the Borough of Luton.

The official version of the impact of the new third floor practical chemistry laboratories, opened in 1860, obviously concentrated on the vast improvements that they presented in terms of up-to-date facilities. Some of the students, such as the "former Square Man" who was at the School in 1880, have more vivid recollections of the top of the new extension: "The glories to be seen from the forbidden region of the roof, the exquisite flavour acquired there by pipe or cigarette, the excitement of whistling for hansom cabs from that point of vantage, are handed down from session to session with unfailing regularity." Students were apparently lifted down from the rooftop on a rope,

> **"At present it is cause for constant regret that our Bell Scholarships do good to all other professions except our own; a Bell Scholarship is too often the lever by which a worthy, clever and ambitious young pharmacist so elevates himself that his talents are lost to pharmacy altogether."**
>
> *Professor Attfield, 1872*

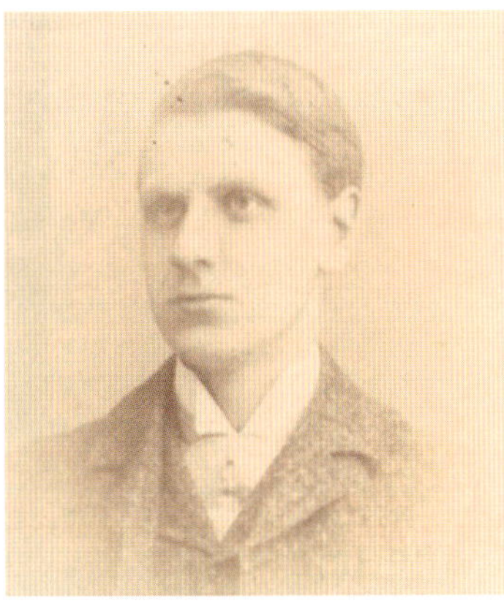

EDWARD FRANK HARRISON (1869–1918)

Royal Pharmaceutical Society Museum

EDWARD FRANK HARRISON (1869–1918)

Edward Harrison began his apprenticeship aged 14. He was awarded the Jacob Bell Scholarship in 1890 and qualified as a pharmaceutical chemist in 1891. In 1892, he became a demonstrator in the Society's laboratory, and later worked as head of the analytical laboratory at Burroughs & Wellcome. He then worked as a consulting and analytical chemist for 10 years before the First World War. During this period he assisted in the compilation of the *British Pharmaceutical Codex*. He also took a great interest in the unmasking of fraudulent proprietary medicines. He carried out a wide range of analyses of "quack" medicines on behalf of the British Medical Association. The results of this work were published in *Secret Remedies: What They Cost and What They Contain* (1909) and *More Secret Remedies* (1912).

When war broke out in 1914 Harrison tried to join the army but was rejected several times on account of his age (45 years). However, in 1915 he was accepted by a "sportsmen's battalion" that took men of any age. In response to the first German gas attack on the Western Front at Ypres in April 1915, the British War Office enlisted chemists to the newly formed Anti-Gas Department. Harrison joined the staff, and from the autumn of 1915 he worked to develop the "large box respirator", the first serviceable British respirator. Around 200,000 were issued. He next worked on the development of the small box respirator, for which he is best known. Incorporating improvements on the large box respirator, it was developed to be effective against all the various poison gases.

Harrison was rapidly promoted through the ranks to lieutenant-colonel. In 1918, he was appointed Controller of Chemical Warfare. He died a week before the Armistice in November 1918. His death was caused by influenza but it was widely believed that it was hastened by overwork and the effects of repeated exposure to poison gas. He had continued to work with a raging temperature for four days before he was taken home to die. A memorial to Harrison was unveiled at the Pharmaceutical Society in November 1921 by Sir Worthington Evans, the Secretary of State for War. Every two years, the Society still awards the Harrison memorial medal to a pharmacist who is judged to have made significant achievement in both the science and practice of pharmacy.

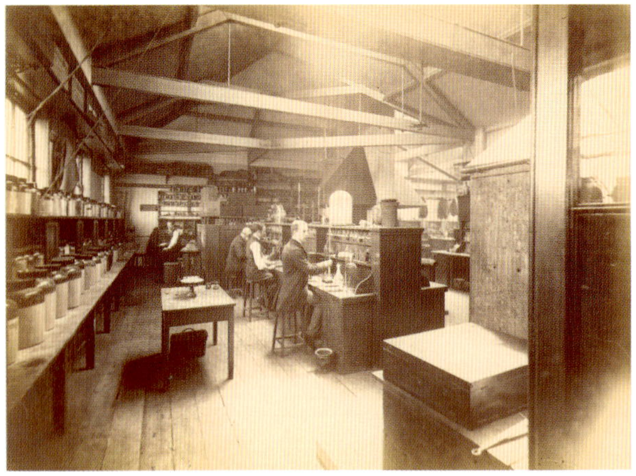

Students posed at their desks in the Major chemistry laboratory on the third floor, in around 1883.

Royal Pharmaceutical Society Museum

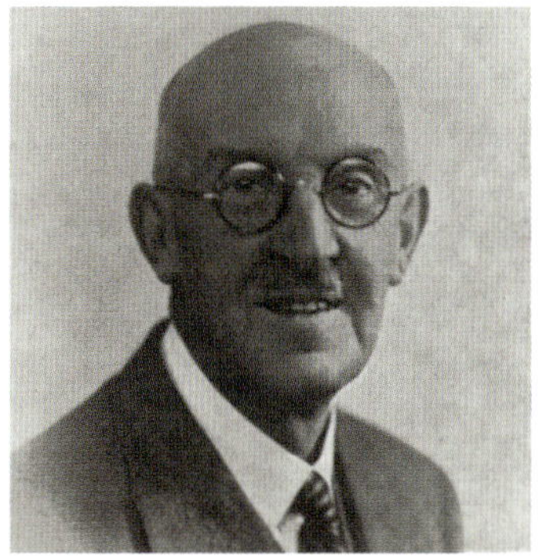

HOOPER ALBERT DICKINSON JOWETT (1870–1936)

Wellcome Library, London

HOOPER ALBERT DICKINSON JOWETT (1870–1936)

Hooper Jowett gained one of the Jacob Bell Scholarships in 1891 having attended the Royal Grammar School in Lancaster. He qualified as both a chemist & druggist and a pharmaceutical chemist in 1892. He was awarded the Redwood Scholarship, and then in 1893, the Manchester Pharmaceutical Association Scholarship to continue for an additional year in the Society's laboratories. He became a Fellow of the Chemical Society and gained a BSc from the University of London. In 1894, he was appointed assistant lecturer in chemistry at the Square and also asked to teach classes in physics and practical physics. In 1895, he took on the role of demonstrator in the Research Laboratory, and also gained his doctorate from the University. In the following year he was elected a Research Fellow of the Society.

In 1897, he joined the staff of the Wellcome Chemical Research Laboratories, and in 1905 he was appointed chief of the experimental department of Wellcome's Chemical Works in Dartford. A year later he became works manager. He oversaw significant achievements at the Works, not least the production of the first British Salvarsan during the First World War, followed by the first British Neosalvarsan. After the war, production of reliable insulin and preparations of digitalis and of ergot were notable successes. Although he often presented papers at conferences and meetings, he was not a published scientist. He was sadly killed as the result of a car accident on his way to work on 10th August 1936, aged 66.

with the notable memory of one who got stuck and had to climb into a bedroom window in Great Russell Street, and follow a workman down the stairs in order to exit the building without being questioned.

> **“probably the best equipped School of Chemistry and Pharmacy in the kingdom.”**
>
> *Michael Carteighe, 5th October 1892*

The experiments carried out by the students did not always follow the approved syllabus: “During the earlier period of the history of gun-cotton, the experiments carried out in the basement with a miniature cannon might well have been attended with serious consequence, as well as those connected with the first applications of anaesthetics.” “Square Man” also remembered a chemistry lecture when the oxygen cylinder tap was turned the wrong way, which caused the thick rubber tubing to burst. Although most students escaped up the stairs, some hid under their seats and tables. “Square Man” vividly recalled other parts of the building: “How distinctly does the picture of the lecture-room in the dull October mornings of 1880 come before me, then and ever since suggesting the arrangement of the sanctum of a mediaeval alchemist.” The fact that the laboratory assistant, Alfred, wore a black skull cap, apparently added to the historical ambience.

THE STUDENT EXPERIENCE

The attitude of staff and others towards the student body at the Square was generally positive, but tinged with the perennial suspicion that they were not devoted enough to their work, or appreciative enough of the benefits that the School offered to them. Frederick T. Roberts, professor of medicine at University

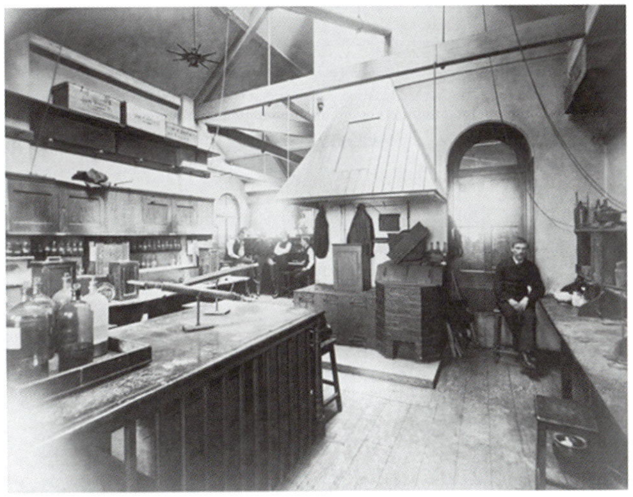

The lab steward's bench was situated next to the fume cupboard. In this photograph taken in around 1883, you can clearly see wooden boxes, presumably full of equipment, stored high up under the beams on the left.
Royal Pharmaceutical Society Museum

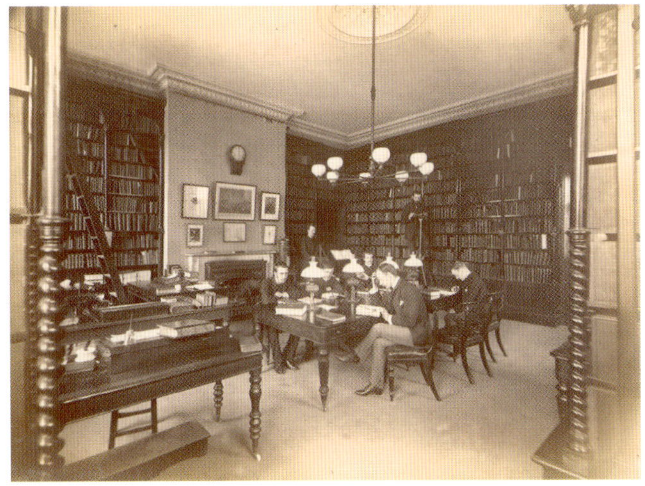

One of the two rooms that made up the Library on the first floor, captured in around 1883. The Society bought the ornate bookcases second-hand from the International Exhibition in 1863.
Royal Pharmaceutical Society Museum

College London (UCL), gave the introductory address to the School's 54th session in October 1895. He had an extremely positive assessment of the School:

> In looking over the Calendar, I have been deeply impressed with the high character, extent, and thoroughness of the instruction which has been provided for you [students]: and with the eminent position and scientific attainments of your professors, lecturers and demonstrators. Moreover, you have a museum and laboratories which are the envy of most medical schools, with an excellent library and reading-room; while your ambition and zeal are stimulated by prizes, scholarships, and valuable fellowships.

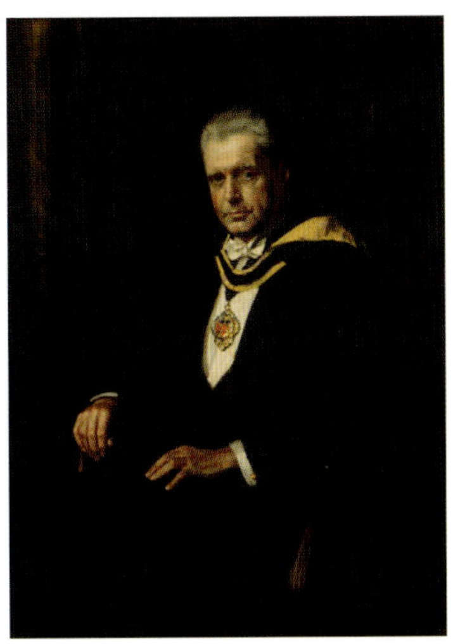

EDMUND WHITE (1866–1928)
Royal Pharmaceutical Society Museum

EDMUND WHITE (1866–1928)

Edmund White was a Senior Bell Scholar in 1886, and passed the Minor exam in 1887 and the Major exam in the following year. After a short time as a demonstrator at the School, he became chief pharmacist at St Thomas' Hospital. He became a Fellow of the Institute of Chemistry in 1892. In 1903, he joined Hopkin and Williams Ltd, manufacturing chemists. He was an examiner for the Pharmaceutical Society for many years, and a member of the Committee of Reference in Pharmacy for the *British Pharmacopoeia* in 1914. He held the post of general secretary of the British Pharmaceutical Conference for six years from 1903, and was its president in 1924 and 1925. He joined the Council of the Pharmaceutical Society in 1907 and served as the Society's president from 1913 to 1918. He was also officially involved with the 1911 and 1923 editions of the *British Pharmaceutical Codex*. He was credited with being a significant source of inspiration for the establishment of the Society's pharmacological laboratories in 1926.

In defence of the student body, especially in the earlier decades of this period, it must be remembered how piecemeal the students' education was. Some students attended for three months, others for 10 months, some registered for the laboratories for two or three days a week, some for two or four hours a week, or even arrangements such as two hours a day for four days a week. Even if a student was registered as full time, he did not always attend full time. It was not unlikely that he could be called back to work in the shop as an apprentice. Of course, a significant minority were not studying to be pharmacists, but were prospective medical students and analysts.

One of the School's strategies to encourage commitment and good performance was the introduction of prizes, described as "stimulants to exertion" in the Calendar for 1870. In 1871, a silver medal was introduced in each of the three subjects in the advanced course, and a bronze medal for each in the elementary course. In 1886, the chemistry and pharmacy medal was replaced by a chemistry and chemical physics medal. In 1888, five silver and five bronze medals were awarded for chemistry and chemical physics, botany, materia medica, practical chemistry, and pharmacy.

Students' associations

In 1875, Council gave permission for the formation of the School of Pharmacy Students' Association. Proceedings of its fortnightly meetings were published in *The Pharmaceutical Journal* alongside other

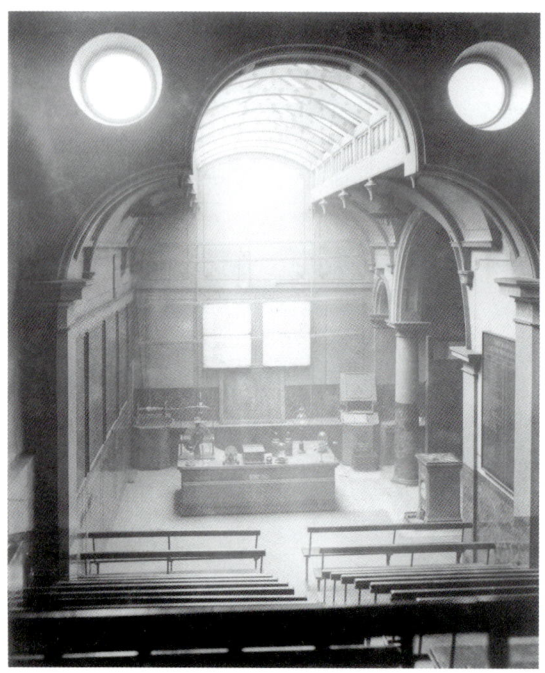

The lecture theatre was created in 1861 when the laboratories were moved to the building's new third storey. Students had to balance their notebooks on their knees until new seating was provided in the 1920s. You can see the boards for prize winners on both sides of the demonstration and lecturing area.

Royal Pharmaceutical Society Museum

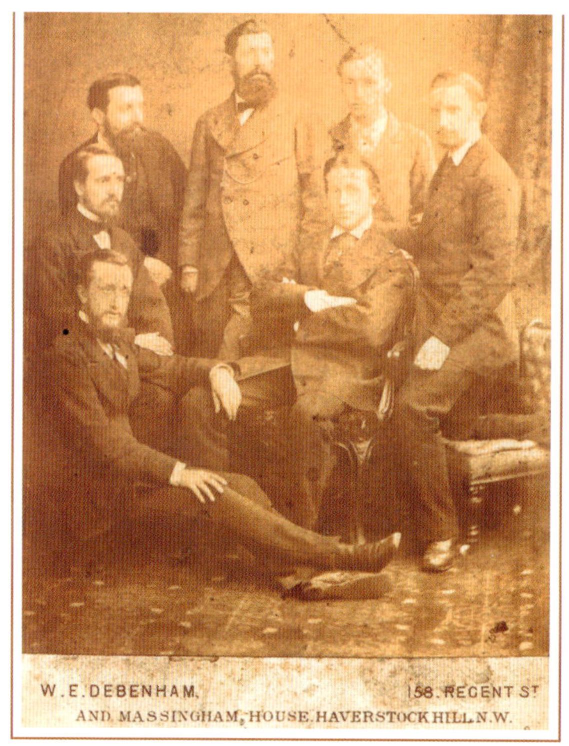

The first committee of the Students' Union were captured for posterity in 1875.

UCL School of Pharmacy Library

"Scientific Societies", as its primary aim was educational rather than recreational. In this sense, it could trace its origins back to the Laboratory Students' Society in the 1850s. Professor Redwood had set up an association for the students in 1870, which seems to have survived for only about a year. According to the School prospectus, the newly formed Association "was founded for the purpose of promoting study and original work in the branches of knowledge allied to Pharmacy, and of furthering social intercourse among its members." Professor Attfield was appointed as the first president, and set the tone with his inaugural presidential address, entitled "On the Best Means of Acquiring Education as Distinguished from Knowledge". At the fortnightly meetings, one member presented a paper which was subsequently discussed. The Association also organised excursions, both botanical rambles and trips to manufacturers and wholesale houses, and visits to London Docks, and initially a small element of social events including the annual dinner and a "smoking concert". A "former Square Man", reminiscing in 1895, remembered the Association as a good place to practise public speaking, and to make friends with students from different sessions.

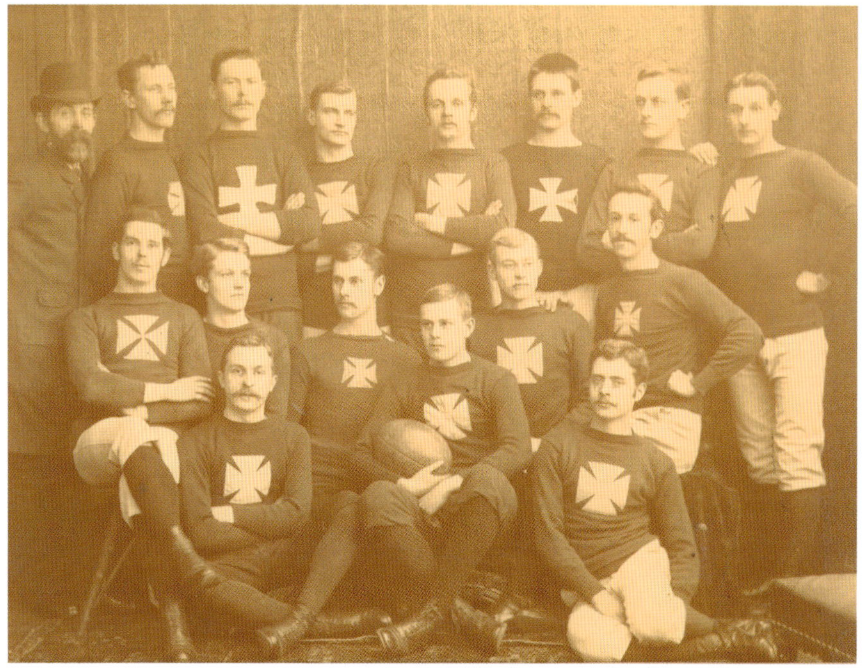

The School rugby team with their distinctive Maltese cross-emblazoned strip and "knickers" (knickerbocker trousers). Is the man on the far left wearing a bowler hat a coach or the groundsman?

UCL School of Pharmacy Library

Sport

A key part of the recreational side of School life was sport, but formal clubs got off to a slow start in the Square's history. In an article in *The Pharmaceutical Journal* in September 1895, a "former Square Man" described how he set up a Pharmaceutical Football Club, inspired by attending a match with a medical student friend and his team. It becomes clear slightly later in the article that he is referring to rugby, not soccer. He remembered that most of the students had never played football before, and that "we were frequently obliged to play men who were more ornamental than useful. A forward who could play on Queen's Park ground without soiling his knickers, was not of much service to his side, yet we had several members who could perform this feat." Of course, "knickers" refers to the knickerbockers that formed part of the strip, rather than the players' underwear. Alongside the matches, the club set up an annual football dinner.

> **"to the new students of the coming session, ... if it is not all 'beer and skittles' at Bloomsbury Square they may justly anticipate a large amount of pleasure, and even good, honest sport and hearty fellowship during the course of study they are about to commence."**
>
> *"A former Square Man", 14th September 1895*

According to surviving minutes, the "Pharmaceutical Football Club" was first formed on Tuesday 12th October 1880, and it was rugby union that was played. The School colours were a dark blue jersey with white Maltese cross in the centre of the breast. In October 1890, Football Association rules were adopted in place of rugby, and the strip colours were changed to a white shirt with a dark blue Maltese cross on the left breast, and dark blue knickerbockers with stockings to match. By the early twentieth century, the strip was a white jersey and shorts with blue stockings and a blue Maltese cross. The apparent reason for the change to association football seems to have been less that soccer was more popular or fashionable (the Football Association had been founded in 1863, so it was not a new trend), but more because the School was finding it hard to turn out 15 players regularly.

Taking advantage of being in London

One of the by-products of attending the Square was its central location in London. This could be viewed as a blessing with lots of opportunities for entertainment, or as a curse with plenty to distract the student from his studies. In 1868, the Council decided to invite someone notable to give an introductory or inaugural address to students entering their studies each year. The first was given on 7th October 1868 by Henry Bowman Brady, Council member and examiner, entitled "Thoughts on the Present Aspect of Pharmacy in its Social and Ethical Relations". Much of its content was to persuade the students to be systematic and thorough. He felt that it was acceptable to take recreation, but that it was an indulgence: "It is the complete unbending that preserves the elasticity of the bow, and the mind requires equally its seasons of relief from strain ... Take amusement in moderation, and of such a sort as leaves the appetite for study unimpaired." His answer was not to take part in sport or leisure, but simply to change the nature of the work that one is undertaking: "When the mind has about it the vigour of youth, change of occupation is of itself relaxation." In contrast, Michael Carteighe, Society president, giving the School's annual address on its 50th anniversary in 1892, remembered attending the theatre as a student in the early 1860s with an actor named Robson playing in burlesque. Three years later, at the same occasion, the speaker was Frederick T. Roberts, professor of medicine at UCL. He was more cautious: "Some of you are so young and inexperienced that I really tremble for you in this great city, probably just removed from the guidance of loving parents and the salutary control of home-life."

Nevertheless, some students went to great lengths to take part in London life. A past student calling himself Verax published some memories in the *Square Chronicle*. He remembered going to the Oxford and Cambridge Boat Race in April 1880. In order to make the 8am start at Putney, they got up at 5.30am and headed to Waterloo to catch a train. After entertainment by "three-card trick men" on the journey, the race was postponed (for the only time in its history) owing to fog.

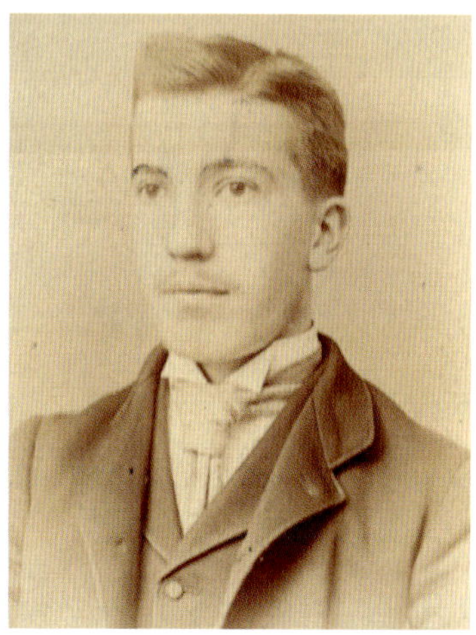

GEORGE SENTER (1874–1942)

Royal Pharmaceutical Society Museum

GEORGE SENTER (1874–1942)

George Senter was awarded the Jacob Bell Scholarship in 1895, having already studied pharmacy in his native Scotland at the Central School of Pharmacy in Edinburgh. He passed the Minor exam in April 1896 and the Major exam in the following July. He gained a scholarship to take the BSc at the University of London, and also achieved the London DSc. He obtained a DPhil at Leipzig in 1903 and worked as a lecturer in chemistry at St Mary's Hospital Medical School from 1904 to 1913. He also served as an examiner to a wide range of institutions including the College of Surgeons, the College of Physicians, Goldsmiths College and the University of Birmingham.

He became head of the department of chemistry at Birkbeck College, University of London, in 1914 and retained that position until 1932. He became principal of the College in 1918. During his principalship, the College was recognised as a school of the University of London in 1920, and in 1926 a Royal Charter was granted. He also played a significant role in the development of a scheme for new buildings for the College. He first became a member of the University's Senate in 1912, and served as deputy vice-chancellor in 1933–4. His publications include *Outlines of Physical Chemistry* and *Text Book of Inorganic Chemistry*.

WOMEN STUDENTS

The minutes of the Library, Museum and Laboratories Committee from 9th October 1861 record that they had been informed that a lady had a ticket of admission to the lectures. They concluded that she was attending upon sufferance. The lady was Elizabeth Garrett, later Elizabeth Garrett Anderson, who attended chemistry and botany lectures by Professors Attfield and Bentley in order to prepare for the medical exams of the Society of Apothecaries. Michael Carteighe, later the Society's president, was a student at the School at the time:

> I remember about the time I became a student here that we had a lady student in this house. I remember exactly where she sat in this theatre, and I remember the envious eyes with which a number of us regarded her. I do not think we regarded her with envy because she was a lady – in fact, we admired her on that account; but we were conscious that when once a lady comes into a class she means to take prizes, and I am afraid we were selfish enough to think of that rather than anything else.

With the knowledge that a female student had entered the School, the Council passed a formal resolution banning the attendance of women.

In his introduction to the first inaugural address in 1868, the Society's president, G.W. Sandford, commented: "As the classes of students are now commencing their work, Mr Brady had kindly undertaken to deliver an inaugural address. He would probably say something of the importance of pharmacy, but hoped he would not draw so glowing a picture as to tempt ladies into the profession." Nevertheless, there were 223 female pharmacists on the first compulsory Register in 1869 (1.9% of 11,638 in total). The majority had taken

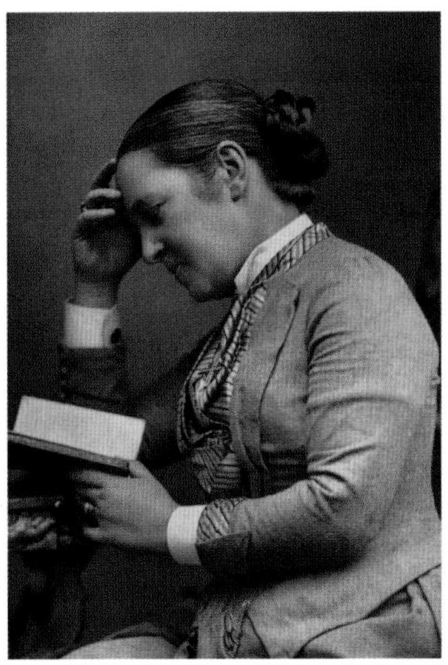

ELIZABETH GARRETT (ANDERSON) (1836–1917)

Wellcome Library, London

ELIZABETH GARRETT (ANDERSON) (1836–1917)

Elizabeth Garrett Anderson was the first female doctor to qualify in England. She began to study medicine in 1860, having been inspired by meeting Dr Elizabeth Blackwell, the first woman to qualify as a doctor in the United States. Both the Royal College of Surgeons and the Royal College of Physicians refused to admit her to their exams, but she obtained permission to attend the lecture course at the School of Pharmacy in 1862 directly from the professors, who were unaware of the Council's attitude towards women. She was studying to obtain the licence of the Society of Apothecaries, which she achieved in 1865. At the same time, she took the degree of MD at the University of Paris. In 1866, she was appointed as a medical attendant at St Mary's Dispensary in London. In 1872, she set up the New Hospital for Women at St Mary's Dispensary, where she held the post of senior physician until 1890. From 1883 to 1898 she was dean at the Hospital, then renamed the London School of Medicine for Women.

In 1876, partly as a result of her campaigning, an act was passed to allow women to enter the medical profession and appear on the British Medical Register. In 1896, she was elected president of the East Anglian branch of the British Medical Association. She retired to Aldeburgh in Suffolk in 1902, and in 1908, she was elected its mayor, the first woman in England to hold the position. After her death, the London School of Medicine for Women was renamed the Elizabeth Garrett Anderson Hospital.

over businesses from their fathers or husbands, an element of the workforce not considered by the male hierarchy of the Society and the profession.

However, if the inclusion of women on this 1869 Register provoked any comment, it was not recorded. Women took the Society's exams alongside their male counterparts (although they were not eligible for the prizes, or to work in the Society's chemical laboratories). Fanny Deacon (née Potter) of Fleckney, Leicestershire, was the first woman to pass the "Modified" exam after the 1868 Act. Alice Vickery was the first woman to qualify as a chemist & druggist by passing the Society's Minor exam in June 1873. However, women were not permitted to become Society members. They could work as pharmacists, but had no rights in the Society and therefore no role to play in the regulation of the profession.

**" A 'Royal charter' you've obtained, and published certain rules
But none of these, I think, excludes the Women from our schools.
If they obey the law laid down, we cannot keep them out,
And, O! they're wide awake enough to know what they're about … "**

"A Valentine to the Council of the Pharmaceutical Society", 22nd February 1873

Robert Hampson, as a member of the Pharmaceutical Society's Council, championed the rights of female pharmacists. He was elected to the Council of the Pharmaceutical Society in 1872, and was an extremely active member. Amongst other issues, he strenuously advocated the admission of women, first to the lectures and laboratories of the Pharmaceutical Society, and then to full membership. Dr Garrett, having gained the Apothecaries' licence to practise medicine in 1865, wrote to the Council in 1872 requesting that more women could attend the School's lectures. The question of women's admission was discussed at both the September and October Council meetings, promoted by Hampson and primarily opposed by Sandford. One Council member reflected that "in 1862 perhaps the admission of lady students to the classes and laboratory might appear a step fraught with great danger, and

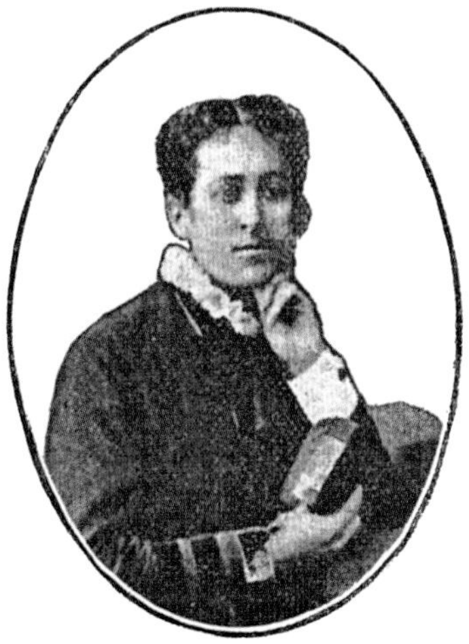

LOUISA STAMMWITZ (1850–1916)

Chemist + Druggist

LOUISA STAMMWITZ (1850–1916)

Louisa Stammwitz campaigned alongside Rose Minshull and Alice Hart to allow female students access to the Society's laboratories. Louisa Stammwitz sat the Society's Preliminary exam in 1873 at the same time as Rose Minshull. She trained at the South London School of Pharmacy at Kennington under Dr Muter, where Isabella Clarke and Rose Minshull trained. Miss Stammwitz claimed later that, if there had been training available for women doctors at the time, she would have chosen that career instead of pharmacy.

Louisa Stammwitz, Rose Minshull and Alice Hart were put forward at the Council meeting in February 1873 as "registered students" of the Society. The motion was rejected. However, Miss Stammwitz passed the Minor exam and registered as a chemist & druggist on 18th October 1877. She passed the Major exam and registered as a pharmaceutical chemist on 12th December 1878.

Her first post was as dispenser at the New Hospital for Women in London, where she stayed for nine years. She then set up in partnership with Annie Neve, another pharmacist, and they opened a pharmacy in Paignton, Devon.

tending to revolution." However, Council agreed at the October meeting to allow female students to attend lectures, but not the laboratories. As Hampson expressed, it seemed strange to allow the women to take the Society's exams, but deny them teaching for them. The female students had seats on the front row of the lecture theatre reserved for them and they had to enter via a special door on a level with the front row.

Hampson continued to keep the debate on the Council's agenda, determined that women pharmacists should have equal opportunities. Having passed the Society's Preliminary exam, Rose Minshull, Louisa Stammwitz and Alice Hart were put forward by Hampson at the Council meeting in February 1873 as "registered students" of the Society. The motion was rejected. In July 1874, Professor Attfield asked if female students could be admitted to his practical classes and was refused by Council. During 1876 and 1877, Rose Minshull, Alice Hart and Louisa Stammwitz petitioned the Council to allow ladies access to the Society's chemistry laboratories. This permission was granted in 1877. After a heavy defeat in a debate on women's membership at the Annual Meeting of 1873, Hampson did not reintroduce the topic until 1878. During 1879, the motion to admit women to full membership was narrowly defeated at both the Annual Meeting and the June Council meeting. However, the motion was carried at the Council's October meeting in 1879. Isabella Clarke and Rose Minshull were elected members of the Society. They had both passed the Society's Preliminary, Minor and Major exams. They made repeated applications for membership from 1875 onwards. Isabella Clarke opened her own shop in 1876, but was still denied full membership privileges. The Council's decision that women could become members in 1879 seems to have come about because some Council members wanted to end the debate, or "to avoid further agitation" as one put it, rather than through any widely held ethical belief that women ought to be allowed equal rights.

> **"It was part of the executive duty of the Council to elect all eligible persons, irrespective of their sex. It would be as reasonable to ask what church they attended as to inquire as to the sex of eligible persons who applied for admission [to the Society's membership]."**
>
> *Robert Hampson, 1st October 1879*

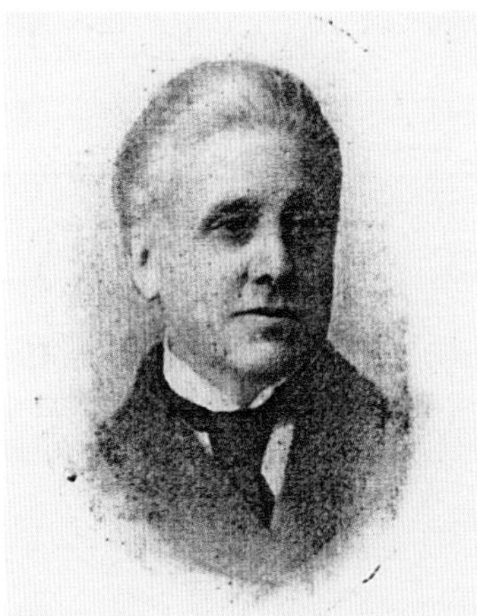

ISABELLA CLARKE (1843–1926)

Chemist + Druggist

ISABELLA CLARKE (1843–1926)

Isabella Clarke (later Clarke-Keer) was one of the two first female members of the Pharmaceutical Society, and the first president of the Association of Women Pharmacists. Isabella Skinner Clarke registered with the Society as a chemist & druggist on 22nd April 1875. She became a pharmaceutical chemist by passing the Major exam on 15th December 1875. She came fourth out of 39 candidates for the Major, 16 of whom failed. Shortly afterwards, she established her own business at Spring Street, Paddington, London, and took female medical students for their dispensing course at her pharmacy. This led to her appointment as tutor in pharmacy at the Royal Free School of Medicine for Women. It was not until 1879 that she was elected as a member of the Pharmaceutical Society.

In 1883, she married Thomas Keer, whom she had met when they were both students at Muter's School of Pharmacy. After her marriage, she gave up the Spring Street business and became her husband's partner in a pharmacy in Bruton Street, Berkeley Square. She later started a home for students at their house in Endsleigh Street. It was at her home here that the first meeting of the Association of Women Pharmacists was held in 1905.

ROSE MINSHULL (1851–1905)

Rose Coombs Minshull was one of the first two women, alongside Isabella Clarke-Keer, to be elected members of the Society in 1879. She was obviously a very talented student. When she passed the Society's Preliminary exam in 1873, she came top of the 166 candidates. She then passed the Minor exam, also with top marks, and registered as a chemist & druggist on 18th October 1877. She passed the Major exam and registered as a pharmaceutical chemist on 19th February 1879. During 1876 and 1877, together with Alice Hart and Louisa Stammwitz, she petitioned the Council to allow ladies access to the Society's chemistry laboratories. This permission was granted in 1877.

By 1884, she became the dispenser at the North Eastern Hospital for Children, Hackney Road, London. Rose Minshull wrote in an article for *The Chemist and Druggist*: "As the result of many years' hospital work, I am decidedly of the opinion that certainly in women's and children's hospitals a lady dispenser is the right woman in the right place." Rose Minshull was described in her obituary in *The Chemist and Druggist* as "not by nature a fighter, but a bright and charming little woman, of an affectionate nature."

Although the battle for recognition at the Pharmaceutical Society and entrance to its School was unquestionably drawn out and frustrating for both sides, the Society was actually extremely pioneering in its admission of women. In 1874, a London school of medicine for women had been opened, and in 1876, an Act had allowed women to be on the medical register. In 1878, women students had been admitted on the same footing as men at UCL. However, after Elizabeth Garrett took the Society of Apothecaries' exams in 1865, it took legal advice and changed its regulations in 1868 to exclude all those who studied privately from its exams, relying on teaching institutions to exclude women students. In 1872, Edinburgh University closed its examinations to female students, and in 1880, the British Medical Association voted not to admit qualified women doctors. It was not until 1910 that women were allowed to become accountants and bankers. Of course, in spite of the very high-profile suffragist and suffragette movement, women did not get the vote until 1918.

> **"what I wish to impress upon those who are interested in the subject is the extreme folly of taking away any remaining barriers to the entry of a profession for which ladies are by their sex eminently disqualified … There is a considerable amount of drudgery connected with it [the profession], which must be repugnant to ladies, and which I should seriously be disposed to think their constitution would not be adapted to endure … there are many cases brought to the notice of an ordinary chemist which would be exceedingly undesirable to bring her in contact with …"**
>
> *Charles Fryer of Scarborough, 17th November 1877*

Historian Dr Ellen Jordan discovered that some of the pioneering women pharmacists were encouraged to go into dispensing via The Society for Promoting the Employment of Women. Elizabeth Garrett Anderson opened the St Mary's Dispensary for Women and Children in Marylebone in 1866, and offered training for other women to become dispensers, probably including Louisa Stammwitz and Rose Minshull. Isabella Clarke gained some of her three years' required experience for registration with Garrett Anderson and some with Robert Hampson. Although small numbers of women qualified by examination in the early days of the Pharmaceutical Society, they were aiming to establish a career rather than inheriting the business from a relative, and believed that they could become independent professionals. In fact, the School enabled some pioneering women to

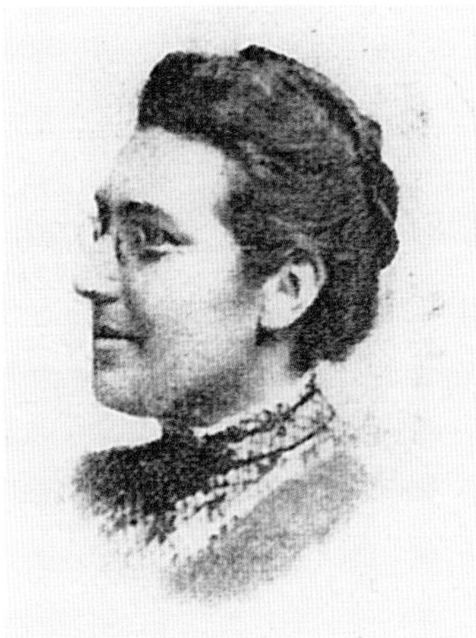

MARGARET BUCHANAN (1866–1940)

Royal Pharmaceutical Society Museum

MARGARET BUCHANAN (1866–1940)

Margaret Elizabeth Buchanan registered as a chemist & druggist in 1886, having served her apprenticeship with her father, and subsequently with Isabella Clarke-Keer and her husband. She was clearly an extremely talented pharmacist: the only female student at the time at the School to take double honours in its exams and the first woman to be awarded its silver medal.

On qualification, she was appointed dispenser to the Westminster General Infirmary. She recognised that what aspiring female pharmacists needed was an opportunity to gain training in running a business. In 1892, she wrote that "it is becoming recognised by the public and the trade that women can be both business-like and well-trained scientifically, the number of lady-pharmacists will doubtless increase as the field further opens up."

The opportunity to try to make a difference came when a pharmacy at 17 The Pavement, Clapham Common became available. Between 1911 and 1914, Margaret Buchanan bought the business, and worked alongside Agnes Borrowman to establish it as a training pharmacy for women. The two women also established a school of pharmacy for women in Gordon Square, a short walk from Bloomsbury Square. Margaret Buchanan was the first vice-president of the Association of Women Pharmacists and later became its president. Miss Buchanan was the first female member of the Society's Council, elected in 1918 and retiring in 1926. "The consternation that arose in certain quarters is one of those things not easily forgotten", according to a report in 1940. She was described by *The Chemist and Druggist* in 1909 as holding "the front rank among the women pharmacists of the British Empire. She is ... a quiet yet effective speaker."

establish themselves in pharmaceutical research. In April 1888, Lucy Boole passed the Major exam and was immediately employed as a research assistant to Professor Dunstan. As such, she was the first woman to undertake pharmacy research in a formal way in Britain. Her interest was tartar emetic (potassium antimony tartrate), including a joint paper with Dunstan in November 1888. The procedure that she proposed to assay tartar emetic was adopted in the *British Pharmacopoeia* in 1898 and remained the official assay method until 1963.

THE SCHOOL'S INDEPENDENCE

At the Council meeting on 2nd July 1873, the Society decided to privatise its School and hand over administration to the professors. Criticism from members of the amount of money spent by the Society on maintaining the School's activities had already led to the decision to reduce the number of professors from four to two by combining subjects, and by separating off the laboratories to be run by the professor of practical chemistry, John Attfield. Up to this point, the course and laboratory fees only contributed to the running costs of the School, which included annual stipends of £300 for the professor of chemistry

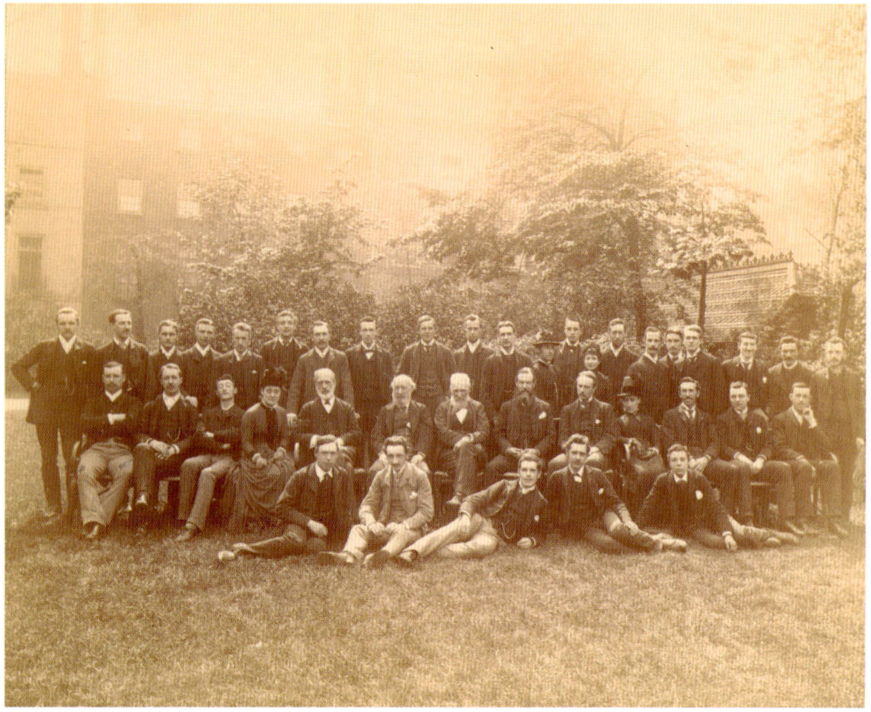

The School year group photograph in 1887 effectively marks the beginning of the end of an era. Alongside the elderly Professors Bentley, Redwood and Attfield sits Professor Dunstan, recently appointed as Director of the new Research Laboratories. Margaret Buchanan, standing behind Professor Dunstan, became an extremely pioneering female pharmacist, and Edmund White sitting on the grass in front of him, became President of the Pharmaceutical Society.

UCL School of Pharmacy Library

and pharmacy (Redwood) and professor of botany and materia medica (Bentley), and of £150 for the professor of practical chemistry alongside a percentage of the laboratory fees. The Society therefore subsidised the School annually by about £500. The financial burden that the School represented, in addition to the competition from the growing number of private pharmacy schools, persuaded the Council that it should be run on a semi-autonomous, self-supporting basis. From 1874, each of the three professors was given an annual endowment of £100 and free use of rooms, but they had to meet all other expenses including materials. In return, they received all of the students' fees. The Council's attitude towards the School was decidedly frosty, as shown by the debate in the August 1873 Council meeting over whether the Society should contribute a positive foreword to the prospectus that the professors had prepared. After much discussion, a copy of this prospectus was sent to each chemist & druggist in the country with a covering letter from the Council.

The Society had hoped to reduce its financial problems by fixing its contribution to the running of the School. However, the School was not fit for privatisation. Not least, the professors were not prepared to focus solely on teaching. As eminent experts in their fields, they undertook other projects, such as research for development of the *British Pharmacopoeia* in the laboratories. This research focus increased when, in 1887, Mr Wyndham R. Dunstan, demonstrator of chemistry under Redwood and Attfield, was appointed to the post of professor of chemistry and director of the Research Laboratories of the Pharmaceutical Society of Great Britain.

RESEARCH

From the start, the Pharmaceutical Society wanted to encourage and promote research. The first official Council address committed to "the establishment of a uniform system of education, which will promote the advancement of science and the elevation of the profession of Pharmacy." However, when the *British Pharmacopoeia* first appeared in 1864, it was under the sponsorship of the General Medical Council (GMC), a situation established by the 1858 Medical Act. There was no pharmacist involved in the first edition, and the finished product was widely viewed as a disaster, with more than half of the 28,000 copies printed destroyed. An invitation for members of the Society to get involved came from the GMC, aware that they needed to raise the next edition's scientific content. Professor Redwood was thus joint editor of the following editions of 1867 and 1885. However, there was no official recognition for this help from the GMC or for other leading Society members who had been involved in raising the standard. As the Society had paid Redwood's salary and costs, they wrote to the GMC in 1874 to ask for an official Pharmaceutical Society of Great Britain (PSGB) position on their *British Pharmacopoeia* committee, but they were refused.

In 1883, a Bill was introduced to amend the 1858 Medical Act, which had brought about the first *British Pharmacopoeia*. The Society's Council prepared a clause proposing the establishment of a British Pharmacopoeia Committee of six medics chosen by the GMC, and five pharmacists, four chosen by the PSGB and one by the Pharmaceutical Society of Northern Ireland. However, at a meeting with the Lord President of the Privy Council, Michael Carteighe, the Society's president, was informed that Professors Redwood, Bentley and Attfield had already accepted an invitation from the GMC to edit the next edition. Unsurprisingly, this caused ructions, including a letter from the professors in *The Pharmaceutical Journal* of 12th May 1883 explaining their situation. The incident left bad relations between the Council and the professors, and was probably a contributory factor towards Redwood's retirement in 1885 – although he was 77 years old.

After Redwood's retirement, Michael Carteighe persuaded the Council to set up a research laboratory. Carteighe as Society president in 1882 had had a primary aim to improve its standing as a scientific body. He was extremely keen that the credit for the research work behind the *British Pharmacopoeia* was recognised as being carried out by the Society. For him, the establishment of a research laboratory would allow work that "would be of extreme value, and the improvement effected in pharmaceutical processes must produce an effect on the medical profession and on the medical council which could not fail to be beneficial." His fellow Council members were not as enthusiastic, feeling that the Society would not gain the recognition that the expenditure merited. They also recognised that there was limited

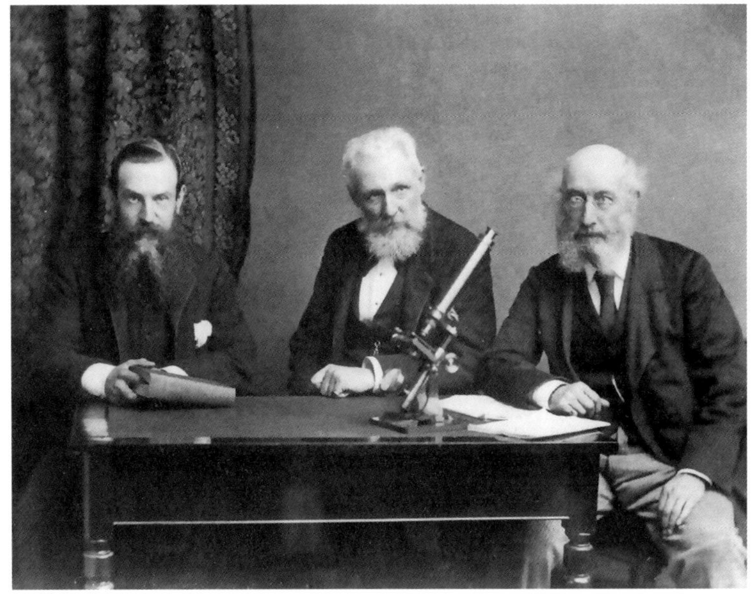

Professors Attfield, Redwood and Bentley had reached their sixth, eighth and seventh decades respectively when this photo was taken in the 1880s. All three still took an active role in the pharmacy profession beyond the School, notably in their controversial joint editorship of the *British Pharmacopoeia* from 1883.

Royal Pharmaceutical Society Museum

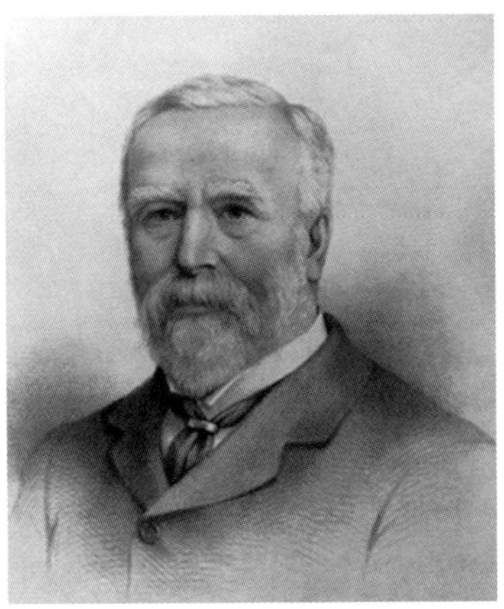

MICHAEL CARTEIGHE (1841–1910)

Royal Pharmaceutical Society Museum

MICHAEL CARTEIGHE (1841–1910)

Michael Carteighe had studied and worked as a demonstrator at University College London before he entered the Square in 1862. He passed the Minor exam in April 1863 and the Major exam three months later. He was an outstanding student, achieving unprecedented high exam marks. He joined the firm of Dinneford and Co. alongside his brother in 1863. He was elected an auditor of the Pharmaceutical Society in 1864, and a member of the Society's Council in 1866. Serving also on the Board of Examiners, he had to step down from the Council in 1869 to prevent a conflict of interest. However, he returned to the Council in 1881. He was elected president in the following year and held the post for 14 years, during which time he was instrumental in intense negotiations over reform of pharmacy legislation which ultimately resulted in the 1908 Pharmacy Act. He also played a significant role in litigation by the Society to protect the status of registered pharmacists.

He was heavily involved in the Society's improvements in education and research, overseeing the establishment of the research laboratories opened in 1888. It was Carteighe's proposal to the Society's Council that led to the first *British Pharmaceutical Codex* in 1907. He served as general secretary of the British Pharmaceutical Conference in 1880 and 1882, and had a significant reputation as a scientist. He was also a member of the Society of the Chemical Industry, a Fellow of the Chemical Society and a founder of the Institute of Chemistry, serving as its vice-president in 1882–1884 and 1890–1893. Although eventual blindness restricted his activities towards the very end of his life, he continued to attend Council and Committee meetings until just before his death.

> **"If such a project could be carried out with spirit, the Pharmaceutical Society might in the future be referred to on all matters connected with the analysis and impurities of drugs."**
>
> *Michael Carteighe, 1882*

room to achieve this at Bloomsbury Square, and also felt that they ought to be promoting research outside the School. However, at the March 1886 meeting, the issue was again discussed and Council agreed to progress tentatively with plans, and also drew up regulations for the operation of the laboratories. In the same year, the Society acquired unoccupied buildings at the back of 15 and 16 Bloomsbury Square which resolved the issue of space.

The Society had already demonstrated its commitment to a research role. By 1881, it was supporting the costs of research work being carried on in its chemistry laboratories, and had agreed the professor of chemistry's £200 annual fee "so long as he is engaged in original research and undertakes the personal direction of the work of advanced students and others in the research laboratory." This was not the case just for chemistry. When Bentley retired in 1886, Joseph Reynolds Green was appointed as professor of botany. He was an established research scientist with a BSc from the University of London and a BA from Cambridge already under his belt, and a track record of research into proteins.

From 1886, the Society had a new building erected at the back of 15 and 16 Bloomsbury Square at a cost of £6,915. The ground floor housed a new examination hall alongside an examination dispensary for 12 students and a chemistry examination laboratory for eight students. In the basement was a lecture preparation room and stores. On the mezzanine floor there was an office for the professor of botany and a waiting room for exam candidates. The first floor housed two research laboratories, a room for the laboratory director and a store room which also contained balances.

At its meeting on 4th January 1888, the Council committed the funding to establish the research laboratory on the top of the new building, alongside £300 to equip the rooms. They also set up a research committee to direct and advise. The leading article in *The Pharmaceutical Journal* of 5th May 1888 stated:

> The establishment of a Research Laboratory, and the appropriation of a sum of three hundred pounds a year to defray the expenses attending the work of that department, are steps which place the Pharmaceutical Society abreast of other institutions that are proceeding in the same direction, and thus giving practical expression to the slowly growing sense of a want that deeply affects our national prosperity.

The new building housing the laboratory was officially opened in May 1888, and in October the District Board of Works renamed what had been called Pied Bull Yard as Galen Place in recognition of its pharmaceutical inhabitants.

Wyndham Rowland Dunstan was appointed as the laboratory's first director, having served as an assistant to Redwood in 1879 and then as demonstrator of chemistry under Attfield. Dunstan was a very capable scientist, and after three years of operation, the laboratory was definitely regarded as a success by both *The Pharmaceutical Journal* and members of Council. Carteighe, unsurprisingly, was delighted. In his president's address at the School's jubilee celebrations in 1892, he claimed that the School is now "probably the best

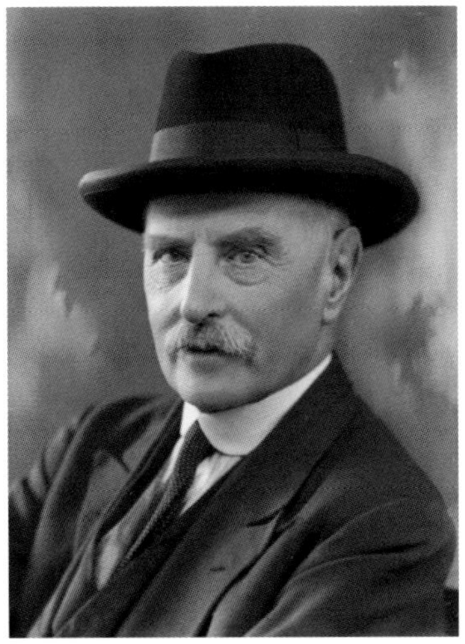

WYNDHAM ROWLAND DUNSTAN (1861–1949)

© National Portrait Gallery, London

WYNDHAM ROWLAND DUNSTAN (1861–1949)

Wyndham Dunstan was educated at Bedford School before becoming assistant to Theophilus Redwood at the Society's School in 1879. He does not appear to have achieved any formal educational qualifications before taking on this post. He went on to become demonstrator of chemistry under Professor Attfield. "Verax", a student in the 1879–80 session, commented that Dunstan's long flowing hair was unusual and that except "for his masculine attire he would easily have passed for a lady student." He went to the University Chemistry Laboratories at Oxford to work as a demonstrator in 1884 and was awarded an honorary MA (Oxon) in 1886. In 1887, he returned to the Society as director of the new research laboratories, which he combined with the post of lecturer of chemistry at St Thomas' Hospital Medical School from 1892.

In 1896, he left the School to take up the position of director of the scientific and technical department of the Imperial Institute. He became full director of the Institute in 1903. He was awarded an honorary degree from Aberdeen in 1904, and was made a Commander of the Order of St Michael and St George in 1913, and a Knight Commander of the Order on his retirement in 1924. His many scientific papers were chiefly concerned with the constituents of aconite, Indian aconite, podophyllum and nux vomica.

equipped School of Chemistry and Pharmacy in the kingdom." The practical pharmacy laboratory and lecture theatre, practical work in botany with cutting-edge microscopes, alongside the research laboratory would allow the School to achieve his aim for the students: "We expect to turn them out, as I think we succeed in turning most of them out, intelligent creatures capable of thinking and acting, not machines that can sell a dose of poison under the regulations prescribed by the law." Carteighe admitted that this meant that some have gone on to wider fields than pharmacy, but this should be embraced as reflecting honour on to the School, the Society and the profession.

This proved to be a telling statement for the research laboratory's director. Dunstan started research work on alkyl nitrates and on alkaloids of monkshood (*Aconitum napellus*). In 1894, he published a paper demonstrating that aconitine was acetyl-benzoyl-aconine. However, *The Pharmaceutical Journal* claimed that this discovery had already been made by German scientists and that Dunstan was a plagiarist. But the Royal Society made him a Fellow and provided him with money from the Government Fund to carry out the research, and the Chemical Society supported the research laboratory with grants. In addition, the director at Kew and the director of the Imperial Institute both asked him to carry out research work. This obvious confidence in his abilities and the legitimacy of his research interests was not shared by his parent body. It appeared that the Society felt that he should not be carrying out work for other institutions. Society members were also highly critical of Dunstan's wide network of research connections. Edward Butt complained:

> We cannot afford to keep an ornamental individual with the title of Director of the Research Laboratory who does nothing but misdirect. What we want is a person who has a knowledge of pharmacy, who knows what the requirements of pharmacy are, and who has sufficient chemical knowledge and

> sufficient enthusiasm for his work to conduct our research laboratory on the lines on which we have always supposed it would be conducted. We want a man who has not fifty other engagements, or even twenty, but a man who will devote his time to the work for which he is paid.

The fact that earlier professors had also supplemented their incomes seemed to have gone unnoticed. Professor Redwood seemed to hold an unachievable number of posts, from public analysis to curator of the Society's museum. Professor Bentley combined his post at the School with chairs of botany at the London Institution and at King's College, London, plus serving as dean of the Medical School at King's College from 1863 to 1883.

Even though the laboratory was very successful in its research, and in attracting external funding, it was attacked by the Society and its members. Carteighe's exasperation at the inability of his colleagues to appreciate its value was very evident:

> What do we want? We want to extend our power and usefulness ... Now, how is that to be done? Not by talking to each other. Some of us want to go to Parliament, and that is right enough. How do we want to make the work of the Society known? It is no use talking to ourselves in our Journal. You want to spread the news far and wide, and everything that is published from our Research Laboratory, which goes all over the world into the hands of persons who are not pharmacists is, to put a vulgar phrase on it, a good advertisement for this Society, and brings with it a respect which you cannot measure. It brings with it in many cases power. In my journey in the [United] States, there was not a single professor of chemistry that I met who did not pay the highest compliment with regard to the work which has come out of the Research Laboratory.

However, in the same year, 1895, the Council considered transferring the laboratory to the Imperial Institute on the suggestion of Sir Frederick Abel, who had been the Government's Chief Scientific Adviser between 1854 and 1888. This transfer was not carried out because of concerns that the Society would have to continue to provide an annual grant, but this was enough for Dunstan. He resigned in 1896 to become director of the scientific and technical department of the Imperial Institute. The fact that Dunstan's replacement, John Norman Collie, was not a pharmacist, did not seem to prompt any negative reaction from members like Edward Butt. Michael Carteighe also stepped down from his position on the Council, marking the end of an educational era.

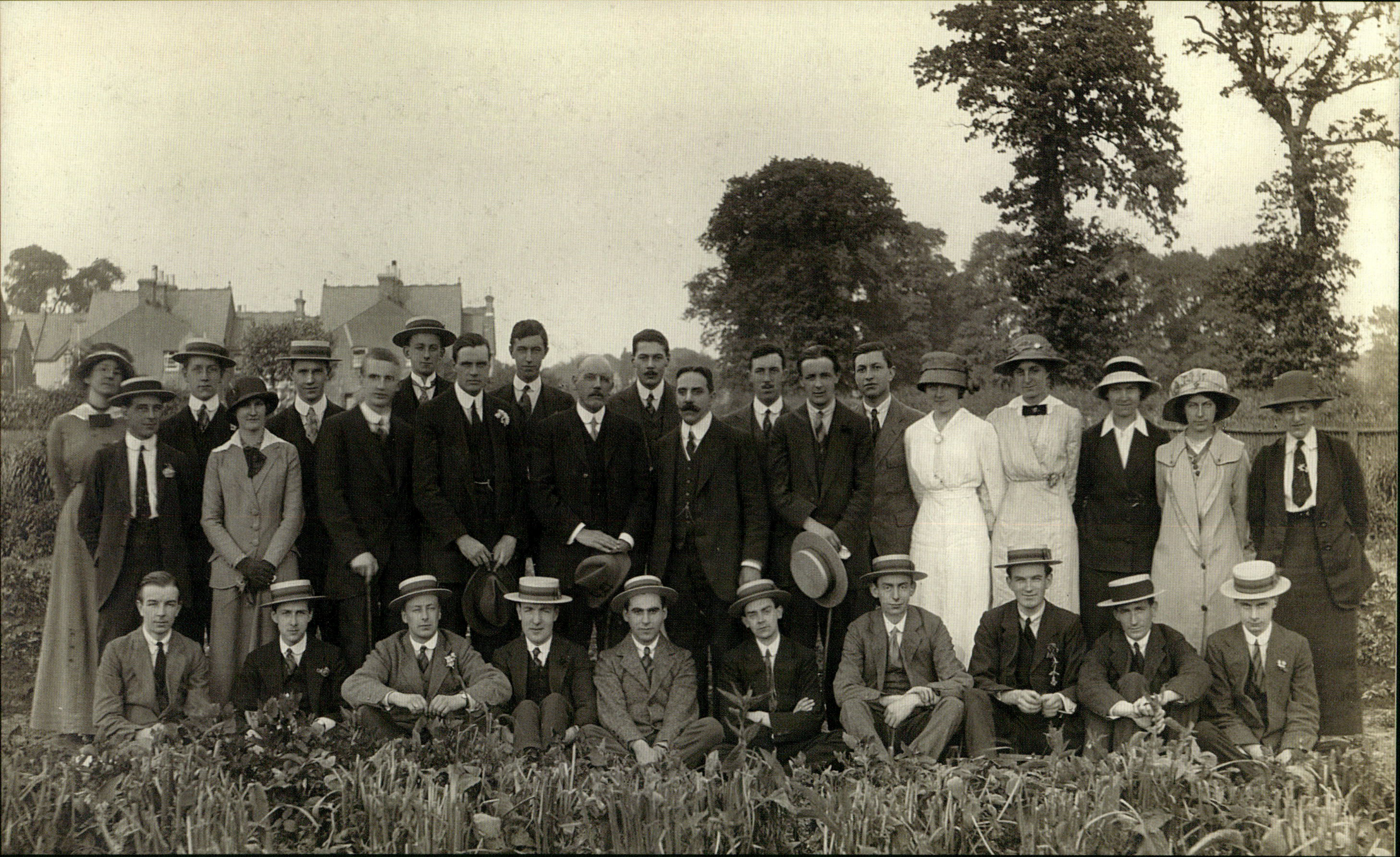

Professor Greenish is shown in the centre of the group of students on a ramble in 1913. He usually accompanied the group on their Saturday outings.

Reproduced with permission from UCL School of Pharmacy Library

MILESTONES

Popular Culture

1908	Model T Ford introduced
1914	Charlie Chaplin's first film
1922	first BBC national radio broadcast

London Life

1899	first motor buses in London
1901	London's population reached 6.6 million
1905	Aldwych and Kingsway opened to traffic
1906	women's suffrage demonstrations in Parliament Square
1908	women's suffrage demonstrations in June in Hyde Park, with up to 300,000 people present
1909	Selfridges opened
1912	women's suffrage demonstrations in May, with windows smashed in West End
1913	Chelsea Flower Show inaugurated
1920	Cenotaph war memorial erected on Whitehall

National News

1901	death of Queen Victoria and accession of King George VII
1911	National Health Insurance Act
1913	Medical Research Council established in the UK
1918	emancipation of women over 30 in the UK
1926	General Strike

The Wider World

1898	Marie and Pierre Curie discovered radium
1899–1902	Boer War
1900	first Zeppelin flight
1900–1901	Boxer Rebellion in China
1901	Marconi transmitted a Morse code wireless signal across Atlantic
1901	Commonwealth of Australia established
1903	Wright brothers made first manned aeroplane flight
1905	Einstein published his special theory of relativity
1907	first manned helicopter flight
1911	Rutherford published his theory of atomic structures
1912	sinking of the *Titanic*
1914	Panama Canal completed
1914–1918	First World War
1917	Russian Revolution
1918	worldwide influenza epidemic
1921	Partition of Ireland

Drug Developments

1897	Ronald Ross discovered that malaria is transmitted by mosquitoes
1898	diamorphine launched as heroin by the German company Bayer, for coughs and pain
1899	aspirin launched by Bayer
1903	Veronal (barbitone) discovered by von Mehring and Fischer
1909	Paul Ehrlich and Dr Sahachiro Hata discovered Salvarsan (arsphenamine), the first "magic bullet" drug, effective against syphilis
1912	"vitamins" named as a concept by Casimir Funk
1913	Medical Research Committee formed in England
1917	heparin, a natural anticoagulant, discovered by Jay McLean and William Henry Howe; introduced commercially from 1935
1921	bacillus Calmette–Guérin (BCG) vaccine against tuberculosis in humans developed in France by Albert Calmette and Camille Guérin
1922	two Canadian researchers, Frederick Banting and Charles Best, used insulin to treat diabetes

An article in the *Square Chronicle*, the Square's alumni magazine founded in 1912, seems to illuminate the concerns of pharmacists about their own profession in the early years of the twentieth century. The article, by E.H. Shields, published in February 1914, imagines the Square in the year AD 2021. The fact that there has been a lift installed for the last 50 years up to the third floor laboratories is the fulfilment of many students' wishes, but it is the courses that are being taught that show the author's anxieties for the profession. The Square is now the headquarters of the "Druggists' Alliance", and the current class in the lecture theatre is where the young druggists in the Academy learn the art of making money. Other lecture topics include candy, soda fountains, tobacco, picture postcards and stationery. The students apparently only read about drugs in their spare time. The museum smells of perfume, tobacco and chocolate, with display cases representing different shop windows. There are a very few old books that no one ever reads in the library. A new facility is a laboratory for show card designing and publicity, and the person giving the guided tour has never heard of examinations. Although the final point may have been greeted with enthusiasm by students, the clear message is that the commercialisation and Americanisation of British pharmacy would take the academic heart out of the profession.

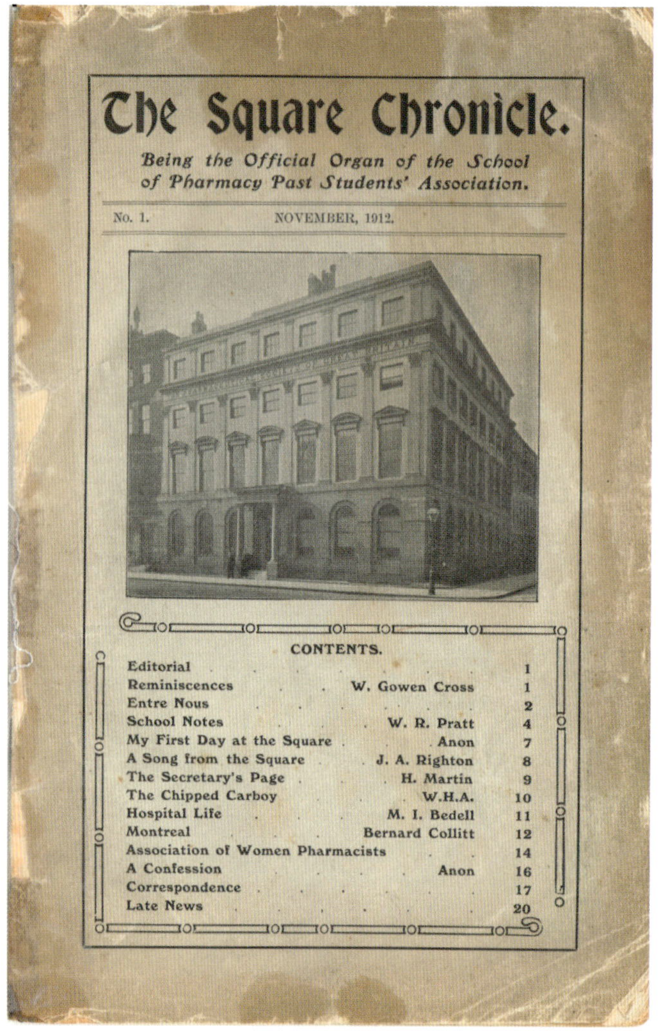
The Square Chronicle.

Being the Official Organ of the School of Pharmacy Past Students' Association.

No. 1. NOVEMBER, 1912.

CONTENTS.

Editorial		1
Reminiscences	W. Gowen Cross	1
Entre Nous		2
School Notes	W. R. Pratt	4
My First Day at the Square	Anon	7
A Song from the Square	J. A. Righton	8
The Secretary's Page	H. Martin	9
The Chipped Carboy	W.H.A.	10
Hospital Life	M. I. Bedell	11
Montreal	Bernard Collitt	12
Association of Women Pharmacists		14
A Confession	Anon	16
Correspondence		17
Late News		20

The first edition of the *Square Chronicle*, showing the School's home at 17 Bloomsbury Square.

UCL School of Pharmacy Library

The reality for the School in the years leading up to the First World War was rather different. By 1896, the attempt at independence was over. At the Council meeting in August, the General Purposes Committee reported that it "deems it expedient that the Council should in future assume the direct control of the Society's School of Pharmacy." Independence of the School had not lifted the need for funding from the Society, and in the last 25 years around £19,000 had been spent on the School and the promotion of research. However, it was clear that a significant overhaul of the teaching, courses and facilities needed to be carried out in order to regain some of the status that the School was felt to deserve. A scathing article in *The Chemist and Druggist* in 1896 damned the School with faint praise: "The Society already has a chemical laboratory which only needs a few touches to make it quite modern. The Botanical Histology department is, we believe, adequate if not complete." It described the practical pharmacy department as "scarcely worthy of the senior school of pharmacy in England." The problem, the editorial concluded, was that the School

Pharmacy Milestones

1896	Proprietary Articles Trade Association (PATA) formed
1905	inaugural meeting of the Association of Women Pharmacists
1909	*Secret Remedies* published by the British Medical Association
1912	*More Secret Remedies* published by the British Medical Association
1912	International Opium Convention
1912	National Health Insurance Act provided free medical treatment to all insured people
1915	medicine stamp duty doubled as a wartime fundraiser
1917	Venereal Disease Act prohibited the advertising of medicines for VD and the selling of mixtures containing scheduled substances: introduced the concept of "prescription only" medicines
1918	Margaret Buchanan became the first female member of the Pharmaceutical Society's Council
1919	Association of Manufacturers of Proprietary Medicines established; became Proprietary Association of Great Britain (PAGB) in 1926
1920	Dangerous Drugs Act regulated the import and sale of potential "drugs of addiction", including the derivatives of opium, cocaine and cannabis
1920	Retail Pharmacists Union (later National Pharmaceutical Union and National Pharmaceutical Association, now National Pharmacy Association) formed after the Jenkins case proved that the PSGB could not act as a trade union, and regulate hours, wages, prices or conditions of employment
1920	Guild of Public Pharmacists (now Guild of Healthcare Pharmacists) founded
1922	Pharmaceutical Society's regional branches formed
1925	Therapeutic Substances Act to regulate biological medicines

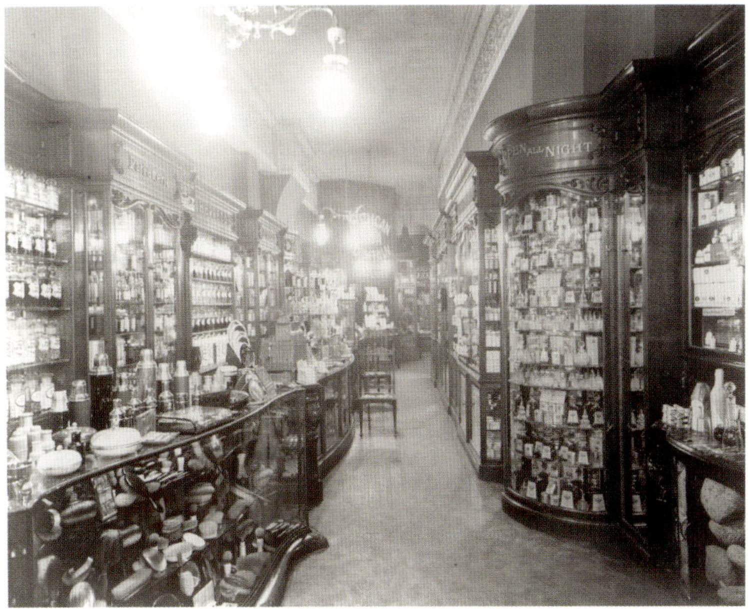

Heppel and Co's high class pharmacy on The Strand opened in the early 1900s. It had an American soda fountain and displayed adverts for Coca-Cola, contrasting with its displays of perfumes, hair brushes and sponges. The shop had a double staff in order to "open all night."

Royal Pharmaceutical Society Museum

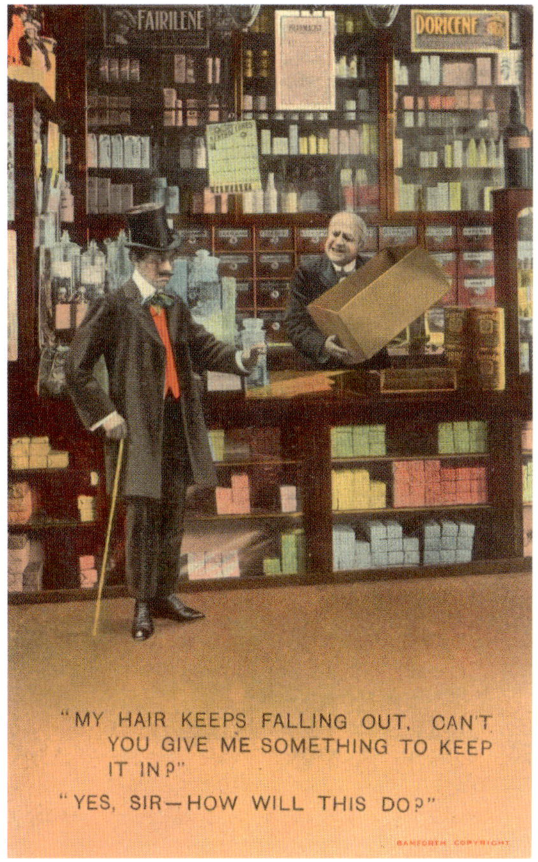
FAIRILENE
DORICENE
"MY HAIR KEEPS FALLING OUT. CAN'T YOU GIVE ME SOMETHING TO KEEP IT IN?"
"YES, SIR—HOW WILL THIS DO?"

Royal Pharmaceutical Society Museum

had not kept up with changes in pharmacy, and had only changed the curriculum in the past to keep up with teaching methods. "It is a school of pharmacy, not of science. Science must be taught thoroughly as far as it goes, but it is absolutely necessary nowadays that theoretical and practical pharmacy should stand in the forefront of the curriculum." The suggestion given was that the changes should come through new staff and courses, and that Council members who have visited schools in Europe and the USA should draw on these experiences to make positive changes.

The new arrangement was that the students' fees went to the Society. Students were no longer allowed to attend single subject classes unless in exceptional circumstances such as to allow dental or medical students to attend materia medica lectures. The Minor and Major courses were extended, the Minor from six to nine months and the Major from three to six months. Teaching was to be carried out by all three professors with demonstrators and assistants appointed by the Council. The professors were paid with a proportion of the fees in addition to annual stipends. They were required to report to Council Committees, and produce an annual written report each year for Council. The Library, Museum, School and House Committee would select one of its members to be a Visitor to the School to attend staff meetings. Michael Carteighe was the first to take this role. Each of the three professors would take the position of dean in a two-year rotation.

The School was back on a tight rein. The Society had had to financially support its activities even during its independence in terms of cleaning, fittings, repairs and around £19,000 in total towards teaching

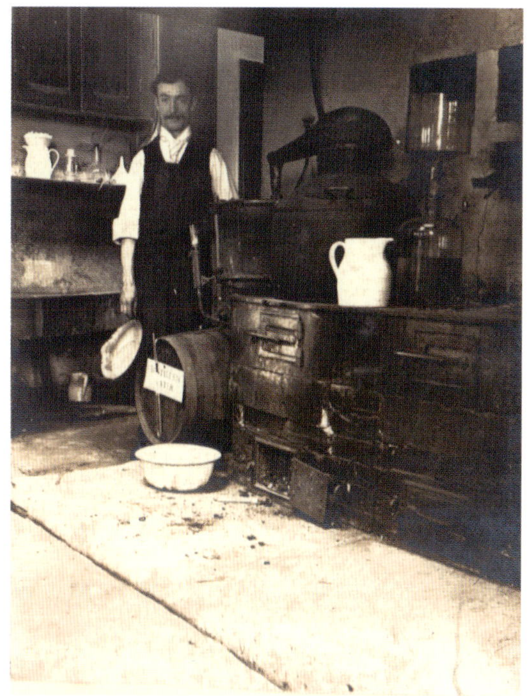

The laboratory assistant, H.Caines, was asked to pose with the old still in the chemistry laboratory in around 1901. Distilled water was made using a copper still on a furnace and a large worm condenser. It was collected in a wooden barrel until this was replaced by an iron tank in 1902.

Royal Pharmaceutical Society Museum

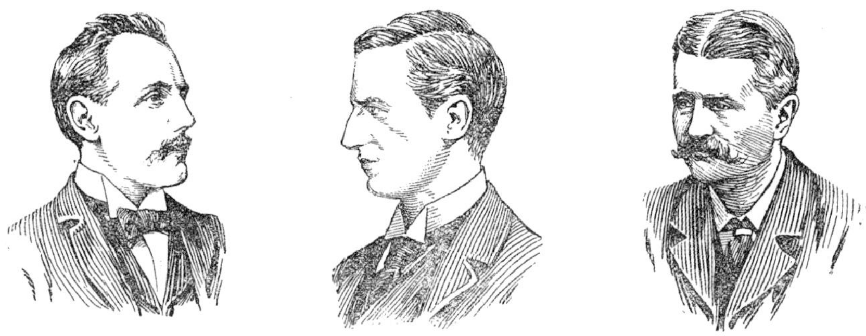

In 1896, *The Pharmaceutical Journal* published a guide to where to study pharmacy. The entry for the School included these drawings of Professors Greenish, Collie and Green, who had recently been appointed, and served as Dean of the School for two years in rotation.

The Pharmaceutical Journal

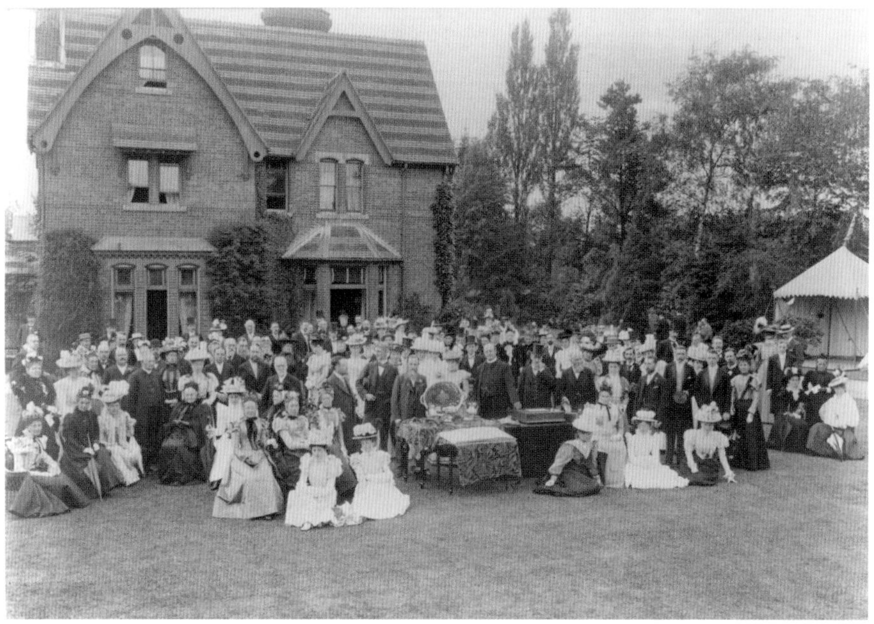

When Professor Attfield retired in 1897, he and his wife hosted an enormous party at their home, Ashlands in Watford in Hertfordshire. This photograph shows the guests in their finery, with Attfield in the centre admiring his retirement presents.

Royal Pharmaceutical Society Museum

and research. It may have been that Society members would have been happy for it to have been less ambitious, and to have competed with the other cramming schools, only educating its students to the level that they needed to pass the exams. However, the Council had higher aims, and still remained committed to the Society's Charter objectives to advance chemistry and pharmacy and to promote a uniform system of education. Even if it was financially risky, they wanted their School to excel, not just to be adequate.

“ We are now making somewhat of an experiment; it rests with our members and friends to make it a success by affording us their help and sympathy. Let us endeavour to make our School as far as possible a model college of pharmacy which may in due time fairly claim to become a recognised part of the teaching University of London. ”

Walter Hills, 5th August 1896

CHEMISTRY

The Council's retaking of control of the School in 1896 brought in a new order in the chemistry department. Professor Attfield was made redundant and the chair of chemistry was completely revised. The professor was put in charge of all chemistry and physics, including delivering lectures to Minor and Major students in physical, organic and inorganic chemistry. This entailed five or six lectures per week from October to July. The professor was also in charge of practical work in the laboratory and supervision of advanced students, and was director of the research laboratory. Stung by their experiences with Dunstan, the Council even went as far as to insist that the professor was present in the department for core hours, and was not allowed to take on any commercial work or any role as examiner to public bodies without the Council's consent. Dr J. Norman Collie was appointed to the role, having previously taught at Cheltenham Ladies' College and University College, London (UCL). The Society's president, Walter Hills, had praise for Professor Collie: his “attainments and past record encourage us to feel confidence as to the future teaching of chemistry, and as to the character of the original work carried out in our Research Laboratory.” He was less confident about the practical pharmacy department: “One cannot but lament that so many of our young men acquire very little of the practical and theoretical knowledge of pharmacy during the time, and under the conditions when it should be best learned. Apprenticeship is, I fear, in many cases, more or less a farce." An assistant lecturer in chemistry, Dr A. Lapworth, was appointed from 1896, the role being taken by T.E. Wallis from 1901 to 1905. Collie's research interests were the study of gases and Röntgen rays (X-rays), and as such the laboratory apparatus was enhanced to include mercury pumps, Ruhmkorff's induction coil and vacuum tubes.

Professor Collie left the Square in 1902 to return to a role at University College. Professor W. Palmer Wynne took over. Although only at the School for two years, he made various changes, not all in chemistry. At his suggestion, common rooms were provided for men and women students, and teaching of practical physics was reorganised. Wynne's interests were in solid substances rather than Collie's gases, particularly derivatives of naphthalene. Professor A.W. Crossley took on the role from 1904 until 1914. He was a more general organic chemist. One of his developments was to add an applied pharmaceutics laboratory in 1904, which was achieved by refitting a private room previously allocated to the director of the research laboratory in Galen Place. His aim was to give students experience in manufacturing processes using apparatus such as percolators, a tincture press and tablet machines. By 1906, the School was advertising that it had one laboratory for Minor students, one laboratory for Major students, one laboratory for women students and one for research.

In July 1914, Professor Henry Llewellyn Smith took over from Professor Crossley. Smith was a pharmaceutical chemist and the first pharmacist to occupy the chair of chemistry since Attfield in 1896. He left in 1918 to

"The practical pharmacy arrangements are scarcely worthy of the senior school of pharmacy in England, and it is here that an attempt should be made to shape the course of instruction so as to lead the way in this country. It is a school of pharmacy, not of science. Science must be taught thoroughly as far as it goes, but it is absolutely necessary nowadays that theoretical and practical pharmacy should stand in the forefront of the curriculum."

The Chemist and Druggist, 1896

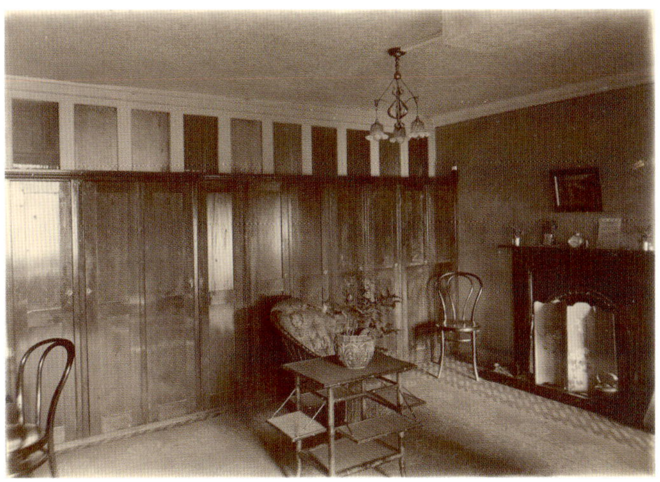

Common rooms for women and men were established in 1903. Although the men's room appears to have decorative wallpaper, the feminine style of the women's room with a comfortable chair, fire screen, potted plant and mantelpiece ornaments shows a gendered difference in approach.

Royal Pharmaceutical Society Museum

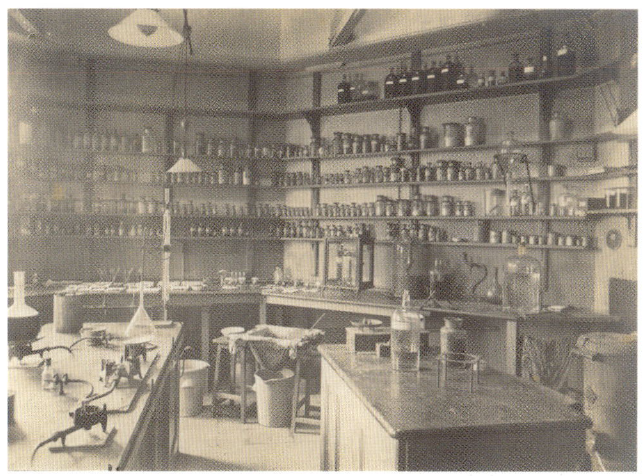

The two-floor Octagon Room had a number of purposes over the years at 17 Bloomsbury Square. In 1896, the lower level was fitted out as a dispensary for 20 students. A spiral staircase could be used to reach this chemistry research laboratory above.

Royal Pharmaceutical Society Museum

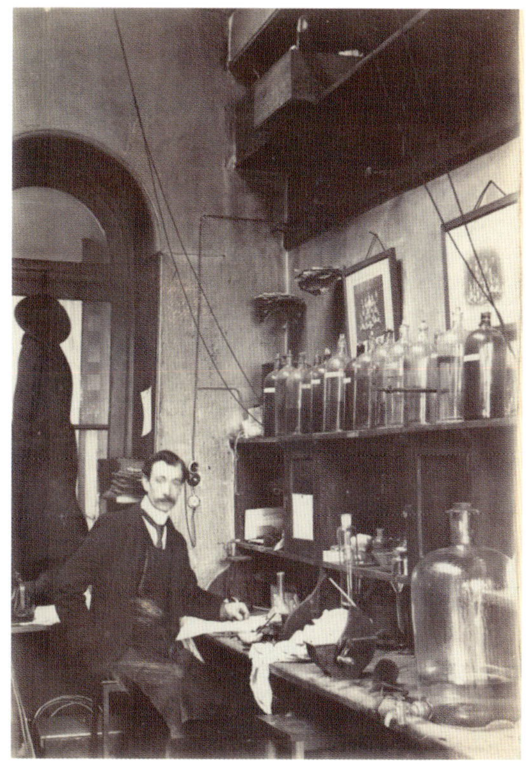

The Chief Laboratory Steward, Mr Caines, was captured in 1901 at his bench. You can see the grindstone for grinding glass tubing on the desk, Mr Caines' coat and bowler hat hanging behind him, and two football team photos above the storage bottles.

Royal Pharmaceutical Society Museum

take up a commission in the Camouflage Section of the War Office. He was replaced by Charles E. Corfield, who had studied at the Square.

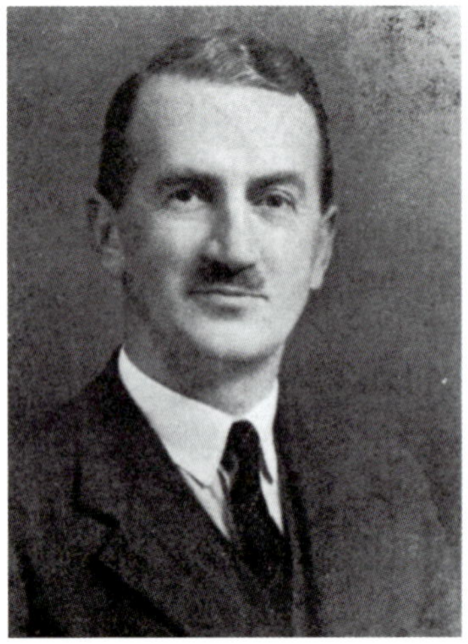

CHARLES EDWIN CORFIELD (1892–1945)

CHARLES EDWIN CORFIELD (1892–1945)

Charles "Flick" Corfield was apprenticed in Ludlow before studying at the Square. He qualified as a chemist & druggist in 1913, and as a pharmaceutical chemist in 1914. He continued as a demonstrator in the chemistry laboratories, and as assistant lecturer in chemistry and physics. In 1918, he was appointed lecturer in chemistry and head of the department, a position he occupied until 1926. He became an examiner for the Society in 1920, and was also an external examiner for London University. In 1925, Corfield joined in partnership with P.A.W. Self in the analytical and consulting practice in Chancery Lane which was founded by Colonel E.F. Harrison. He published numerous scientific papers including those on the assays of belladonna, cinchona and opium, as well as on organic compounds of bismuth, and on the stability of ammonium carbonate. He was appointed editor of the *British Pharmaceutical Codex* in 1923. In 1933, he was put in charge of the *Extra Pharmacopoeia*, recently acquired by the Pharmaceutical Society, and was responsible for the production of the next two editions. He was also responsible for the twelfth, thirteenth and fourteenth editions of *The Pharmaceutical Pocket Book*. From 1924 to 1944, Corfield was honorary secretary of the British Pharmaceutical Conference. In 1921, he married Ella Caird, who was also an outstanding student at the Square, a Fellow of the Royal Institute of Chemistry and a hospital pharmacist. She served as the president of the Past Students' Association in 1930, and after her husband's death, she carried on his analytical practice for several years.

The School's first microbiology lectures started with two each week from April to June 1917, taught by Dr Edward Burnet. The plan was to follow these lectures with practical work from the following October. About 100 students attended the lectures, but after only three entries were received for the practical course, the plan was abandoned. The attempt to introduce microbiology was revived in April 1920 when students who had passed the Major exam were encouraged to take an evening course of about 10 lectures and practical work during the summer term on Wednesday and Friday evenings, conducted by Albert E. Parkes. A small class was held for two years, but did not last.

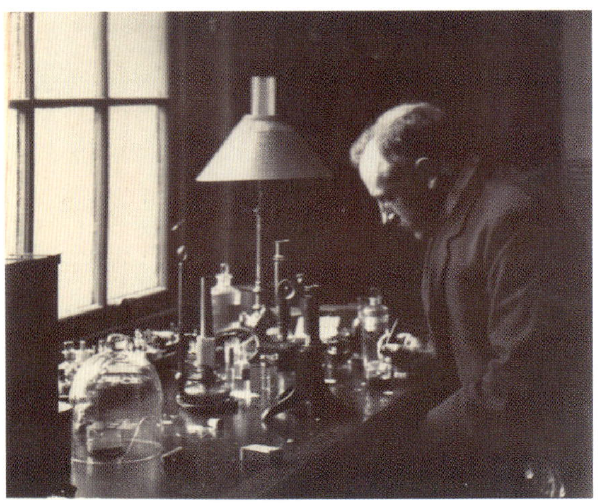

Professor Greenish took over a waiting room for exam candidates in 1895, and kept it as his office until 1927.

Royal Pharmaceutical Society Museum

MATERIA MEDICA AND BOTANY

Materia medica remained a key part of the courses taught at the School throughout this period, and the introduction of microscopical studies gave it a new lease of life from the 1890s. The School was fortunate to continue to have professors with high levels of expertise, and as leaders in the field, teaching and research in the subject remained at the cutting edge of the subject. Holmes in the late nineteenth century and Wallis from the early twentieth century continued to develop what became known as pharmacognosy. Teaching remained joined with botany, with a shared exam.

After taking back control of the School in 1896, the Society's Council persuaded Joseph Ince, lecturer in pharmacy, to retire, aged 70. Greenish was promoted to professor of materia medica and pharmacy, and was informed that he could not take any other roles without the Council's consent. In the same year, the Council gave a general indication of the Minor's materia medica syllabus in *The Pharmaceutical Journal*. Applicants needed to have knowledge of all drugs in the *British Pharmacopoeia*, plus some in an additional list. However, the requirements of the Major exam were still quite vague until 1898, when the question papers were published regularly in the *Journal*. In 1899, an article gave more of an idea of what exactly the Minor students needed to know about all of the drugs in the *British Pharmacopoeia*. It explained that they needed to be able to recognise specimens and commercial varieties, identify their botanical, geographical and commercial sources, and understand the natural orders of plants, and their modes of collection and preparation for market. They also had to be able to identify the morphological features of organised plants with a hand lens, identify unorganised drugs, name the chief constituents of these drugs and understand the qualitative tests used for the *British Pharmacopoeia*. For the Major exam, students needed to know the drugs' chemical constituents, alkaloids, glucosides, resins, fixed and essential oils, and to know the methods of evaluation used for the *British Pharmacopoeia*.

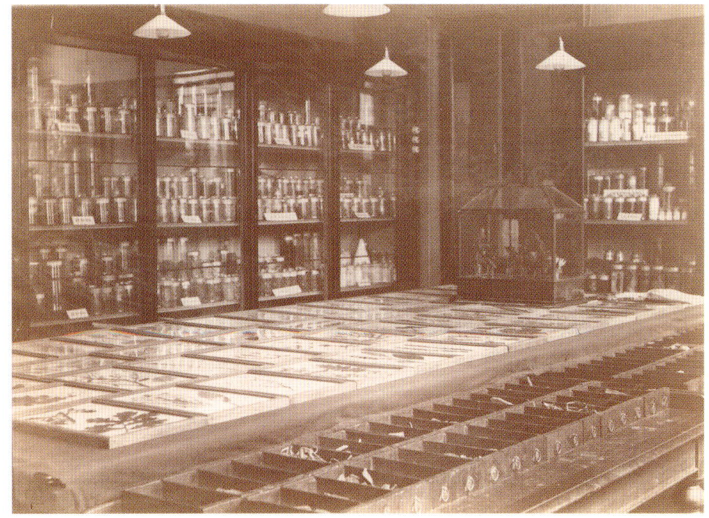

Museum Room 1 was set out with specimens in open drawers and herbarium sheets on the table for students to practise their identification skills.

Royal Pharmaceutical Society Museum

From 1897, a new feature appeared in *The Pharmaceutical Journal*, a students' page. The first article was entitled "What the Microscope Does". Between 1897 and 1900, there were 54 different articles in the *Journal* of all the commonly used crude drugs, meaning that pharmacy students across the country had access to this information. The resulting requests to the museum for study samples led to a decision by the Council to allow Holmes to send specimens to local associations and schools of pharmacy. Students could also supplement their use of the Society's museum or local collections by buying their own student collection. From 1869, Southall, Son and Dymock of Birmingham started producing their student materia medica collections. The entire collection of 138 specimens was sold for 30 shillings initially.

CHARLES HORNE WARNER (1883–1945)

Charles Warner was brought to England by his American parents when he was a baby. After his apprenticeship, he entered the School in 1903 and qualified as a pharmaceutical chemist in 1905. He became a demonstrator in chemistry and gained his BSc in 1908. He was lecturer in botany at the School from 1912 to 1917. Although he enlisted in the First World War, he was recalled to finish his medical training at the Middlesex Hospital and returned to the Royal Army Medical Corps. During the Second World War, he assisted in the organisation of the Air Raid Patrol Casualty Services and was assistant director of Medical Services for Nottinghamshire. He had a large and popular medical practice at Southwell in Nottinghamshire.

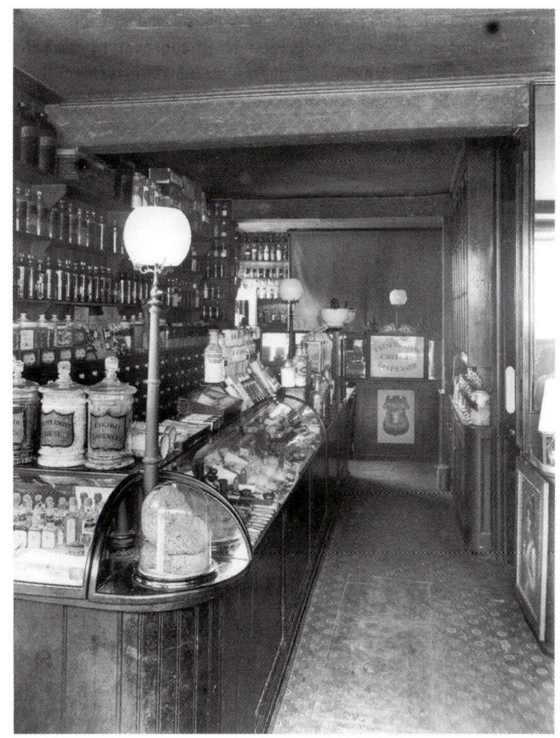

T.E.Wallis became Senior Demonstrator in Chemistry at the School in 1901. At about the same time, he took a series of photographs of his father's pharmacy, J.T.W.Wallis, at 78 Essex Road in Islington, north London. With the packed shelves, decorative lozenge jars on the counter and the sign stating "prescriptions carefully dispensed" at the rear, the shop was a typical small pharmacy of the era.

Royal Pharmaceutical Society Museum

EXAMINATIONS

A catalyst to raise the level of pharmaceutical education emerged in 1896 when the Institute of Chemistry rationalised its exams for its associateship to provide a recognised qualification for prospective public analysts. The Society's Major exam had previously served this purpose. More generally, the standards

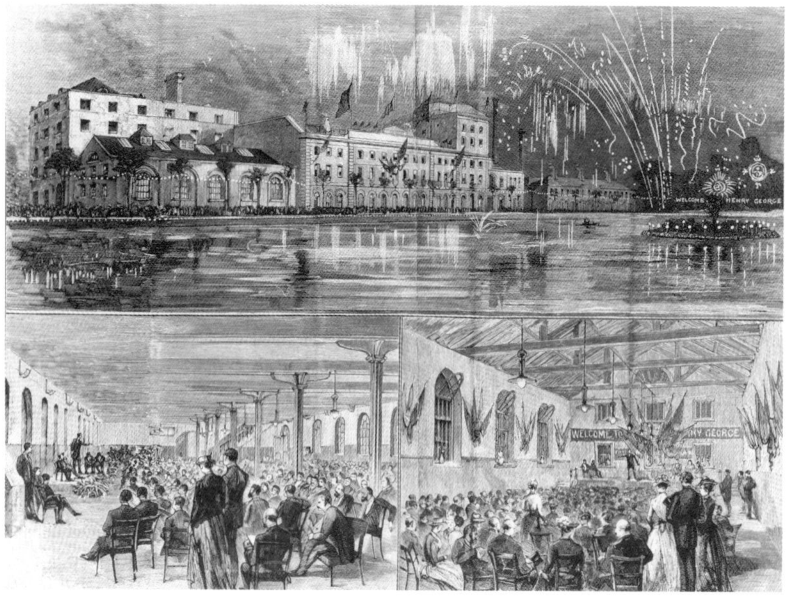

The opening of Burroughs Wellcome and Co's new factory at Dartford in 1889 was marked with a fete and fireworks, as depicted in *The Pictorial World*. The company's use of tabletting machinery, and its pioneering approach to marketing led to great success. In 1894, it established Physiological Research Laboratories followed in 1896 with Chemical Research Laboratories, the first company in Britain to have this level of scientific research and development underpinning its products.

Wellcome Library, London

of scientific education were increasing, with newly created technical schools, the polytechnic movement from 1881 onwards, and within the pharmaceutical industry. In 1896, Henry Wellcome set up a chemical research laboratory as part of his company, a first in Britain. One of the first two directors of Wellcome's laboratory was Dr H.A. Jowett, Dunstan's chief assistant in the Society's research laboratory. Another research assistant at the Society, Dr F.H. Carr, became head of the chemical department at Wellcome in Dartford in 1898.

The syllabus was expanded around 1900 to recognise new developments including experimental pharmacology and bacteriology. Pharmacy's academic reputation was also enhanced by reports from the British Pharmaceutical Conferences, School of Pharmacy research papers, and Recognised Teacher status at the University of London, awarded to the professors in 1901. However, in 1904, a Society conference was held on pharmacy education owing to the continued high failure rate in Minor exams. The conclusions drawn were that the voluntary nature of the courses and the lack of a compulsory syllabus were the main problems.

The Pharmacy Act of 1908 allowed the Society to put some improvements into action. For many years, the Society had been making approaches to Parliament for a Bill to amend the Pharmacy Acts of 1852 and 1868 and specifically to add by-laws to improve pharmaceutical education. Privy Council had already advised that the powers conferred on the Society under the 1868 Act referred to the conduct of the exams and not the means of preparing for it. The Act, when it was finally passed in 1908, included in its Section 4 an extension of the Society's powers to make by-laws relating to the examination and registration of pharmacists. This meant that they no longer had to go to the Privy Council or Parliament to make changes to courses or exam and registration requirements.

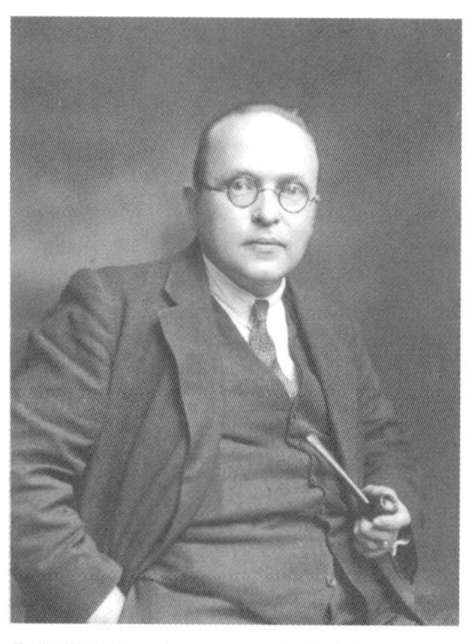

JAMES SMALL (1889–1955)

Royal Pharmaceutical Society Museum

JAMES SMALL (1889–1955)

James Small served his apprenticeship in his native Brechin, Scotland, before taking up his place at the School as Jacob Bell Scholar and Herbarium Medallist in 1910. He passed the Minor exam in 1911 and the Major exam in 1912. In the following year, he became a demonstrator in botany at Armstrong College in Newcastle upon Tyne. He took the London BSc in 1913. He enlisted in the First World War and was wounded twice. He was invalided out of the army in 1916 and took the MSc (London). He was promoted to lecturer in botany in Newcastle in the same year. In the following year he was appointed lecturer in botany at Bedford College for Women in London, and also at the Pharmaceutical Society. He gained his doctorate in 1919. In 1920, he became professor of botany at Queen's University, Belfast, and stayed in the post until his retirement in 1954. Small wrote a number of books including *Textbook of Botany*, *Practical Botany* (1931) and *Pocket-Lens Plant Lore* (1931). His speciality was the study of geological history based on pollens and diatoms. He was one of the university representatives on the Pharmaceutical Society of Northern Ireland's Council from its inception.

A fascinating insight into the experience of taking the Minor exam was provided by Bernard Gill in an article published in *The Pharmaceutical Journal* in 1955. Mr Gill had taken the Minor in April 1913. The fact that he immediately wrote up his experiences and posted them for publication, only to have the envelope charred because the following parcel to be posted in the letter box had been filled with phosphorus by militant suffragettes, serves to put his experiences in their historical context. Of course, Gill served an apprenticeship, and relates that his articles of pupillage included not being able to haunt taverns or playhouses, not to play at cards, dice tables or any other unlawful games, not to contract matrimony, nor to absent himself night or day from the service of his master. In return, his master had to instruct him in the art of a chemist & druggist, and supply meat, drink, clothing, medicine, books and lodging. They were bound for a three-year term. During the first and second years, the weekly wage was two shillings and sixpence, and in the final year it was increased to five shillings. He received 10 days' summer holiday, but worked hard, including 8am to 11pm on a Saturday.

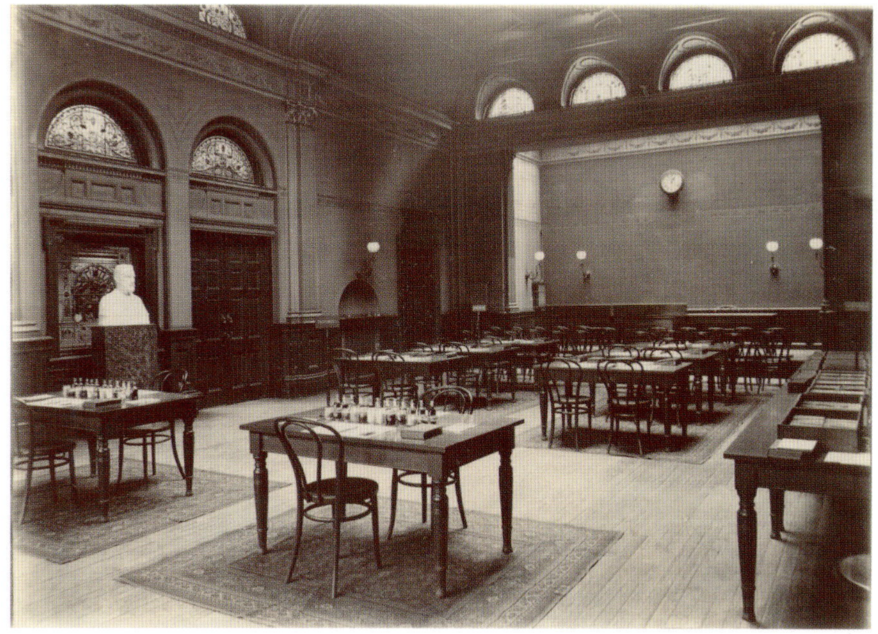

The exam hall, set out for an exam, in 1903. The bust of William Martindale oversaw proceedings from this year onwards.

Royal Pharmaceutical Society Museum

The fee for taking the Minor exam at a first attempt was 10 guineas, plus Gill had to pay for the bed and breakfast that he had booked nearby in Southampton Row. It was his first visit to London, and he went to the theatre on the night before the exam. The following morning, the first task on arriving at the Square was to address an envelope to himself, in which the results would be posted.

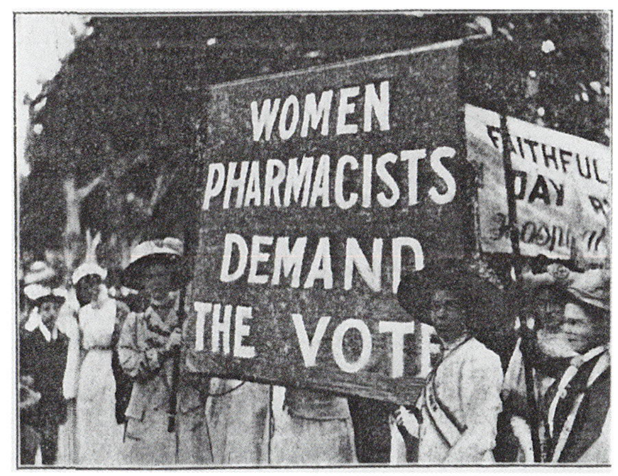

A short illustrated report of a march of over 40,000 women from Victoria Embankment to the Albert Hall was published in *The Chemist and Druggist* on June 24th 1911. The suffragette demonstration included a group of women pharmacists with a banner stating "Women pharmacists demand the vote." One of those involved was Elsie Hooper who had started her pharmacy career as a research student at the School.

Chemist + Druggist

The first exam was dispensing, where he had to make a mixture, pills, suppositories, an inhalation and a draught. There was practical chemistry in the afternoon. He had to undertake a qualitative analysis of a powder (a mixture of cupric oxide and glucose) and examine dilute hydrobromic acid for strength and specific gravity. This was followed by having to write a report of what had been done. The remainder of the curriculum was assessed via an oral exam. Gill remembered that "The ordeal was accompanied by few of the terrors with which imagination had invested it; the examiners were courteous and fair, and showed every consideration." He was first given 20 minutes to translate an English prescription into Latin, plus carry out some simple calculations involving percentages. Then he had to read out badly written prescriptions, translating them into English and pointing out any overdoses. This was followed by questions on the posology of potent drugs. The chemistry and physics section included discussions on atmospheric pressure, constituent gases of the air, and commercial production of oxygen, which Gill described as "a happy tête-à-tête." He also had to talk about the effects of lightning on a manufacturing process, and the "electrolysation" of an aqueous solution of common salt. He was also asked if he knew anything about diazo-salts, and when he said no, the subject was dropped. "A chat on formaldehyde, hydrocyanic acid, and the compounds of benzene with chlorine completed the [chemistry] interview."

Following this, he was given a list of 12 preparations from the *British Pharmacopoeia* and told to write down their strengths. He was then asked how to make various syrups, an extract and wine of ipecachuana, phosphorus pills and menthol plasters, and how to use a thermometer. He was shown various bits of apparatus used to make galenicals and asked to name them and describe their use.

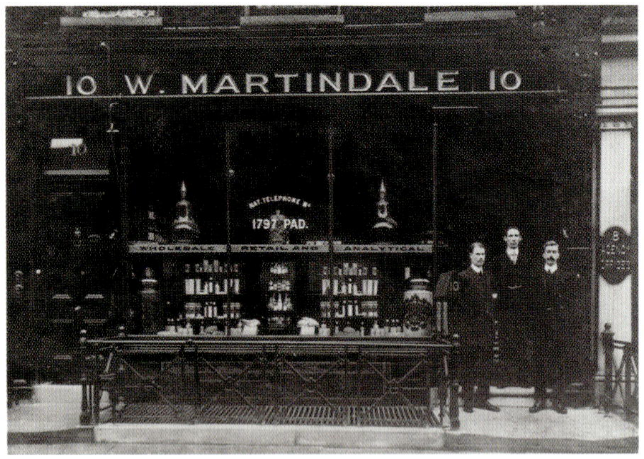

William Martindale's pharmacy, 10 New Cavendish Street, London, in 1913.

Royal Pharmaceutical Society Museum

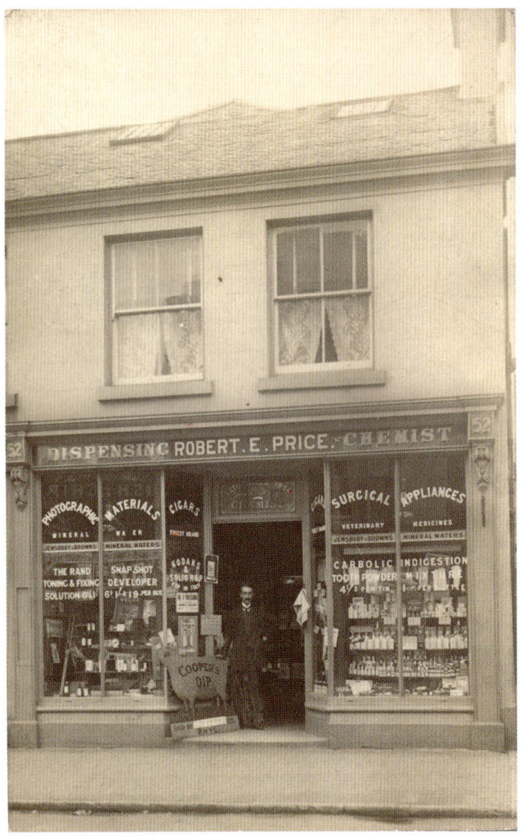

Captured in 1909, Robert E.Price stocked an impressive range of products at his shop on the High Street in Rhyl, North Wales. The sheep-shaped advert for Cooper's Dip at the door complements the advert in the window for veterinary medicines. Price's windows show that he also sold photographic materials, mineral water, surgical appliances, carbolic tooth powder and indigestion mixture.

Royal Pharmaceutical Society Museum

He described the materia medica element as a "comprehensive interrogation on the sources, botanical and geographical, and the constituents of various drugs." In botany, he was required to use a microscope to look at the transverse section of a stem, and then was given an inflorescence of broom-rape to describe and classify. On completion of all sections, the candidates returned to the Hall, and were called up one by one for a short interview with the president, who gave them their result.

After waiting so long for the powers provided under the Pharmacy Act of 1908, it is perhaps surprising that the Society did not have the amendments that it wanted to make, waiting in the wings for immediate implementation, and only published draft proposals in 1911. As Ernest Saville Peck, Society president, recalled in 1935, the situation up to 1910 meant that two candidates for the Minor exam could have markedly different experiences. One might have registered as an apprentice or student by passing the Junior Local exam while at school, followed by three years' apprenticeship, and attendance at a school of pharmacy for three months. The other might have passed the College of Preceptors' exam while doing an apprenticeship and attended night classes whilst working, but otherwise studied on his own. This was not true for the Major exam, which very few candidates entered without a comprehensive training course. A small prewar change was made by the Society in 1913 to the regulations governing registration as an apprentice or a student. As there was a significant decrease in the number of secondary schools where Latin was taught, this was no longer a compulsory part of the Preliminary exam, although candidates were advised to take it if possible.

PROVINCIAL EDUCATION

By 1900, there was a number of public institutions offering pharmacy courses: Mason's College, Birmingham, Owen College, Manchester, Hartley College, Southampton, and University Colleges of Nottingham, Liverpool and Bristol. The Technical Instruction Act of 1889 had encouraged county councils to provide technical and scientific education. By 1899, pharmacy courses were available in 15 new technical schools. For example, the first prospectus of the South West Polytechnic (later Chelsea Polytechnic) in 1895 included courses in pharmacy within the chemistry department. Evening classes were organised soon afterwards in pharmaceutical chemistry, botany and materia medica. The session of 1899–1900 marked the peak in institutions offering pharmacy courses, with 45 available across the country. However, the high failure rate in the Minor exam persisted. The issue seemed to be the variable standard of the courses, as the Society was unable to enforce any kind of compulsory curriculum.

THE FIRST WORLD WAR

The First World War had a significant impact on the School, both as an institution based in central London, and on its student body, past and present. The February 1913 edition of the *Square Chronicle* makes the impending situation clear, describing the current time as "these days of wars and rumours of wars ...", alongside a description of students who had already entered the volunteer regiments, and a separate article about the Territorial Army.

Not least as a London-based institution, the experience of the war would have been life-changing. The first bombs fell on London in 1915, and around 700 people died, mainly as the result of Zeppelin raids during the war. Blackouts and food rationing, normally associated with the Second World War, became a daily annoyance in the First World War.

By the November 1914 edition of the *Chronicle*, the editor found himself "in the middle of a three-month-old war of horrible intensity, involving the greater portion of the world." The publication worked hard to keep track of present and past students who were serving in the forces, but also noted in this edition that someone who had served for four years in the Territorial Army had been refused permission to enlist by his firm, who did not want to recruit to fill his place. The *Chronicle* points out that a qualified woman could have taken his place. The students also approached the University in order to form an officers' training corps at the School, but because most students were only there for a year, and the training was held over two years, they were informed that it was not possible. Some students joined the company at King's College instead. This edition also included a "Roll Call" listing past students who had enlisted, alongside short pieces on "Britain in War Time" with reports from areas as diverse as Clacton-on-Sea, North West London and York.

"We are bound together now, as we never were before, by the common interest of serving our country in her hour of need. Some are on active service across the Channel, others are mobilised for home defence, while the bulk of us are doing the necessary though less romantic work of keeping the business end going, and we all need to be in conscious touch with one another."

John C. Umney, March 1915

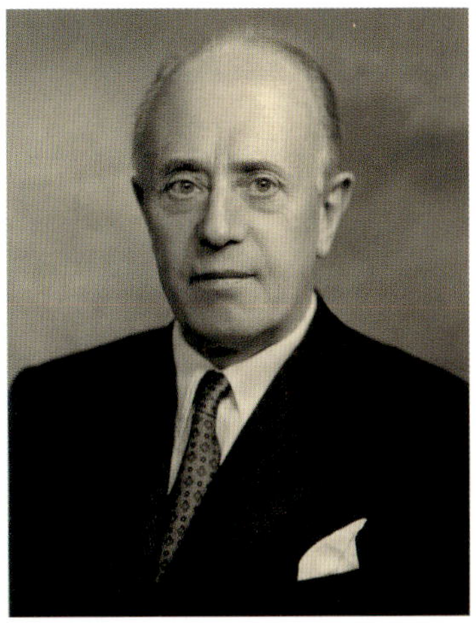

WILFRED HERBERT LINNELL (1894–1983)

UCL School of Pharmacy Library

WILFRED HERBERT LINNELL (1894–1983)

After an apprenticeship in Newcastle upon Tyne, Wilfred Linnell entered the School and qualified as a pharmaceutical chemist in 1916. He then joined the Royal Engineers and was wounded at Passchendaele. He returned home in 1918, and studied chemistry at Durham University. He was awarded the Earl Grey Memorial Fellowship with which he attended Lincoln College, Oxford, where he obtained an MSc and a PhD. He was then employed as a research chemist for HM Fuel Research Station in Greenwich. He was appointed lecturer in pharmaceutical and general chemistry at the School in 1926, and was recognised as a reader in chemistry by the University of London in 1927. In 1925, Linnell played a key role in the division of pharmacy into pharmaceutics and pharmaceutical chemistry at the School. He was later awarded a DSc by London University in recognition of his work in chemotherapy. He became professor of pharmaceutical chemistry in 1944, and dean of the School from 1956 to 1961. He was also a member of the *British Pharmacopoeia* Commission and the *British Pharmaceutical Codex* Revision Committee. He was president of the British Pharmaceutical Conference in 1960.

Linnell was a renowned lecturer at the Square, and was also known for the fact that, because he kept full scripts of his lectures in notebooks, an assistant could deliver them if he were unavailable. He also had his own set of wooden and wire molecular models which he used to illustrate his organic chemistry lectures. One of his students commented: "In a way which I wish I could emulate, Linnell managed to unfold the magic of organic chemistry which gave me a permanent interest in twisting the tail of chemical science for potential therapeutic advantage."

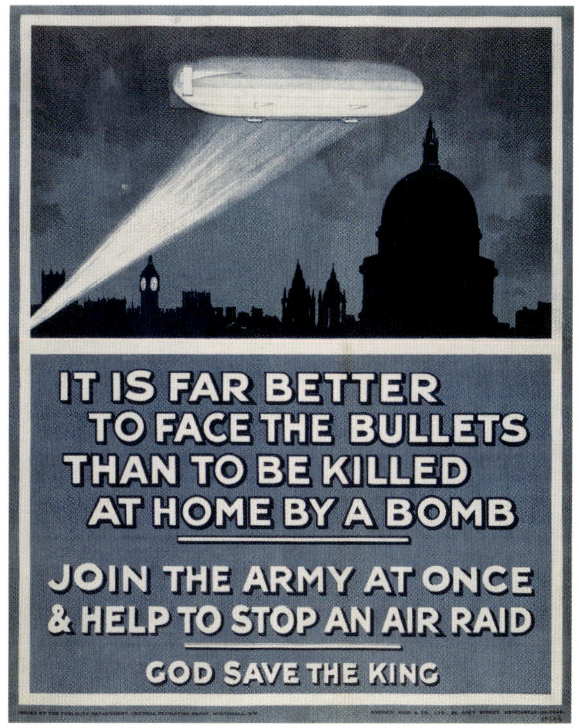
IT IS FAR BETTER
TO FACE THE BULLETS
THAN TO BE KILLED
AT HOME BY A BOMB
JOIN THE ARMY AT ONCE
& HELP TO STOP AN AIR RAID
GOD SAVE THE KING

© *Museum of London*

The Students' Association president, John C. Umney, addressed the student body in the following edition of the *Chronicle*, published in February 1915:

> We are bound together now, as we never were before, by the common interest of serving our country in her hour of need. Some are on active service across the Channel, others are mobilised for home defence, while the bulk of us are doing the necessary though less romantic work of keeping the business end going, and we all need to be in conscious touch with one another.

The Association suspended the football "smoker" and the school dinner, but produced three editions of the magazine in this year, presumably in an attempt to fulfil Umney's aims. The students still kept their sense of humour: "Since our last issue, London has been brought into the war zone by the advent of Zeppelins, and pharmacists have experienced a considerable boom in the sale of respirators, and Anti-Zeptic solutions." However, they also took every opportunity to take practical action, and started a Pharmacists' Volunteer Training Corps in August 1915, based at the Square. Their training focused on first aid, ambulance work and field sanitation, presumably felt to play to their strengths. However, pharmacy was not classified as an essential occupation, and so men had to enlist. The *Chronicle* of November 1915 included a poem entitled "The Unessential Chemist" by W.H. Allen, passing comment on this decision by Harold Tennant, Under-Secretary of State for War, between 1912 and 1916:

> But now I hear that I am unessential
> And Mr Tennant grants me a reprieve;
> He sees in me a khaki-clad potential,
> With stripes and decorations on the sleeve.

The School did, however, continue to operate during the war, although with a smaller number of students. There was also an increase in the number of women students, which marked a milestone in their participation in the School's academic and social life. As a result of the war, the *Chronicle* closed down from 1915 until 1921, and the main social events at the School were dances and dinners, where possible. The first edition of the revived *Chronicle* in February 1921 had the events of the war still firmly at the forefront: "In taking up the task of setting before past and present students this chronicle of events at the 'Square', we cannot help thinking of the gallant gentlemen, cut down in the flower of their manhood, who will never again grace our functions."

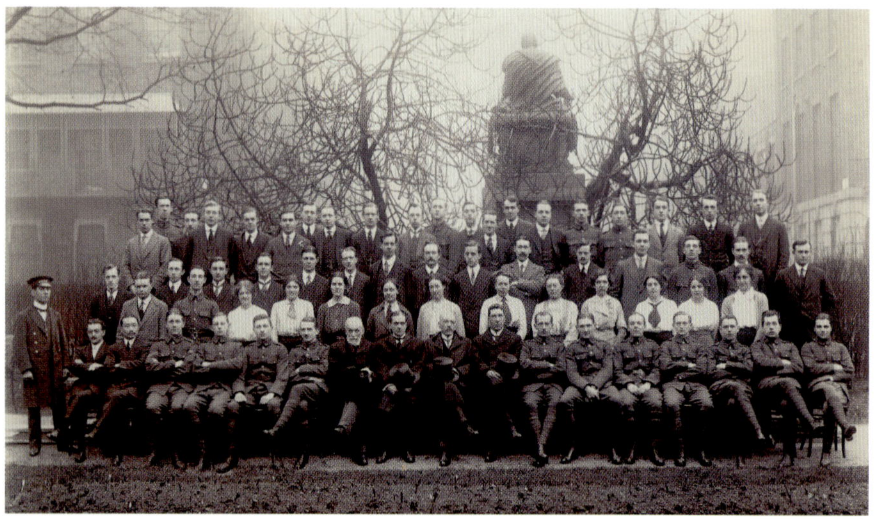

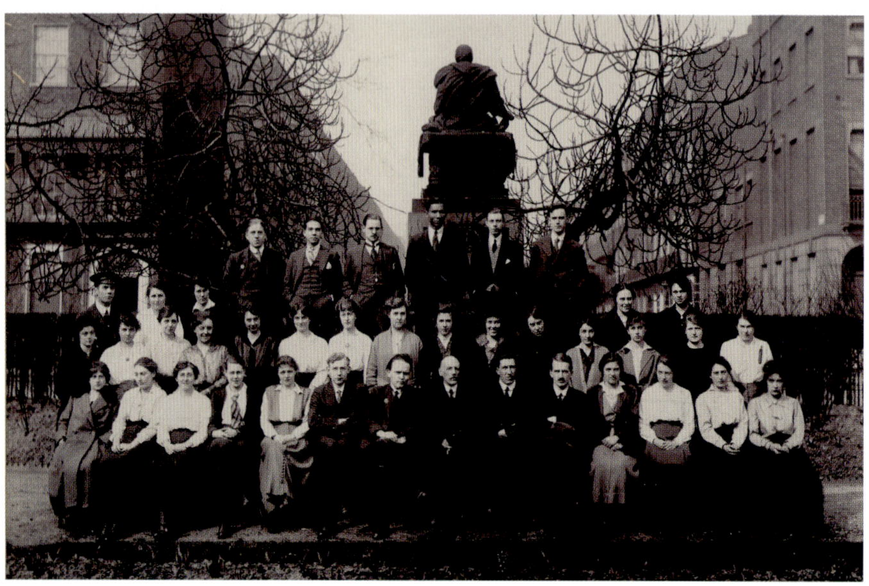

Unsurprisingly, the School's year group photograph for 1914–15 shows a large number of male students in military uniform. By 1917–18, the majority of students were women, although a small number of men in uniform were pictured. As Dean, Professor Greenish was the constant figure at the centre.

UCL School of Pharmacy Library

Across the broader profession, the war had an inevitable impact, not least on the development and supply of medicines. Germany had led much of the drug development work from the end of the nineteenth century. Now at war with a major supplier, Britain closed down subsidiaries of German companies, suspended German trademarks and patents, and ceased to import German products. British companies were prompted by the Government to produce chemicals to fill the gaps, particularly with newly discovered products such as the "magic bullet" arsenical, Salvarsan, which had been discovered by Paul Ehrlich in Germany in 1909. As a key weapon in the battle against syphilis, it was an important drug for both military and civilian use. Burroughs Wellcome and May & Baker were licensed to produce arsenical products during the war. Meanwhile, Boots and other companies started to make aspirin and other synthetic drugs which had previously been imported from Germany. These developments provided an impetus for these British companies to build up their expertise, alongside their facilities. However, the postwar period was one of limited drug development, and so these developments did not have an immediate impact on the British pharmaceutical industry.

"During the last ten years women in pharmacy have proved by their college careers that they have enthusiasm, that they intend to take first place, that nothing less will satisfy them. Unless I am very much mistaken, the same enthusiasm and determination will carry them through in the business world into which this war [the First World War] has given them the entry."

Agnes Borrowman, 10th December 1917

The shortage of pharmacists available to work in the First World War meant, as in other professions, that women were able to increase their representation in the profession. An estimated one million women entered the British workforce between 1914 and 1918, enabling them to gain financial and social independence for the first time. The war also made the female workforce more visible. As a letter to *The Pharmaceutical Journal*, printed on 3rd January 1916, put it:

> To say that only now women are coming to the forefront in usefulness sounds like the sudden awakening of a slumberer to economic consciousness. They have for a long time played in most large pharmacies a great and successful part, and the abnormal demand arising, as it naturally does in war time, does so in the first instance principally because they have been ready and eager and fit to step into the breach …

Although many women returned to their domestic roles at the end of the war, this period did mark an increase in the number of female pharmacists and female pharmacy students that did not disappear entirely.

The impact of the First World War understandably delayed any meaningful developments in pharmacy education, and it was the return of demobilised servicemen at the end of the First World War for the School session of 1919 that enabled the Society to put significant changes into action. In 1918, the principle of a compulsory course of study for the Minor exam was introduced. By 1920, the Minor exam was split into two parts: pure science (chemistry, physics and botany) and an applied pharmaceutical section [materia medica, pharmacy including posology (study of dosages), the translation and dispensing of prescriptions, and poisons laws]. It was possible to take the parts together or separately. Students also had to attend approved courses of instruction in order to enter the exam, and an apprenticeship of 4,000 hours was essential. This could be served either wholly in retail, or half and half in retail and a hospital setting. Council also agreed preliminary scientific syllabuses in chemistry, physics and botany, which had been

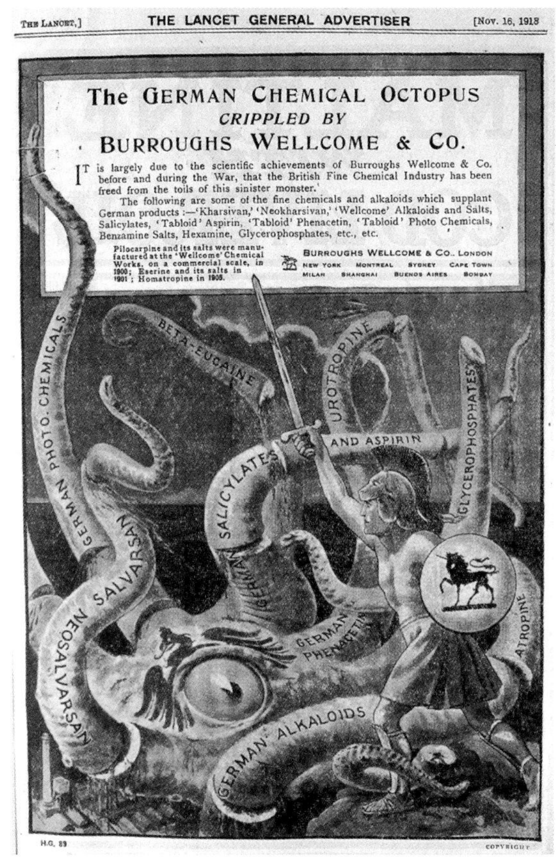

As this advert in *The Lancet* makes clear, Burroughs Wellcome were able to profit from the interrupted supplies of German drugs during the First World War by developing existing and new products to replace them and thus build up their own techniques and expertise.

Wellcome Library, London

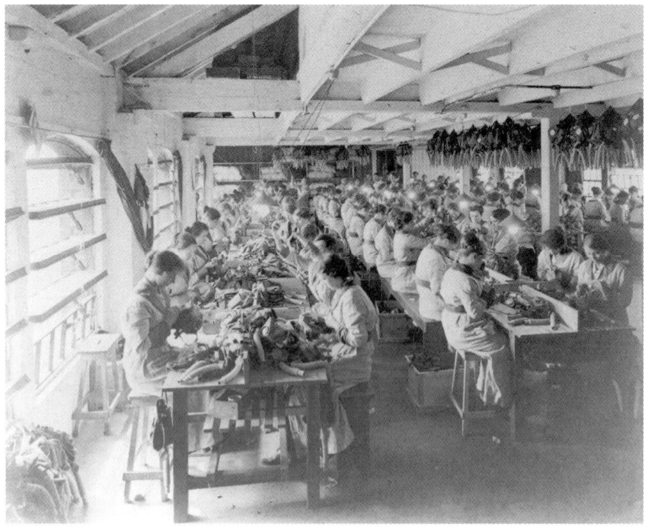

John Bell, Hills & Lucas & Co were a wholesale pharmacy manufacturing company. However, during World War 1, they hired a large workforce of women to produce anti-gas respirators at their works on Tower Bridge Road in London.

Royal Pharmaceutical Society Museum

devised to bring them in line with first year syllabuses in those subjects at university level so that the pharmacy students could be hosted by existing science courses. This tied in with a proposal that Schacht had made way back in 1881, that pharmacy students could take advantage of university courses for medics where the subject matter was common.

The impact of the National Insurance Act of 1911 was also only fully felt after the First World War. Its implementation in July 1912 meant that free medical treatment was supplied to all insured people. This had a significant impact for retail pharmacists who were part of the "panels" that were authorised to provide National Insurance prescriptions. Before 1913, 90% of dispensing took place in doctors' surgeries, and one provincial pharmacy reported dispensing only 43 prescriptions in nine years. Now, pharmacists were a key part of a system that marked the first step towards today's welfare state in Britain. As the Act required that National Insurance dispensing had to be carried out by contracted pharmacists, this allowed the introduction of a compulsory course for qualification officially related to the dispensing of medical prescriptions as well as to the supply of scheduled poisons as an element of the applied pharmaceutical section of the new Minor exam.

After the First World War, the Society also gained the opportunity to approve schools of pharmacy. The number of servicemen who had been accepted by the Central Grants Committee to enter the profession after the war meant that the Ministry of Labour asked the Society in 1919 to arrange for and approve schools to train them. The capacity of the existing schools of pharmacy was about 500 students, but 4,000 ex-service men had applied for State-aided pharmaceutical training. The schools of pharmacy that were approved by the Society in this postwar period were in Aberdeen, Birmingham, Brighton, Cardiff, Dundee, Edinburgh, Exeter, Glasgow, Leicester, Manchester, Newcastle, Nottingham, Portsmouth, Sunderland and Swansea. The formation of these schools made it much easier to insist on a compulsory curriculum. By 1920, there were 25 institutions with approved teaching for the new split Qualifying exam. An unlimited number of schools were allowed to teach Part I of the new exam in order to facilitate these numbers, but the number allowed to teach Part II was restricted to allow a level of control over the purely pharmaceutical elements so that they remained up to date. Schools that were going to train ex-servicemen received a government grant. This official recognition of courses, combined with the compulsory course of study, led to the end of most of the private schools.

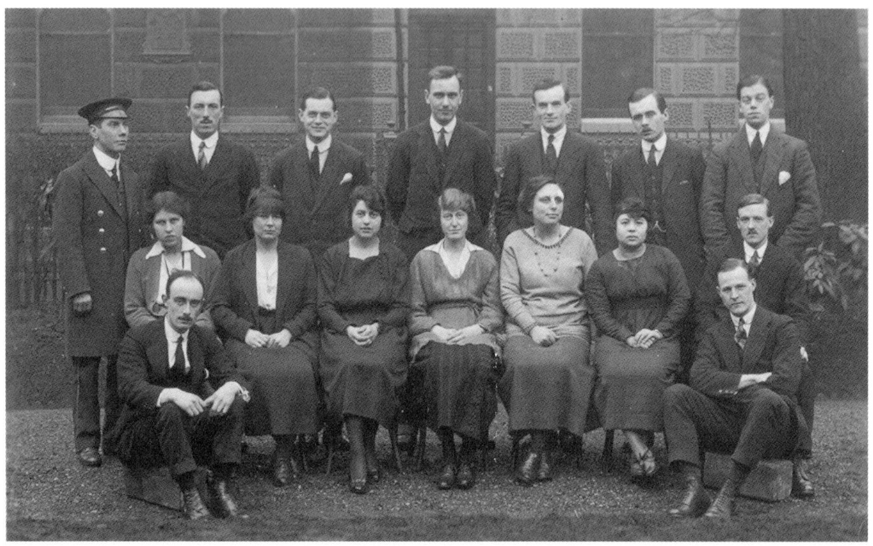

This group studying for the Major exam, taken in March 1920, are nearly evenly male and female students. Romance blossomed in this year: on the photo's reverse it is noted that Miss Saunders at the left end of the front row became Mrs Williams, marrying the student standing directly behind her.

Royal Pharmaceutical Society Museum

The impact on the Square was also felt with the massive increase in the number of students. Demobilised troops so swelled the numbers that some lectures were held during the evening in the early 1920s, and the examination hall was used as the common room so that everyone could fit in. A student during the 1920–1 session remembered: "It was a stimulating atmosphere for study, copying out and enlarging lecture notes, using that famous oval table, with the portraits of former famous people gazing down at you."

UNIVERSITY OF LONDON, AND THE BACHELOR OF PHARMACY DEGREE

The School forged its first formal links with the University of London in 1901 when the three professors were given the status of recognised teachers. This meant that the School was recognised as an educational institution at which students could study prior to sitting the University's Bachelor of Science. However, as Professor William Ramsay, chair of inorganic chemistry at UCL and discoverer of helium, had pointed out in a speech in October 1900, the fact that pharmacy was not available in British universities put it way behind continental Europe.

University of London regulations allowed it to set up a board to supervise studies in pharmacy, but it had not done so. In 1903, the Society's Council resolved to press the Senate to do so. Michael Carteighe led the charge, and explained at a Council meeting in January 1904 that he did not want to make entrance into pharmacy by degree compulsory, but that those who were able to achieve this level should be able to do so and as such immediately qualify for Society membership.

In May 1904, it was reported in *The Pharmaceutical Journal* that the Court of Victoria University in Manchester had adopted an ordinance for a BSc in Pharmaceutics. Although there was suggestion that the Society saw this as a potential degree for their authorisation, its imminent arrival had prompted them to organise a special afternoon meeting on education on 20th January 1904. At this gathering, Carteighe explained that to set up a BSc in Pharmacy, the relevant university needed to set up a pharmacy board. Professor Robert B. Wild from Manchester also spoke at this meeting on "University Education for Pharmacists."

In 1907, the University of Birmingham approached the Society's Education Committee regarding the establishment of a school of pharmacy and the potential to award pharmacy degrees. The Committee responded by saying that it wanted to keep the awarding of pharmaceutical qualifications in the hands of the Society. In the same year, it was reported in the *Journal* that the Privy Council had approved regulations for the institution of a degree of BSc in Pharmacy in Glasgow. Although there was no current funding available to institute the course, the organisers were hopeful that money would be forthcoming in the next 12 months. A letter to the *Journal* published on 30th March 1907 stated that this degree would be the first in the country.

In 1912, Henry George Greenish, professor of pharmaceutics, and A.W. Crossley, professor of chemistry, were appointed professors at the University of London. However, in 1913, a Royal Commission on education commented that no pharmacy students had been students of London University. This was in fact not true as some had gone on from the Square to study there. The issue was that only botany and chemistry were recognised as university degree subjects, not pharmacy, in contrast to the rest of Europe. The Royal Commission recommended that University of London staff and students should have access to the Society's library and museum, but not that the School should be part of the University. The University did have a brand new pharmacology department, opened at UCL's medical complex in 1912, funded by Carnegie.

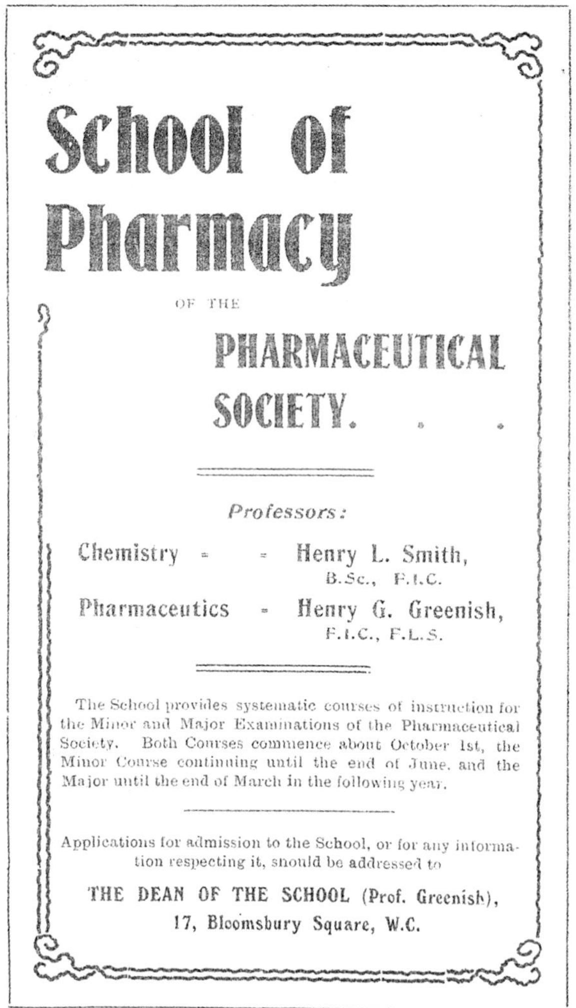

School of Pharmacy

OF THE

PHARMACEUTICAL SOCIETY.

Professors:

Chemistry - - Henry L. Smith, B.Sc., F.I.C.

Pharmaceutics - Henry G. Greenish, F.I.C., F.L.S.

The School provides systematic courses of instruction for the Minor and Major Examinations of the Pharmaceutical Society. Both Courses commence about October 1st, the Minor Course continuing until the end of June, and the Major until the end of March in the following year.

Applications for admission to the School, or for any information respecting it, should be addressed to

THE DEAN OF THE SCHOOL (Prof. Greenish),
17, Bloomsbury Square, W.C.

This advert for the School featured in the ***Pharmaceutical Pocket Book*** **in 1915.**

Royal Pharmaceutical Society Library

In the same year, the School received a grant from the national Board of Education. This had first been raised as an issue in 1911, but it needed the Council to resolve that the institution could not be dissolved in order to gain a grant. The grant continued annually until 1926, when the School became part of the University of London. In 1914, the Board of Education recommended that the Major course be extended to a full academic year so that the School could be registered as a technical college and be eligible for a bigger grant. These changes were made and registered for the 1915–16 year.

In 1919, Margaret Buchanan called for the Society's Library, Museum, School and House Committee to approach the appropriate authorities to establish a degree in pharmacy at the University of London.

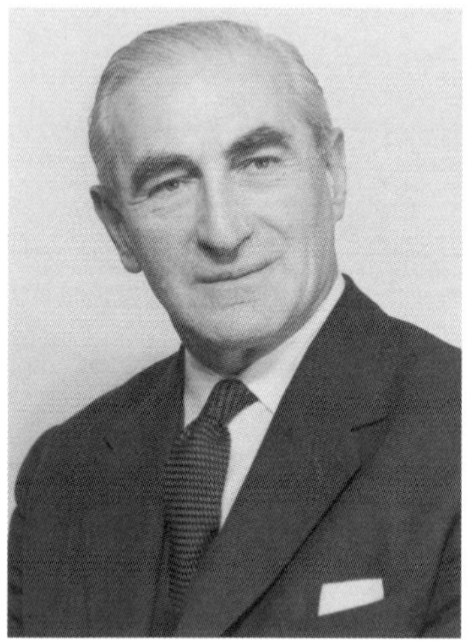

SIR HUGH LINSTEAD (1901–1987)

Royal Pharmaceutical Society Museum

SIR HUGH LINSTEAD (1901–1987)

Hugh Linstead was the son of a pharmacist and entered the Square as a Jacob Bell Scholar in 1921. He registered as a chemist & druggist in 1922 and as a pharmaceutical chemist in 1923. Having spent six months in retail pharmacy, he returned to the School as a demonstrator in pharmacy. However, in January 1924 he was appointed assistant secretary of the Pharmaceutical Society. He became its secretary and registrar in 1926, aged only 26, and continued as secretary until his retirement in 1964. He oversaw the transfer of the School and its partially completed building to the University of London.

He was deeply involved in the negotiations that led to the 1933 Pharmacy Act. He was called to the bar in 1929. In 1942, he became Conservative MP for Putney in London and stayed in Parliament until 1964, holding a number of committee roles, particularly in the areas of health, social and educational affairs. He took an active part in the passing of the Education Act of 1944 and the National Health Service Act of 1946. He was a member of the Poisons Board from 1935 to 1957 and of the Medical Research Council from 1959 to 1964. From 1938 to 1946 he was secretary of the Central Pharmaceutical War Committee. He was made an honorary member of the British Dental Association to recognise his work in chairing a committee set up in 1947 to consider the possibility of merging the three dental bodies into one organisation. In 1952, he chaired a committee to examine the hospital pharmaceutical service, and in 1970, he chaired a committee to consider the NHS pharmaceutical services. He was president of the International Pharmaceutical Federation (FIP) from 1953 to 1966.

Sir Hugh was made OBE in 1937 and was knighted for political and public services in 1953. He also received many foreign honours. After his retirement from the Pharmaceutical Society he became vice-chairman and then chairman of Macarthy Pharmaceuticals Ltd and director of Savory and Moore Ltd. He served as a commissioner with responsibility for training of Scout officers for the Boy Scout movement from 1932 to 1941.

In his presidential address at the British Pharmaceutical Conference in 1922, Professor Greenish explained that a number of advanced students from the Square, having passed the Major, were proceeding through the University of London's Intermediate Examination in Science to the degree of Bachelor of Science. They were able to carry on working in the Society's research laboratories and to proceed to the degree of Doctor of Philosophy. However, they were unable to proceed to become a Doctor of Science until the University of London recognised pharmacognosy as a subject for the BSc, as had already happened in Manchester and Glasgow.

In October 1922, H.J. Waring, vice-chancellor of London University, gave the School's inaugural address. He had been invited to speak on "The value of a university training for the pharmacist", and stated:

> I can assure you, however, if the Pharmaceutical Society brings forward a concrete scheme in which they ask that either pharmaceutical chemistry should be made the chief subject for a science degree or that a new degree such as Bachelor of Pharmacy should be instituted, the University will explore the entire question and try to meet you in every way, provided that whatever is done is for the progress of science, the good of the nation, and the improvement of the vocation of pharmaceutical chemists and pharmacists.

Subsequent negotiations led by Sir William Glyn-Jones meant that a proposal was accepted by the Senate, and a joint committee of the University and the Society's Council was set up.

By 1924, final regulations had been drafted and submitted to the University for approval to set up an internal degree with the possibility of setting up an external degree immediately afterwards. The primary issue from the Society's side was to work out how the course would qualify graduates to be admitted to the Register. As a result, the Society altered the pharmaceutical chemist qualification so that applicants had to study a three-year academic course and a 2,000 hour apprenticeship before or after the university exam. The intermediate BPharm was the Preliminary Scientific exam and the BPharm was the pharmaceutical chemist exam. The Society continued to conduct the forensic pharmacy exam, which had to be passed before the PhC diploma was awarded. As such, the University of London degree was the first to be recognised by the Pharmaceutical Society, followed by the degrees in Manchester, Glasgow and Wales.

It was reported in *The Pharmaceutical Journal* of 18th October 1924 that:

> At a meeting of Convocation held in the Great Hall of the University [of London] on Tuesday, October 14, which was largely attended, the resolution of the Senate for the amendment of Statute 108 by the addition of the words "(9) Bachelor of Pharmacy" to the list of degrees that may be granted by the University, was considered, and the motion that the amendment adopted by the Senate should be approved was carried almost unanimously.

The School was formally recognised to teach the degree course from 1st January 1925, as a school within the University's Faculty of Medicine. The resolution of the Senate on accepting the School into the University was:

> That the Court be informed that the Senate consider that it is of the greatest educational importance that the College of the Pharmaceutical Society should be maintained and extended as a

"The School of Pharmacy of the Pharmaceutical Society is now, as regards pharmacy, a recognised school of the University of London, and for the first time in its history the students of the School are University students."

Professor Greenish, 7th October 1925

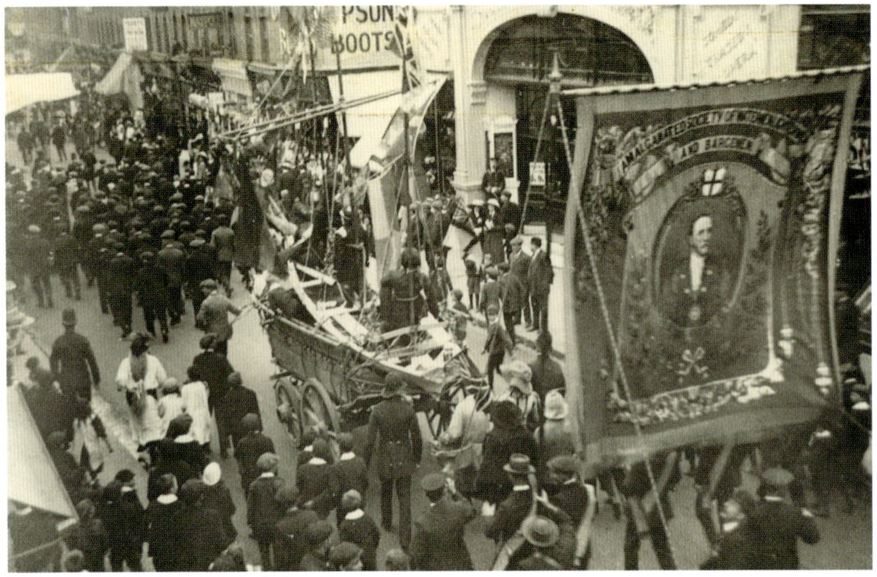

Dockers, watermen and lightermen demonstrated with their union banners on the High Street in Grays, Essex in 1926. The Trades Union Congress had called a General Strike of all industrial workers in support of miners who walked out in May 1926.

© Museum of London

School of the University, both on account of the high value of the work that is being done there and of the necessity, emphasised by the Faculty of Medicine, for highly trained pharmacists, whose training will in future involve a three-year post-Intermediate course for the BPharm Degree.

Students would study pharmacy and pharmacognosy at the School, and chemistry and botany at any recognised school of the university. In his Dean's Report for the opening of the School's 84th session on 7th October 1925, Greenish stated: "The School of Pharmacy of the Pharmaceutical Society is now, as regards pharmacy, a recognised school of the University of London, and for the first time in its history the students of the School are University students."

As Chelsea Polytechnic also had recognised teachers, students could read for the two-year internal BPharm University of London degree at the Square's great rival.

"Future historians may, perhaps, speak of this session as forming part of a transitional period ..."

Square Chronicle, June 1926

POSTWAR EXAMINATIONS

On 2nd December 1924, a Council committee reported on meetings to improve the standard of the Preliminary exam and to ensure the Council's control over the two parts of the Qualifying exam. The committee suggested that the standard of the Preliminary exam should be raised and that the Preliminary Scientific exam should be separated from the Qualifying exam so that the two could not be taken at one sitting. It also proposed separating the Major or pharmaceutical chemist exam from the Minor or chemist & druggist exam. Once a student had obtained the Preliminary Scientific exam, they had to decide whether to do a one-year course to become a chemist & druggist or a two-year course to become a pharmaceutical chemist. They suggested an apprenticeship of 4,000 hours to be completed before the Minor exam, or one of 2,000 hours for the pharmaceutical chemist course, which could be taken before or after the final exam. There was significant opposition to these suggestions from the membership. William Glyn-Jones and the president, F. Pilkington Sargeant, went to meetings to present the rationale behind the changes, and each branch was sent an explanatory memo. The two main objections were the suggested difference in apprenticeship hours between the chemist & druggist and pharmaceutical chemist regulations, and the fact that you would be able to become a pharmaceutical chemist without first being a chemist & druggist. But the new regulations were passed by a Special General Meeting and the Privy Council then gave its approval.

The new regulations came into force in August 1925. They resulted in Part I of the Qualifying exam becoming the Preliminary Scientific exam and including practical exams in physics and botany. Part II became the chemist & druggist Qualifying exam. The Major exam became the pharmaceutical chemist Qualifying exam. Apprenticeships had to be served under articles of pupillage. Students were not allowed to enter for Preliminary and chemist & druggist exams at the same time. The pharmaceutical chemist exam also had a compulsory course of study. A student could enter for this exam without passing the chemist & druggist exam if they had attended an approved course over two years after passing the Preliminary exam. The other major change for candidates was that written exams were instituted in all subjects, and practical exams were required in all subjects apart from forensic pharmacy. Oral exams were discontinued in everything apart from the pharmacy paper for the chemist & druggist Qualifying exam.

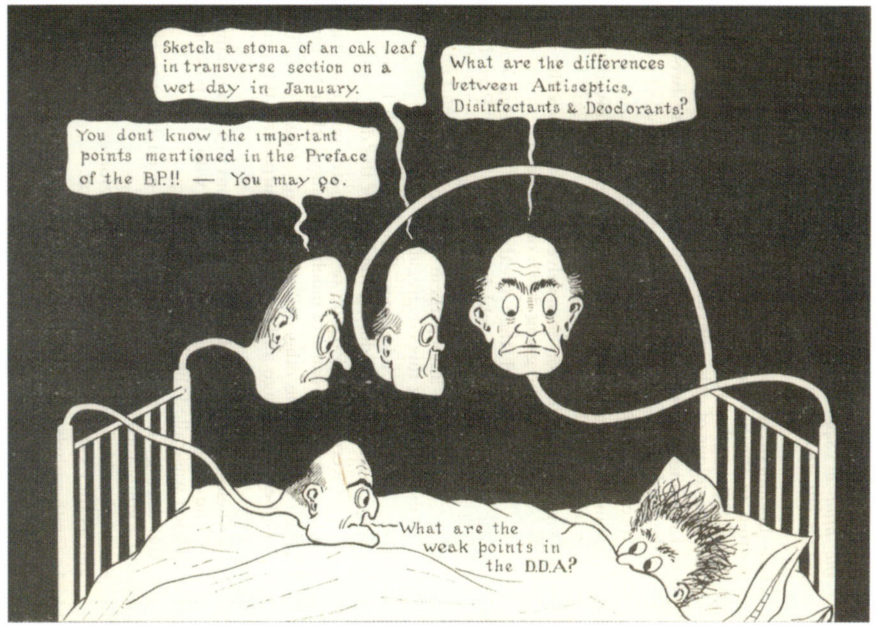
You dont know the important points mentioned in the Preface of the B.P.!! — You may go.
Sketch a stoma of an oak leaf in transverse section on a wet day in January.
What are the differences between Antiseptics, Disinfectants & Deodorants?
What are the weak points in the D.D.A?

The School's lecturers loom over this poor student suffering from examination panic, published in the *Square Chronicle* in January 1925.

UCL School of Pharmacy Library

The impact on the Square was primarily due to the decision not to teach any courses for the preparation of the Preliminary Scientific exam. Students at the Square had to have already achieved this and would start courses for the chemist & druggist Qualifying exam, the Major/pharmaceutical chemist Qualifying exam or the BPharm degree. This meant a decline in the number of students at the School and an associated decline in income for the Society. In the *Square Chronicle* in 1925, it was pointed out that this also meant less income for the Students' Association.

The other major change for the Society was that it needed to be able to inspect the schools teaching the external BPharm (Lond) degree and the PhC course. For the first time, a body of inspectors was set up for this purpose, jointly between the University of London and the Society's Council.

The course content was also updated. When the BPharm degree course was introduced, general chemistry teaching was transferred to University College. However, in order to keep a lecturer of chemistry post at the School, parts of the old pharmacognosy syllabus (chemistry of constituents, chemical tests for unorganised drugs and chemical assays of crude drugs) were moved into a new pharmaceutical chemistry course which was taught from 1925 onwards. The course also included the study of chemical processes underlying the preparation of chemicals used in medicines (inorganic and synthetic organic substances), and the study of fixed and volatile oils, fats and waxes. However, Corfield left to become an analytical and consulting chemist in 1925, and the new chemistry post was taken by Dr W.H. Linnell from October 1926.

As for botany and pharmacognosy, Holmes had retired in November 1922, having had an accident in 1921, which had kept him away from the museum and resulted in the use of a prosthetic leg. Professor Greenish took over and reorganised the museum on a morphological scheme, with specimens grouped as to whether they were leaves, flowers, barks and so on. Holders of the Ransom scholarship, first awarded in 1917 as a two-year research award in the Society's laboratories, were then given duties and the title of part-time curator. C.W. Maplethorpe was the first in 1922, then G.R.A. Short in 1924.

The introduction of the BPharm degree course in 1924 transferred botany teaching to University College, and kept pharmacognosy at the Square. Transferring botany to UCL meant that T.E. Wallis, who had returned to the Square as lecturer in botany in 1919, could concentrate purely on materia medica. The pharmacognosy content in the BPharm was almost exclusively botanical, primarily macroscopical and microscopical description, which was a backward step and not up to date with the research going on at the School. Although there had been much debate about the subject, it was not until 1924 and the BPharm that the term "pharmacognosy" was used for the course. Wallis, as the main pharmacognosy lecturer in this period, published a series for students on "practical pharmacognosy" in the *Journal* from 1922 until 1925.

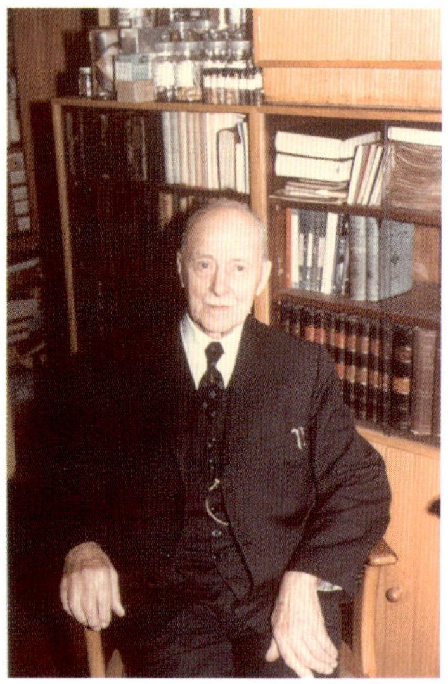

THOMAS EDWARD WALLIS (1876–1973)

Royal Pharmaceutical Society Museum

THOMAS EDWARD WALLIS (1876–1973)

T.E. Wallis served his apprenticeship with his father before studying at the Square from 1895. He passed the Minor exam and was awarded bronze medals in botany, chemistry and materia medica in 1898. He became a pharmaceutical chemist in the following year and a junior demonstrator in chemistry. In 1900, he passed the final BSc (London) exam, and was appointed demonstrator in pharmacy and materia medica at the School. He became senior demonstrator in chemistry, and lecturer in physical chemistry and physics in 1901. After a period away from the Square teaching science in Tunbridge Wells, and assisting another Square alumnus, Thomas Tickle, as a public analyst in Exeter, he returned to the School as lecturer in botany in 1919. He was appointed reader in pharmacognosy in 1926 and curator of the Society's museum in 1927. He was the author of three standard textbooks used internationally: the *Textbook of Pharmacognosy* (1946), *Practical Pharmacognosy* (1925) and *Analytical Microscopy* (1923). He received the Hanbury memorial medal in 1939, and gained a Doctorate from the University of London in 1943. His expertise in pharmacognosy was inextricably tied to his leading role in the use of microscopy in the field, and his publication record reflected both areas of research. He worked on every edition of the *British Pharmaceutical Codex* from 1933 until 1971. He also contributed to the pharmacognosy content of the *British Pharmacopoeia*, and was an examiner for the PSGB, the Pharmaceutical Society of Northern Ireland (PSNI), the University of London, the University of Wales and Queen's University, Belfast.

Dr Wallis was president of the Square Association in 1935 and 1936, and chairman of the British Pharmaceutical Conference in 1942 and 1943. He was appointed emeritus curator to the Pharmaceutical Society on his retirement in 1946, and was appointed as the first ordinary Fellow of the School of Pharmacy, University of London in 1957. He wrote *History of the School of Pharmacy, University of London*, published in 1964. On his retirement, one of his past research students wrote that he was "at once a specialist, and yet catholic in his knowledge and experience of the Sciences generally ... No man in modern times has brought a more mature experience to the advancement of pharmaceutical knowledge. His influence upon the development of Pharmacognosy will be felt long after all who know or knew him have passed into the night. His love of accuracy and hatred of pretence ensure for his own work and that of his students an enduring place in the advancement of Pharmaceutical Science."

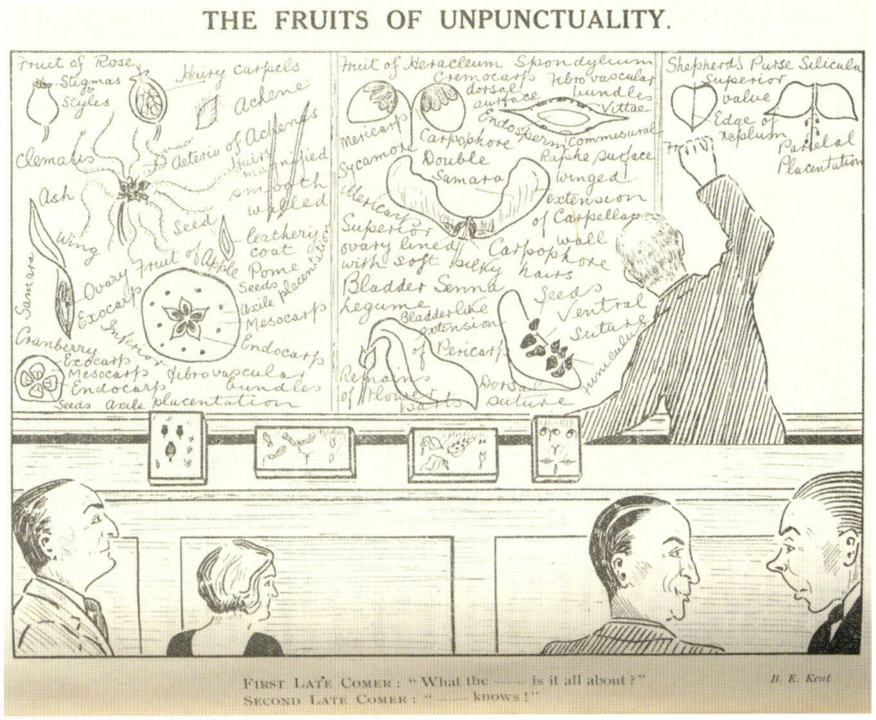
THE FRUITS OF UNPUNCTUALITY.
First Late Comer: "What the —— is it all about?"
Second Late Comer: "—— knows!"
B. E. Kent

This cartoon from the *Square Chronicle* of January 1925 suggested that missing the start of Wallis's botany lectures was unwise.

UCL School of Pharmacy Library

On 7th August 1925, the Therapeutic Substances Act was passed. By the 1920s there existed a number of substances for medicinal use that were neither poisons nor dangerous drugs, which were both covered by existing legislation. The Therapeutic Substances Act regulated by licence the manufacture, but not the sale, of a limited number of products, the purity or potency of which could not be adequately controlled by chemical means. Such products included vaccines, sera, toxins, antigens and insulin. However, although from 1925 biology was one of the subjects which could be offered up by a prospective student wanting to register with the Society, it did not feature in the syllabuses other than for the pharmaceutical chemist, which mentioned an "elementary knowledge of vaccines and sera." The students were well aware that their curriculum was not keeping pace with developments in the wider world. As early as November 1913, an article by a C.T. Allen had appeared in the *Square Chronicle*, attempting to persuade his peers to take the Major exam rather than stopping at the Minor, but with the recognition that to encourage people, the syllabus needed to be modernised to include subjects such as bacteriology and the preparation of vaccines. At the School dinner that year, Mr E.T. Neathercoat, later to become Pharmaceutical Society of Great Britain (PSGB) president, proposed a toast to the School of Pharmacy and mentioned the possible inclusion of optional Major subjects including botany, optics, bacteriology and photography in the near future. By 1925, the *Chronicle*'s editor had no doubt that the staff should go ahead with plans for a menagerie in order to provide animals for physiological research, and that changes were needed to the materia medica course to cover more modern therapeutic agents.

The School had also attempted to keep its students up to date with other developments. Radium, discovered by the Curies in 1898, was first isolated in its metallic state in 1910. By 1921, according to the *Square Chronicle*, it was "now so much discussed in the papers." The students were given a lecture on the topic on 9th March 1921, by Mr F. Browne. Described as "rather deep", the report claimed that the lecturer did well to explain its effects and its discovery, and got cheers at the end.

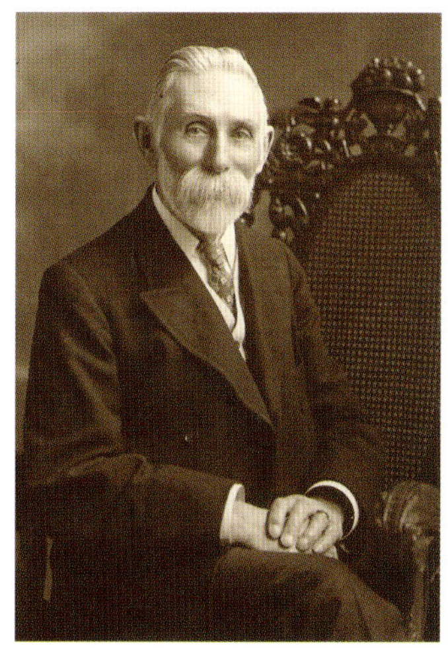

Gilbert E.Jones was Chief Cashier for the Pharmaceutical Society for 52 years. This photo was taken on his retirement in 1921.

Royal Pharmaceutical Society Museum

“The qualification, so far as the public is concerned, is regarded as the hallmark of skill and qualification to carry on the whole business.”

William Glyn-Jones, 1924

THE STUDENT EXPERIENCE

An article in *The Pharmaceutical Journal* in 1896 was realistic about the students' use of the School. It gave a detailed overview of the facilities, presumably prompted by the fact that it was back under full Society control, and so was unsurprisingly glowing about the laboratories, equipment and staff. It described the lecture theatre in promotional terms:

> here have sat several generations of British pharmacists, to listen to and criticise their leaders as the latter expounded the policy of the Council for the time being, or again to drink in scientific and technical knowledge as it has been skilfully dispensed in a fit state for ready assimilation by experts in pharmacy and the kindred sciences and arts.

Student use of the museum was summed up:

> The department specially arranged for the use of budding pharmacists serves its purpose well, when once those who resort to it realise that knowledge of the macroscopic appearance of drugs cannot be gained by walking round the room, gazing for a few moments at some of the specimens in the cases, and then moving on again, repeating the process at irregular intervals, and continuing such peregrinations during the half-hour or more available for the purpose. Other objectionable methods of study (?) that have been observed are to sit down daily week after week, before the drawers of specimens upon the table and casually glance at the contents to see if they can be recognised, or to use knife and lens in a desultory fashion just before an examination, after calmly ignoring the existence of the museum as a place of study for months past.

The library was also described, and the reality seems to have been that it was used in the later decades of the nineteenth century as a common room of sorts, with students coaching each other on various areas of study. Even the area used for the Hanbury collection of historical books “is invaded at times, despite the efforts of the patient and long-suffering librarian to preserve its holy calm.”

“Students are more luxurious in their habits now, and apparently require more rest.”

Joseph Ince, 1903

E.M. Holmes, curator of the museum, was equally realistic about the students' use of its collection. He wrote an article of guidance for the museum in the *Journal* in September 1899. One of the features he pointed out was that prunes, almonds, figs, liquorice, manna and other edible specimens are not in the open drawers like the majority of the items because they “are apt to disappear, and with which students are evidently too familiar to need to examine.” Presumably certain students were dropping in for a snack. G.E. Trease reminisced in the *Journal* in 1982 about the museum whilst he was a student at the Square in 1924. The collection included cannabis, coca leaves and opium, all available to be handled. The only supervision on many occasions was the elderly hall porter who glanced through the door. However, the only security incident that Trease recalled was on a Saturday morning when students from a South London college of pharmacy held the porter, while others transferred the bust of Jacob Bell into a taxi. The marauders were stopped before Bell was taken away.

> **" the fame of many past students is not confined to the British Isles, but has travelled to all parts of the civilised world. "**
>
> *The Pharmaceutical Journal*, 1906

In October 1912, the School of Pharmacy Past Students' Association was formed with Professor Greenish as its first president. Its publication, the *Square Chronicle*, started in November 1912, subtitled "Being the Official Organ of the School of Pharmacy Past Students' Association". The first editor began in a humble tone: "We ask for a friendly reception for this little journal, which, though of modest dimensions, may by the co-operation of our readers grow with each number in size and quality, and form an interesting history of the school ..." On the first secretary's page, it was stated that the subscription for the association was half a crown, and its aim was to communicate with past students, not to debate politics or science. During the first six months of the new Association's existence, nearly 500 past students had been approached, and over 160 had joined. The aim was very much to bring present and past students together both in print and in person:

> Every prominence will be given to school news, and we feel sure that when the present students realise that the past students, many of whom figure in the honours lists on the walls of the lecture theatre, are now following their careers with interest, rejoicing in their successes, whether scholastic, social, or athletic; it cannot but be for the good both of the students, and the grand old school which we all love and honour.

By the second edition in February 1913, nearly all of the 300 copies of the first edition had been distributed. The key social event on the horizon was the School dinner, to be held on 26th February in the Gordon Room of Holborn Restaurant. This was not a new development, but the presence of past and present female students for the first time, including Margaret Buchanan, Nora Renouf and Elsie Wardle, was seen as a significant milestone: "and once the ice is broken, we trust that this innovation will become a regular feature."

By February 1914, the Past Students' Association had amalgamated with the School's Students' Association with a joint executive.

Although still not a significant number, a small number of students came from overseas to spend time at the Square. In the June 1915 edition of the *Chronicle*, there is an article on China by Shung-Lai Chang, a Chinese student, who was shortly leaving the Square to return to China. It would be fascinating to know his thoughts on his experiences. The first international student to gain a PhD was Jamaican Professor Herbert C. Kassner (1899–1934), who did so in 1924. He went on to work at the Albany College of Pharmacy, Union University, and the New York College of Pharmacy in the United States.

Rambles

Some of the most memorable activities in this period were the botanical rambles organised from around 1900 by the Students' Association and encouraged and supported by Professor Greenish and Mr Wallis. A "former Square Man" remembered earlier Saturday trips in 1880 to "happy hunting grounds" including

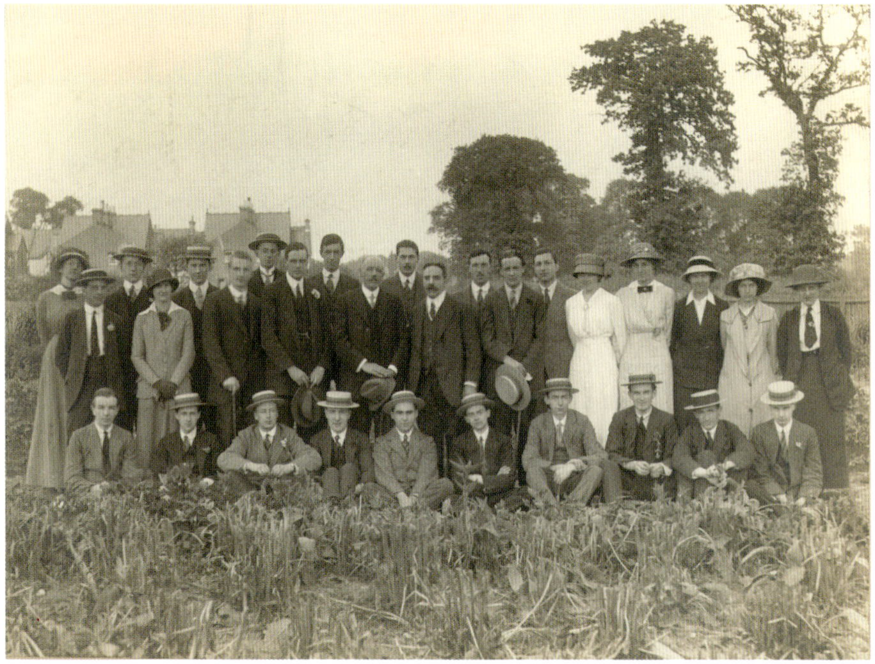

Professor Greenish is shown in the centre of the group of students on a ramble in 1913. He usually accompanied the group on their Saturday outings.

UCL School of Pharmacy Library

Hampstead Heath, Willesden, Acton, Penge and Highgate. By the time he was writing in 1895, other destinations were "now covered with bricks and mortar, or protected by the County Council." He recalled a particular incident of a student trying to obtain "treasures" from a bog on Hampstead Heath "to secure a prize in this quagmire, which to all appearance was as firm as a bowling green, a rash student once made a rush to anticipate his comrades, and was speedily engulfed to the waist." They had to take him to the nearby hostelry, Jack Straw's Castle, where he had bucketfuls of water poured over him by the ostler.

From around 1900 until 1927, the rambles were combined with instruction in botany, followed by a high tea, and were held on Saturday afternoons in May and June. There are many happy reports of these outings in the *Chronicle*, and in reminiscences from past students. The outings usually took advantage of the developing public transport system to explore rural areas outside London. The idea was to combine a social event with an opportunity for the students to familiarise themselves with the 40 or so plants that they were supposed to be able to recognise for their exam. From 1920 onwards, the professors issued notes to support their teaching. For example, in June 1915, Professor Greenish and Mr (later Dr) Wallis took a group on the train from Charing Cross to walk at Hayes Common in Kent. Wallis's report in the *Chronicle* named some of the species they had found and discussed the nature of the soil. The group returned to Keston village for tea, and came back on the bus to Liverpool Street. In 1922, Wallis supported the students to form a natural history club. The inaugural meeting was a trip to Totteridge Lane by train, where they walked around Mill Hill. The report concludes: "the party afterwards entrained for St Pancras."

Nevertheless, the taught botany course remained a recurrent target for students' attention. As pharmacy practice started to move away from a reliance on drugs of a botanical origin, the course seemed irrelevant and out of date. A detailed article appeared in the *Chronicle* of June 1913 entitled "How to Brighten Botany", by W.H. Allen. He complained that the subject had been spoilt by the pedantry of the professors and the insistence on Latin terms, and proposed new terms should be introduced such as "spuddate", meaning shaped like a potato. Botany was also unexciting: "Botany lacks the explosiveness of chemistry and its entrancing uncertainty. The chemical student mixes things in a test tube, applies heat, and hey presto, he is on his back with his eye-brows and other face trimmings burnt off."

Allen makes the more serious point that the textbooks are dated, not using the latest technology such as photography and colour printing. More jokingly, he remarks that "Text-books on Botany are silent too on many points of practical interest, for instance it would be vastly entertaining to know what happens, other than the green-keeper's bad language, when Suffragettes pour vitriol on gold greens." He also suggested that the garden in the middle of Bloomsbury Square could be used by students to create a rock garden, and to grow vegetables. "Yankee tourists from Southampton Row would hang over the railing saying: 'Gee whizz, ain't it Bully?'"

Perhaps the students were actually looking for a different kind of excitement. In the first edition of the *Chronicle* in 1912, under the heading "Common Room Notes", it is reported that "It is rumoured that Botany lectures are no longer what they were. Gone are the days when sponges and calabar beans used to hurtle across the theatre ..."

Sport

By 1912, the football report by W.R. Pratt in the first edition of the *Square Chronicle* reveals that the School had their own ground in Shepherds Bush, the Home Ground, No. 1 Pitch, Wormholt Farm. In fact, this was next to the Queen's Park Rangers' ground on Loftus Road. Wormholt Park itself opened as a public park in 1911, having previously been farmland. The White City Lido opened nearby in 1923, completing a set of public amenities. However, the ground was almost six miles from Bloomsbury Square. The team at this stage was playing mainly other pharmacy schools including the London College, South of England College and Westminster College, but also "Casino FC" and "Lloyds United Sports Club". It seems that they took full advantage of any opportunity for practice. According to a student's account of his first day at the Square, also published in the first edition of the *Chronicle*, he arrived three days after term began, and entered the common room: "Inside a football match was in full swing; but someone scored a goal by demolishing an electric light globe, the game ended one to nil, but one and six to pay." At another point in the same magazine, there is a suggestion that staff had become wise to the sporting activity going on: "It is said that the new position of the table in 'our room,' has been long premeditated. It considerably limits the area formerly used by the football team for practice matches." A further comment suggests that the common room saw a lot more sporting activity than intellectual development: "Newspapers and periodicals adorned the tables, chairs, mantelpiece, and floor, I actually saw someone reading one."

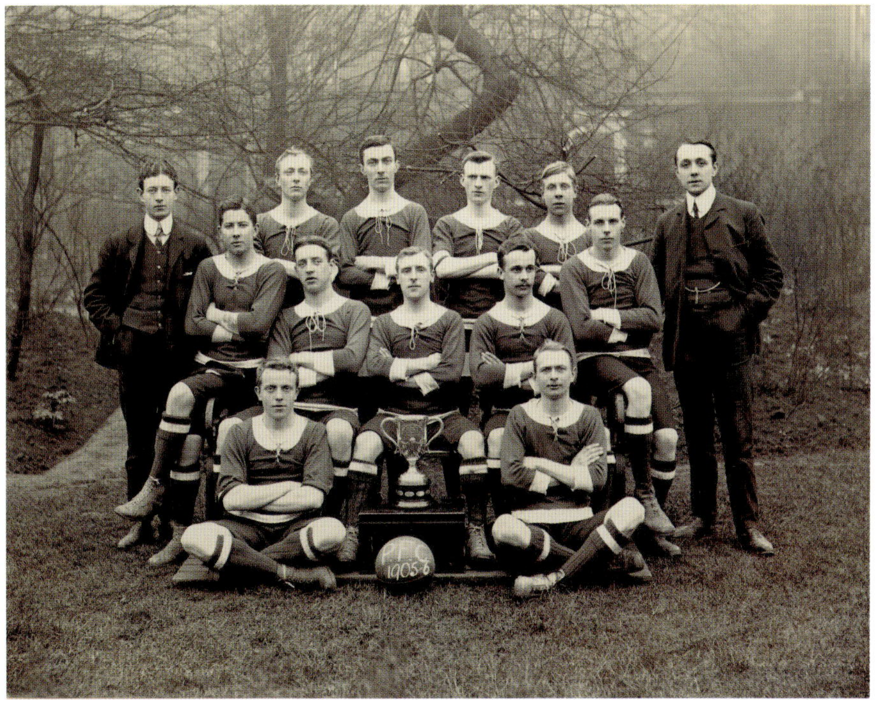

In 1905–6, the School's football team were winners of the Inter-Pharmacy League Cup, under captain, J.T.Bellamy.

UCL School of Pharmacy Library

However, the sporting facilities available at other institutions also seemed to be of dubious quality. A report of a football match played on 23rd November 1912, against Westminster College, stated: "the Square played down the hill against the wind" in the first half. At least we can assume that they were playing uphill with the wind in the second half! Clearly football was very popular, and well supported by the other students. In February 1914, the football report in the *Chronicle* stated that "it is comforting to be able to take three 'bus loads of leather-lunged adherents to cheer the Square to victory."

An annual old boys' football match was started around this time, with current students against a team of past alumni. The first game was played on 8th March 1913, with the plan to follow with an inexpensive dinner somewhere in the West End.

There is no mention of a long-lasting cricket club in the historical record until July 1924. However, it seems to have been a popular pursuit. In the *Chronicle* in November 1913, a report of a botanical excursion to

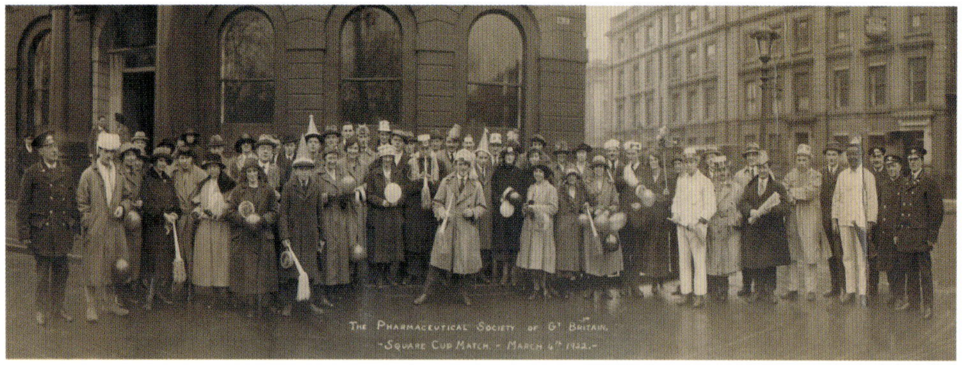

On March 4th 1922, this group were ready to enjoy the Square cup match between past and present students.

UCL School of Pharmacy Library

Caterham includes details that the students had persuaded the dean that they needed money to buy a cricket bat and ball to take with them, and he had obliged. The report states that they did not see many plants, but they played cricket with a ladies' team against a gentlemen's team, who handicapped themselves by playing left handed and allowing the ladies a "lackey" to run for them.

By 1914, students were also playing tennis on three pitches made available to them in Edgware. That same year marked the choice of official colours for sports teams, to be worn as a tie for men or a hat band for women. The choice of red, blue and gold, taken from the Society's coat of arms, was described in the *Chronicle* as "rather too sensational for everyday wear." By 1922, it was also possible to buy a School blazer in red, blue and gold stripes for sports occasions.

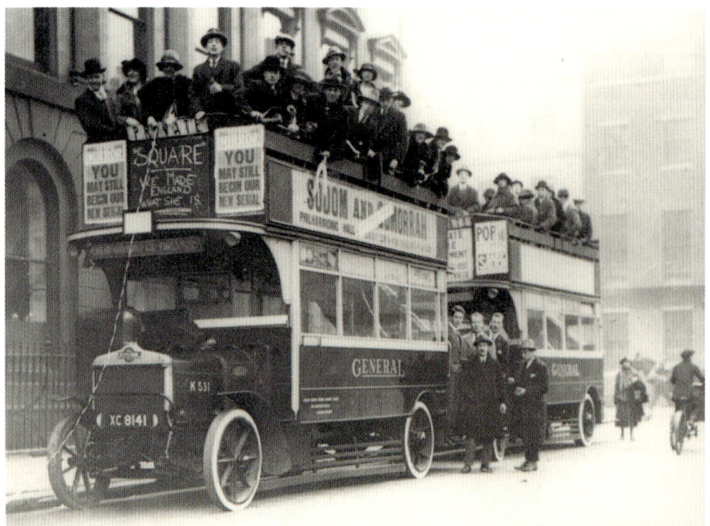

The supporters' bus was decorated for the annual Square cup match in 1924.

UCL School of Pharmacy Library

By the years just before the First World War, the Square also had a second eleven, and a hockey club with a ladies', men's and mixed team. It was reported in the *Chronicle* that the hockey club became more popular as the number of female students grew. But there were still issues with the pitch. The *Chronicle* complained that the groundsman:

> appeared to think that the excitement of the game was added to if the ground were only marked out once in four weeks, and who, in spite of many tactful financial hints to the contrary, clung desperately to a firm belief that an inch of dead leaves all over a hockey ground was a great improvement and added to the zest of the game.

By December 1922, the editor of the *Chronicle* reflected the students' desperation: "*Wanted.* – A scheme to persuade the Society of the School's need for playing fields of its own – and the necessary action, please!"

In 1923, the pharmaceutical company Maws came to the rescue for tennis and cricket with the offer of the use of two tennis courts and the cricket nets at their company facilities at Monken Hadley Estate in New Barnet. A past student recalled that, in the 1920s, the School used to hire a double-decker bus to take them to football matches on Saturday afternoons in the winter, "with rattles and vocal stimulation proceed via Oxford Street and Edgware Road to more playing fields at Barnet." In 1924, the Golders Green branch of what became the Northern Line was extended to Edgware. The *Chronicle* in January 1925 expressed a hope that this tube extension would improve access to the playing fields that they were using there.

Of course, there were other sporting pursuits available outside the school teams. A very excited poem in the *Chronicle* of June 1925 advocated the mixed bathing available at the Baths in Great Smith Street!

THE BUILDING

The majority of students appeared to have a love/hate relationship with 17 Bloomsbury Square in this period. A piece written as a guided tour by a ghost in the *Square Chronicle* of February 1914 had the guide describe the building thus: "The general impression is that it, like the dog kennel, was built rather to keep the rain off the inmates than for show … There are no lofty towers or echoing quadrangles, no marbled entrance or refreshment tent …"

The chemistry laboratory and the lecture theatre are the two areas that seem to have prompted most comment, not least because presumably this is where students spent most of their time. In 1914, the laboratory is introduced to new students as "the Crystal Palace, glass roof, bottles and test-tubes. All windows made to keep closed and so prevent any chance of the obnoxious fumes escaping." From the early twentieth century, there were also numerous complaints about the fact that students had to climb so many stairs to get to the top of the building and there were repeated calls for a lift. In 1926, the editor of the *Chronicle* felt that a new species of Minor student had entered the building as there were no calls for a lift – although did that mean that the students were not eager enough to go up to the laboratory?

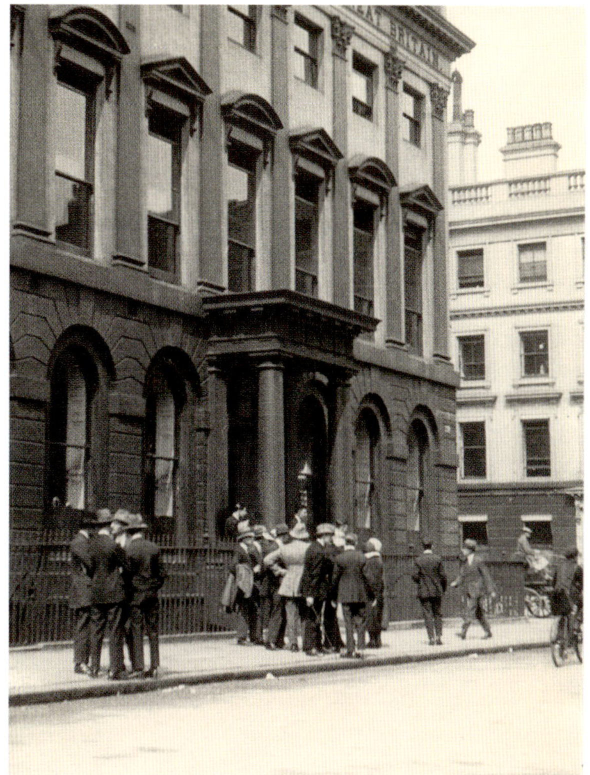

Was this group of students in 1923 waiting to go into a lecture, or catching up on gossip before heading home? Note that hats were still universally worn.

Royal Pharmaceutical Society Museum

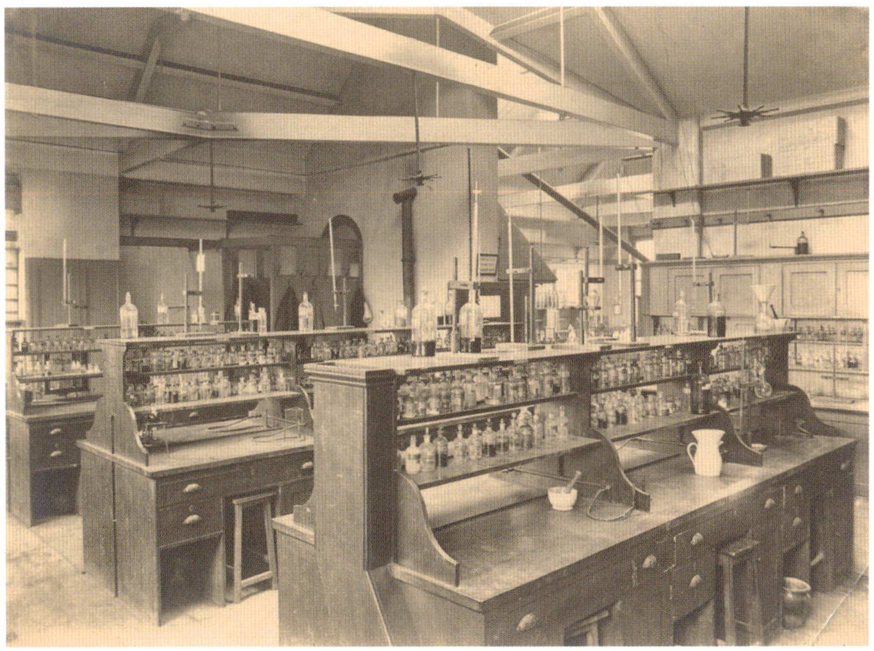

Although the top floor lab for Minor students was re-arranged in about 1900, the benches still had no water or sinks, but they did have a gas supply.

Royal Pharmaceutical Society Museum

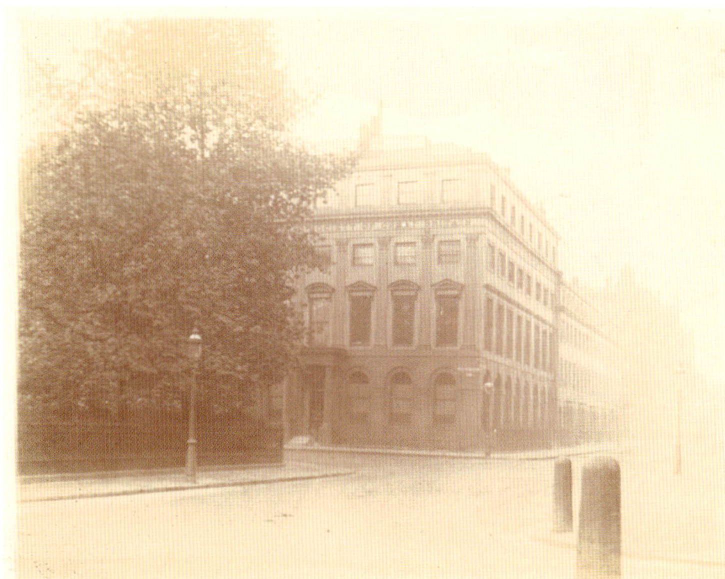

17 Bloomsbury Square in the late 1800s.

Royal Pharmaceutical Society Museum

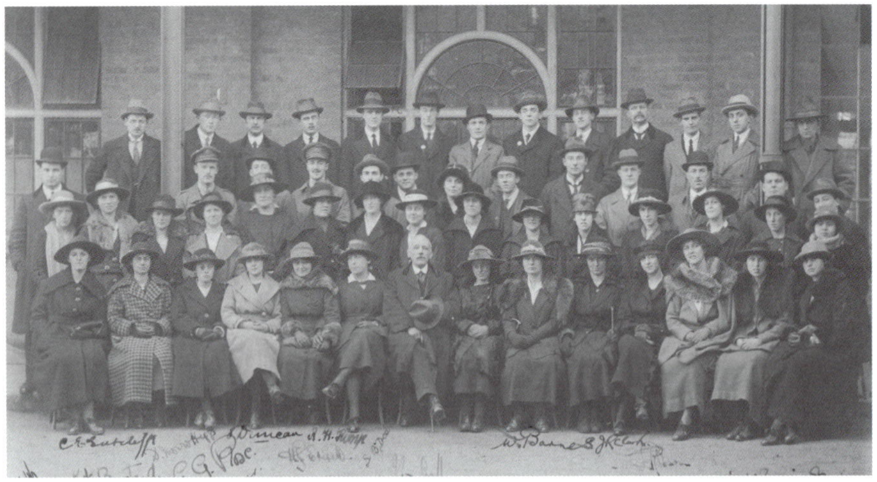

The regular visits to Parke, Davis and Co's Laboratories in Hounslow were commemorated with a souvenir photograph, this one from 13th March 1919.

UCL School of Pharmacy Library

In June 1922, an article in the *Chronicle* described the lecture theatre as "the coldest, most uncomfortable and uninviting room ever constructed ... The whole place is undoubtedly constructed on a 'keep you awake system', and is exceedingly efficient yet we have known of students having even more than forty winks." It goes on to advise: "Students, when ordering new suits, would be wise in having two or three extra pairs of trousers, as the continual shuffling about, trying to find a soft spot on a hard seat, does the lower portion of one's apparel no great amount of good." However, by January 1925, new central heating had been installed and produced a different effect for those attending lectures: "Although at first it threatened to be a universal floor washing system, it is now functioning well, especially in the lecture theatre where it produces a marked soporific effect." The same edition of the *Chronicle* saw the irony in the call from the PSGB president for "a School housed in the finest pharmaceutical building in the world" whilst they were grappling with Victorian facilities at best.

In 1921, the roof had fallen down in the Major laboratory. The joke amongst the students seems to have been that this was because of the deep thinking going on in the room, explained by psychology: "According to some exponents of this now popular science, thoughts are of the nature of vibrations. We are aware, of course, that the Major syllabus is conducive of much cerebral commotion – but, so early in the term!"

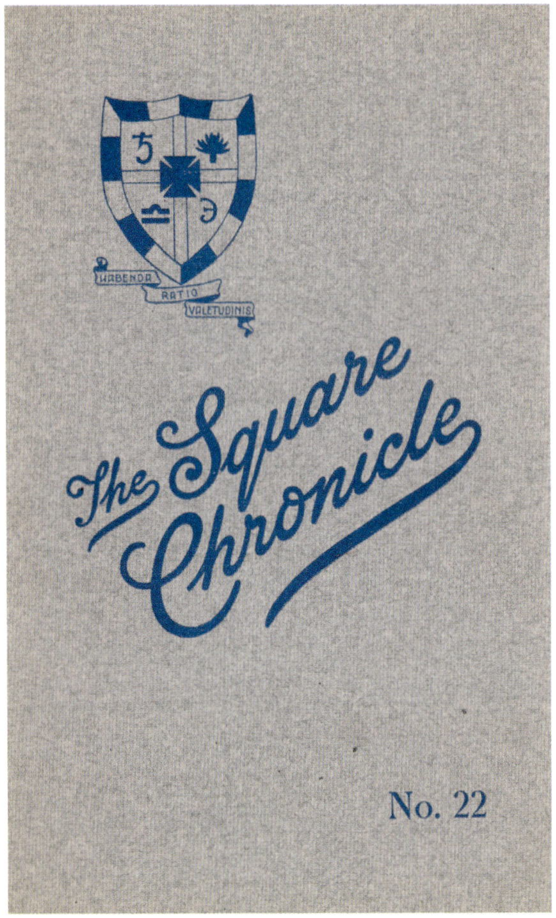

The *Square Chronicle*'s cover did not change from 1926 until the shortages of World War Two.

UCL School of Pharmacy Library

WOMEN PHARMACISTS

From the 1880s, the number of women in the pharmaceutical workforce increased, with many working as dispensers in hospitals and other institutions, or as assistants in shops. However, the number of women on the statutory register fell in the late nineteenth century. By 1905, there were only 195 female pharmacists on the Register (1.2% of 15,948 in total). However, on Thursday 15th June 1905, a group of women pharmacists met at 5 Endsleigh Street in London. Their aim was to establish an Association of Women Pharmacists. The group's objectives would be to discuss questions relating to women's employment, establish a locum register and a register of all qualified women, and the "furtherance of social intercourse". Members had to hold one of the Society's certificates and pay a membership fee of five shillings if they were a Society member, or 10 shillings if they were not. Fifty women joined immediately. Isabella Clarke (by now Clarke-Keer) was the Association's first president, with Margaret Buchanan as vice-president.

This first meeting, described in *The Chemist and Druggist* as "a meeting both historical and novel", was particularly focused on the problems of women trying to find pharmacy employment. Although women were now able to become members of the Pharmaceutical Society, there were still concerns about the availability of suitable employment for them, and about the conditions under which they were expected to work. The Association held its first public meeting on 17th October 1905. One-hundred women and 12 men heard Mrs Louise Creighton, who had been the first president of the Union of Women Workers, speak on "The present responsibilities of women."

"Where to settle! … The woman pharmacist has something else to weigh besides expense: it is the question of her sex, and the fact that at present she is a pioneer in her profession, and must naturally turn to where she thinks an enterprising woman will be respected and her ability made use of rather than to a locality that appears very 'Early Victorian.' … The places to avoid are centres, such as cathedral towns, where anything new is looked upon with suspicion, and must stand the test of time before it can be trusted."

E.L.B. Forster, 12th August 1916

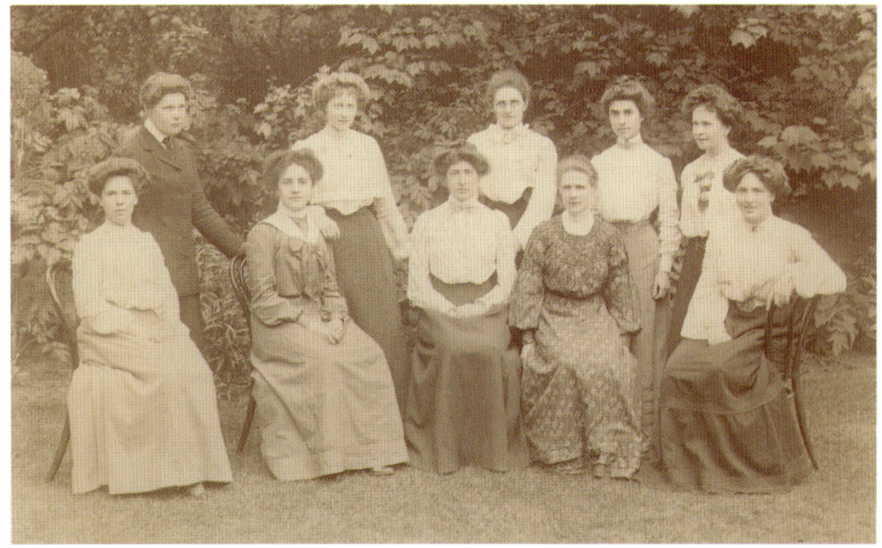

The women students at the School were recorded in 1904, including Elsie Hooper in the centre of the front row with Hilda Caws to her left. They became the first joint secretary and the first treasurer, respectively, of the Association of Women Pharmacists, formed in the following year.

UCL School of Pharmacy Library

Although the issue of female membership of the Society had been resolved, women still had to work hard to achieve within the pharmacy profession. This was not because they were less able academically. In fact, by 1925, there had been five female winners of the Society's Pereira medal, seven Redwood scholars, five Jacob Bell scholars and 15 Burroughs scholars. What was difficult was that women's pay and job opportunities were still limited by their gender. The majority of women in the early twentieth century seem to have been working in hospitals and institutions as dispensers, or as managers or assistants in retail pharmacy. Very few were running their own businesses. Female pharmacists' pay was lower than that of school teachers, bank clerks or civil servants at a clerical grade. The Association of Women Pharmacists, particularly through its employment bureau, was able to begin to put pressure on employers to improve salaries and conditions of employment.

By 1923, of the 15 girls trained at the pharmacy at 17 The Pavement, Clapham Common, who studied at the Pharmaceutical Society's School of Pharmacy, 14 had taken prizes and scholarships. The business had been set up by past Square student Margaret Buchanan and her business partner Agnes Borrowman. As *The Pharmaceutical Journal* of 15th December asked: "Is there another pharmacy in the country that can beat this record?" Under Miss Borrowman's leadership, the business was staffed entirely by women, and as far as possible, everything was made on the premises, rather than holding large stocks of proprietary medicines. She believed firmly that if women were given the opportunity, they could achieve just as much as male pharmacists.

"It is easy to understand that men, and especially unemployed ex-Service men, in the drug trade should object to female competition, chiefly on the ground that competition tends to depress the wage standard … There is no more reason for excluding women from earning a livelihood in pharmacy than there is for excluding men who are less than 5 ft. 4 in. in height … let marriage be the gilding of a full life, not the end and object of an empty one. Even now the

happiest marriages are those in which each partner works for the common home – a menage not unknown in pharmacy – and we are emboldened to hope that the problem of women in pharmacy may in the future be largely solved on these lines.

"

Letter from "A Free Woman", The Pharmaceutical Journal, 13th November 1920.

The same was true of the student population. The *Square Chronicle* of December 1915 noted that for the first time on record, the number of lady members of the School equalled the number of men. There was a female Bell Scholar, Fairchild Scholar and Hewlett Exhibitioner. An article later in the magazine entitled "The Ladies' Year" outlined the female successes, notably all drawn from students nurtured by Margaret Buchanan. Dora White had won the Pereira medal, plus bronze and silver medals in botany, the silver medal in chemistry, and certificates of honour in elementary and advanced chemistry, and materia medica. Ella Caird, the Hewlett Exhibitioner, was the second woman to hold this post. She had gained medals in botany, chemistry and pharmacy in the Minor course, plus certificates in materia medica and practical chemistry, and was now an undergraduate at the University of London. In the same year, Dorothy A. Bills was the first woman to hold a Bell Scholarship, and Doris Gregory the first woman to hold a Fairchild Scholarship.

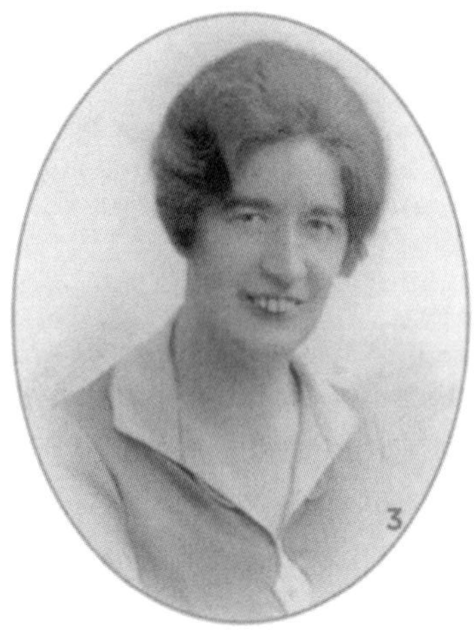

HOPE CONSTANCE MONICA WINCH (1894–1944)

School of Pharmacy, University of Sunderland

HOPE CONSTANCE MONICA WINCH (1894–1944)

Hope Winch qualified as a chemist & druggist in 1917 and was awarded the Hewlett Exhibition. She passed the Major exam in the following year, when she was Pereira medallist. She then spent two years as a Redwood Scholar in the research laboratories, and in 1920 she became an associate of the Institute of Chemistry. In the same year she took up a post as lecturer in pharmacy at Sunderland Technical College, and became head of the department in 1930. Having spent a short time at Rutherford College in Newcastle upon Tyne, she was convinced that Sunderland had more potential as a pharmacy school, and on her request, the Pharmaceutical Society approved the transfer of all pharmacy teaching in the north-east to Sunderland.

The Sunderland pharmacy department began with three fee-paying students and 25 ex-servicemen and consisted of one double-sided bench in the chemistry school. Miss Winch taught the whole course. In 1926, two lecturers joined her and she was able to equip a purpose-built dispensary. In 1928, a laboratory for drug preparation became the second room to be dedicated to pharmacy teaching. In 1930, Sunderland Technical College was recognised by London University for the teaching of its external BPharm degree.

Miss Winch played a significant role in the establishment of the Society's local branch in Sunderland and served for 20 years as its secretary, and then its chairman. She was a keen mountaineer and achieved difficult climbs in Switzerland and Italy. She died tragically as the result of a fall when climbing Scafell in the Lake District, aged only 49.

However, the women of 1915 were following in distinguished footsteps, with a number of previous female students at the School achieving high awards and some continuing into academia. In 1893, Annie Tilson was awarded a Council silver medal, and in 1899 Frances Morgan also achieved this accolade. The year

1902 could have been viewed as another "Ladies' Year", with Certificates of Honour in elementary courses gained by Georgina Barltrop, May Burt and Hilda Caws.

Although there was a spate of opposition to the growing number of women pharmacists in the 1920s, their position was getting firmer. The women students at the Square were achieving consistently highly, and since their entry into the School in 1872, their numbers gradually increased from around half a dozen up to 1914, to around a third of each year's intake from the start of the First World War onwards. However, as an article in *The Chemist and Druggist* in 1925 pointed out: "there remains the consoling fact that though women have been demonstrating their capabilities in pharmacy for thirty years or more, it is still men who teach them, men who examine them, and men who hand them out their medals."

RESEARCH

In spite of the problems caused in the past, the Society continued to allow the professors and other researchers in the School to take part in production of the *British Pharmacopoeia*. For the 1898 edition, Professors Greenish, Bentley and Attfield led research in the Society's laboratories, and Professor Attfield acted as editor. They also brought in other members of the School's staff and alumni to act as referees for different sections, such as E.M. Holmes and W.A. Tilden. From 1900, Society staff started reviewing

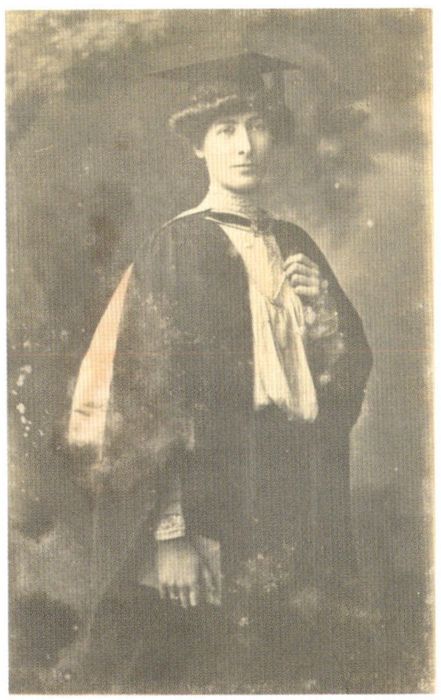

ELSIE HOOPER (1879–1969)

Royal Pharmaceutical Society Museum

ELSIE HOOPER (1879–1969)

Elsie Seville Hooper passed the Minor exam in 1901, and passed the Major exam and registered as a pharmaceutical chemist in the following year. She was then awarded the Redwood Research Scholarship, the first woman to achieve this since its foundation in 1888. She was awarded a Burroughs Scholarship by the Society in 1903, also the first woman to do so. She undertook her research with Professor Greenish, including a joint paper in 1904 on barks. Her later papers were on belladonna root and on chinchonon. Meanwhile, in the evenings she worked for a degree in botany and chemistry at Birkbeck College, which she gained in 1905. She then worked on the first *British Pharmaceutical Codex* (1907) and studied for her Institute of Chemistry qualification, which she passed in 1906. She became a Fellow of the Institute of Chemistry in 1909. After a year's analytical work at King's College, she worked on *Secret Remedies*, a publication produced by the British Medical Association to expose the previously unknown formulae of popular medicines. After a year, she left to join the chemistry department at Portsmouth Municipal College, where she was given responsibility for setting up a course in pharmacy subjects. During the First World War, she worked as an analyst for Ucal in Cheltenham.

After this, she remained London-based for the rest of her working life. From 1920 to 1942, she worked as lecturer then proprietor of the Gordon Hall School of Pharmacy, the place where she had trained under Margaret Buchanan. Whilst at the school, Elsie Hooper owned two pharmacies in Hampstead: from 1936 until 1945 at Belsize Terrace, and at 1 Flask Walk until 1961. She was keen to apprentice female pharmacy students from the Gordon Hall School in her businesses. Elsie Hooper was one of the Association of Women Pharmacists' first joint secretaries, from 1905.

the content of the 1898 edition ready for the next one. Still the General Medical Council questioned the propriety of recognising the Society's role, but nevertheless wanted its staff and laboratory facilities to check several areas, for example, the boiling points of various substances.

The success of women pharmacy students in this period led a significant few to follow a career in pharmaceutical research, with the School's laboratories an obvious continuation of their work. Elsie Hooper was a significant pharmacy scholar, the first woman to hold the Redwood Research Scholarship since its foundation in 1888, and the first woman to gain the Burroughs Research Scholarship in 1903. She undertook her research with Professor Greenish, including a joint paper in 1904 on barks. Her later papers were on belladonna root and on chinchonon.

In 1904, Norah Renouf, from Jersey, took the Redwood Research Scholarship. In both 1905 and 1906, she was the first woman to be awarded one of the Salter's Research Fellowships. She worked with Professor Crossley on the chemistry of camphor derivatives, giving joint papers at the Chemical Society and the Pharmaceutical Society.

In 1908, Gertrude Wren became the first woman to win the Pereira medal, having been the first woman to win a silver medal in the Society's Herbarium Competition in 1906. In 1908, she was awarded the Redwood Research Scholarship and was appointed demonstrator in chemistry at the Square. Dorothy Braithwaite, who gained the Minor in 1909 and the Major in 1910, took a role as research assistant to Professor Greenish. They wrote a joint paper on the drug room beetle in 1910. Braithwaite went on to become a pharmacist at Guy's Hospital in 1912, and then joined the Central Checking Bureau for National Health Insurance dispensing. She was promoted to responsibility for all staff engaged in this work by the Retail Pharmacists' Union (later the National Pharmacy Association).

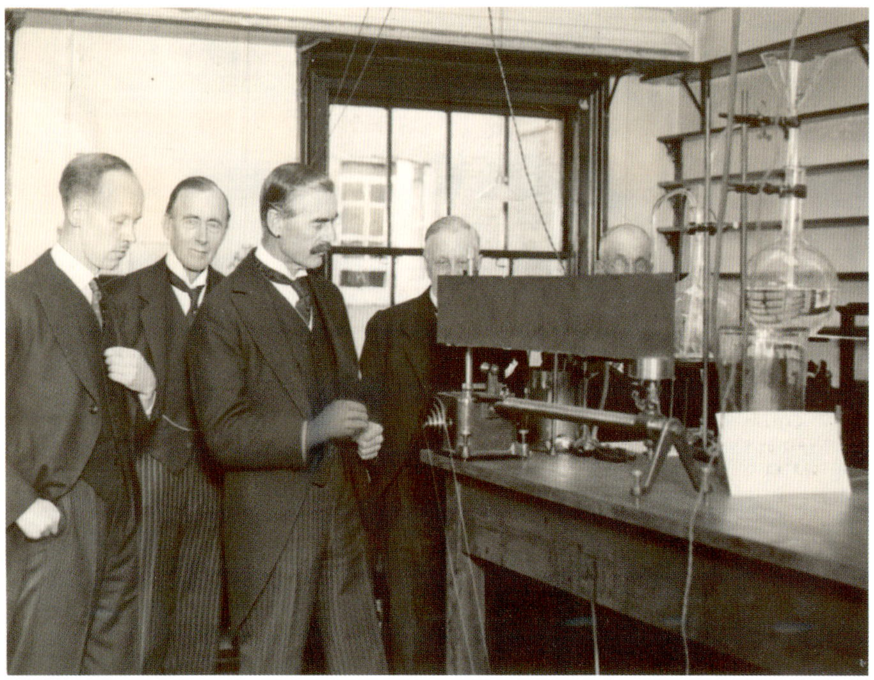

Neville Chamberlain, Minister of Health, opened the new pharmacological laboratories on 16th June 1926. He is shown with Dr J.H.Burn, head of the laboratories, F.E.Bilson, PSGB President 1926–7, Sir H.Rolleston, President of the Medical Society of London and Physician-in-Ordinary to King George V, and P.F.Rowsell, PSGB President 1925–26.

Royal Pharmaceutical Society Museum

Pharmacognosy research in this period was primarily based on the identification and quality control of crude drugs that were botanical in origin. T.E. Wallis concentrated on microscopical research including counting discrete particles, measuring lengths, and calculating areas or volumes of plant cells and tissues to determine extent of adulteration in powdered drugs. He was appointed reader in pharmacognosy of the University of London in 1925.

A new era in pharmaceutical research at the Society began in the 1920s when it established a laboratory for pharmacological research and assay in 1925. The facility was formally opened in 1926 by the Minister of Health, Neville Chamberlain. The development sat neatly alongside the Therapeutic Substances Act, passed on 7th August 1925. The leading article in *The Pharmaceutical Journal* of 19th June 1926 explained that recent discoveries of the therapeutic value of extracts or products of animal tissues and other chemical compounds had prompted the Therapeutic Substances Bill. As a result, the Council had decided that it needed to undertake testing and standardising work for manufacturers, and had set up a laboratory for this purpose, fully titled the "Laboratory for the Biological Examination and Standardisation of Remedial Substances." Dr J.H. Burn was appointed to direct the work.

At an event to mark the Laboratory's 50th anniversary, Burn recalled the reasons for setting up the laboratory. First, William Glyn-Jones felt that pharmacy needed taking from a craft into a medical science. Secondly, there was still much criticism of the *British Pharmacopoeia*, especially from the leading pharmacologist Dr Henry Dale, who was director of the department of biochemistry and pharmacology at the National Institute for Medical Research. Thirdly, discussions primarily between Dale and Edmund White about other areas of pharmacology research that could be achieved suggested the need for a dedicated facility. White, PSGB president from 1913 to 1918, steered the decisions through the Council. Burn also explained that the laboratories were necessary because of the growing number of medicinal substances that could not be chemically tested for purity and potency. These included substances from pharmaceutical firms who could not test the substances themselves. In addition, in 1926, Burn recommended adding a vitamin-testing and nutrition laboratory, under Dr Katharine Coward, to the facilities. This laboratory worked on requests for cod-liver oil and margarine tests, vitamins A and D having been added to the margarine. Dr Coward's research established dose–response curves for the action of vitamins A, B_1, C and D. The work relied heavily on animal testing, and a large room in the basement was kitted out to house the animals required. The main pharmacology laboratories achieved many successes including establishing methods for the biological assay of vitamins, digitalis and ergot alkaloids. Quantitative biological methods developed in the laboratories also led to the isolation and identification of the form of calciferol (ergocalciferol) then believed to be the only form of vitamin D active for prevention of rickets.

The laboratories started with research and testing, but there was also a direct impact on the School as Burn later drew up the first syllabus for teaching pharmacology. However, this impact was relatively slight initially as students had not been taught biology and there were no biologists on the staff of any existing schools of pharmacy at the time. The development of pharmacology teaching increased in pace from 1933, when Professor Burn became dean of the School.

The establishment of a nationally important scientific research laboratory, serving a rapidly increasing pharmaceutical industry and a growing body of pharmaceutical and pharmacological research, was just one aspect of change that staff and students at the School experienced in this period. Looking back to the opening of the research laboratories on the new third floor in 1861, the contrast is enormous. The development of increasingly accurate equipment, the standardisation of processes and the understanding of medicinal action may have been built on nineteenth century foundations, but now the work was being carried out by both male and female students, who were able to achieve a degree qualification from one of the world's greatest universities. The School had arrived at a significant milestone in its history.

CHAPTER 4

"THE WHOLE QUESTION OF THE FUTURE": 1927–1948

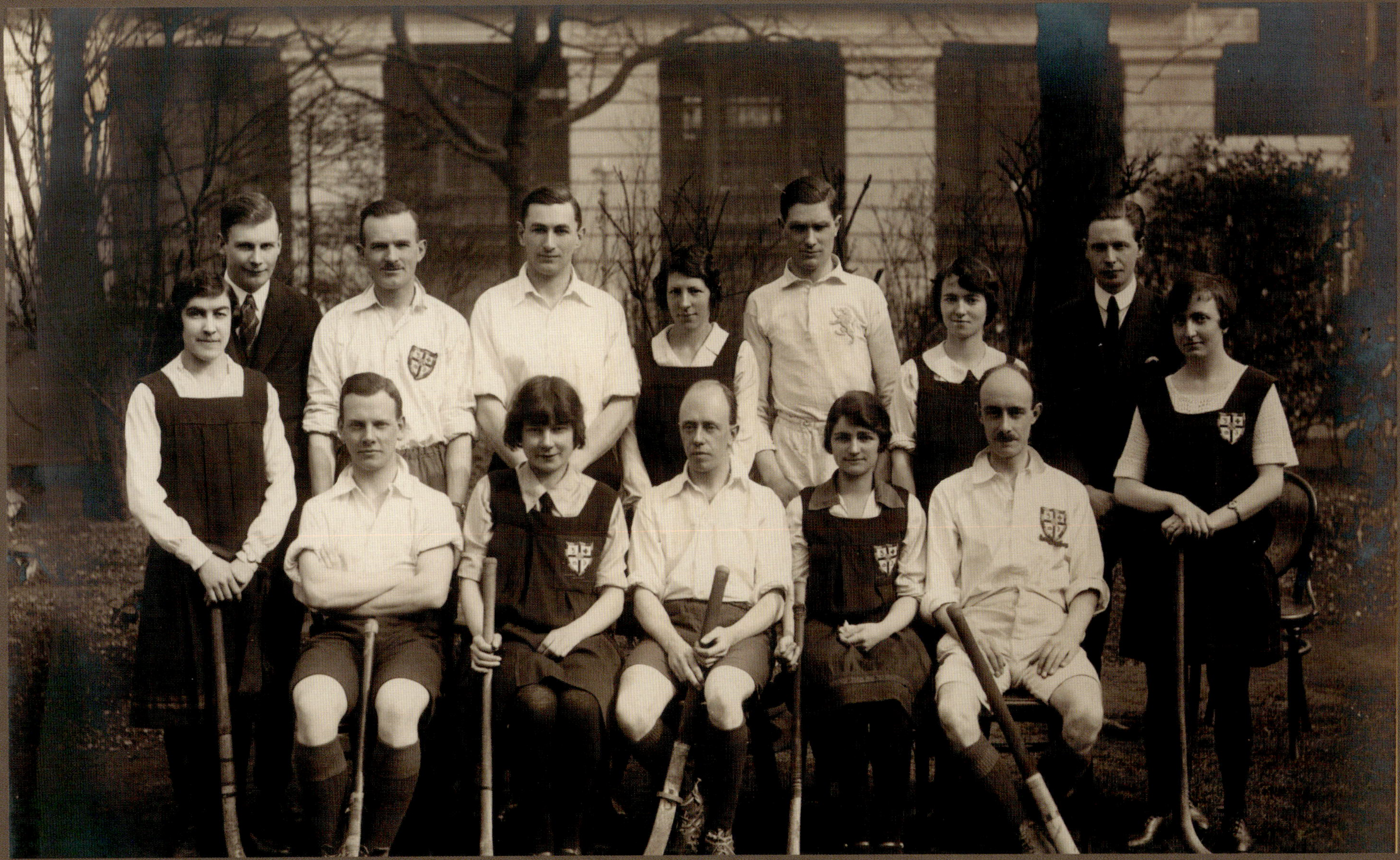

The 1926-7 hockey team went on to produce a professor and dean at the School, W.H. Linnell, and two people who became Pharmaceutical Society Secretary and Registrar, F.W. Adams and H.N. Linstead.

Reproduced with permission from UCL School of Pharmacy Library

MILESTONES

Popular Culture

1927 *The Jazz Singer*, the first talking film
1932 Chadwick discovered the neutron
1938 creation of Nylon
1941 first mechanical computer
1941 first jet aircraft
1942 splitting of the atom
1947 transistors demonstrated
1947 Christian Dior's "New Look" fashion collection launched

London Life

1936 Battle of Cable Street clash at British Union of Fascists' march
1937 999 emergency calls introduced in London
1940 London Blitz began on 7th September
1948 Olympic Games held in London

National News

1936 crisis over abdication of King Edward VIII
1937 King George VI crowned
1940 start of rationing
1945 VE (Victory in Europe) Day celebrated on 8th May
1947 exceptionally hard winter
1948 National Health Service established

The Wider World

1929 Wall Street Crash, followed by Great Depression
1932 Frank Whittle's patent for the jet engine was granted
1936–1939 Spanish Civil War
1939–1945 Second World War
1947 India and Pakistan gained independence from Britain
1948 World Health Organization established

Drug Developments

1928 penicillin discovered by Alexander Fleming
1928 Albert von Szent Gyorgi isolated vitamin C
1932 Gerhard Domagk, director of research for German company Bayer, found that Prontosil red, a dye, cured mice that had been injected with a lethal dose of streptococci
1935 sulfanilamide identified as the active principle in Prontosil
1944 streptomycin discovered; initially used for tuberculosis
1948 cortisone used to treat rheumatoid arthritis

Pharmacy Milestones

1933 poison bottles had to be distinguishable by touch, by law
1933 Pharmacy and Poisons Act: Privy Council became pharmacy's central authority and three Privy Council nominees were to serve on the Pharmaceutical Society's Council. Membership, with an annual fee, became compulsory for all registered pharmaceutical chemists and chemists & druggists. The Statutory Committee was established as a disciplinary body and the inspectorate was set up. Registration of premises was proposed, and

Pharmacy changed dramatically in the period between the wars, predominantly because of the pace of drug development, but also owing to changes brought about by the Pharmacy Act of 1933. In spite of the economic depression, the 1920s and 1930s were a time of growth for the pharmaceutical industry globally, with the discovery and development of vitamins, insulin, hormones and the sulpha-drugs. Gerhard Domagk's discovery of Prontosil in 1932 opened up an exciting new area of antibacterial treatments. Meanwhile, pharmacy legislation in Britain further regulated both the drugs and the profession. The Pharmacy and Poisons Act of 1933 established a Poisons Board to advise the Secretary of State, and introduced four schedules of poisons including those that were "prescription only." The Act also gave the Pharmaceutical Society the powers to enforce the Act, which led it to set up its inspectorate and Statutory Committee. For the public, the pharmacist's role may not have seemed that different, but their advisory position was vital for people to navigate their way through the new medicines available, whether in the shop or in the hospital.

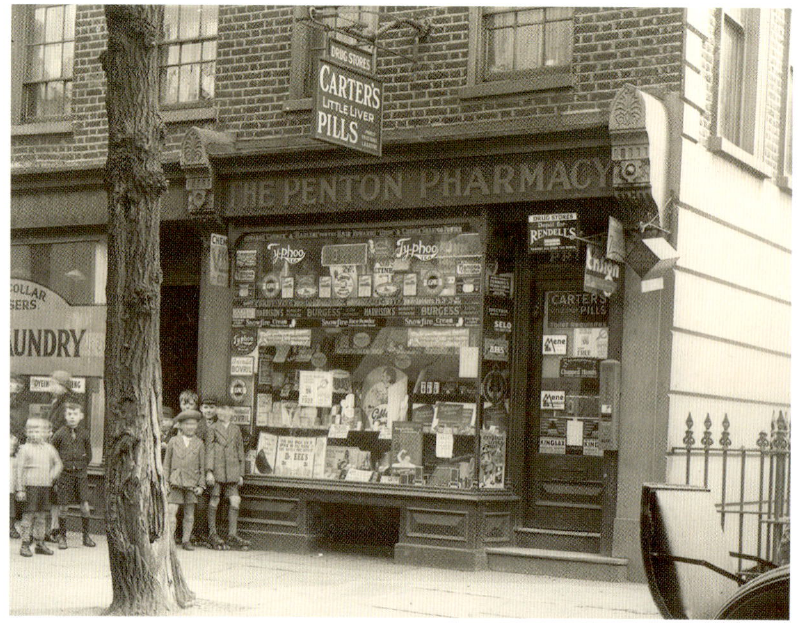

The Penton Pharmacy in north London had a window display packed with advertising from Typhoo Tea to Burgess' Lion Ointment, and Bovril to Snowfire Cream. The children trying to get into the photograph, taken in about 1930, include two boys wearing roller skates.

Royal Pharmaceutical Society Museum

> **"Requiring something from the chemist, I entered a chemist's shop where I knew a lady assistant was employed … I think where women chemists are employed a notice should be put in the window, and this would attract the women shoppers who are sometimes a little sensitive about their personal requirements."**
>
> "Pharmacista", *The British and Colonial Pharmacist*, May 1938

THE BUILDING

At the Society's annual general meeting (AGM) in May 1927, the president announced that the Council was considering moving from Bloomsbury Square. The leases on the various buildings would run out by 1948. "It is, therefore, not too early for us to be considering the whole question of the future of the Society's premises." He also reported that the Council had put aside £5,000 to form the nucleus of a building fund in preparation for a new property. Bloomsbury Square had ceased to function effectively as a modern school of pharmacy, and the space needed for the administration of the Society was also

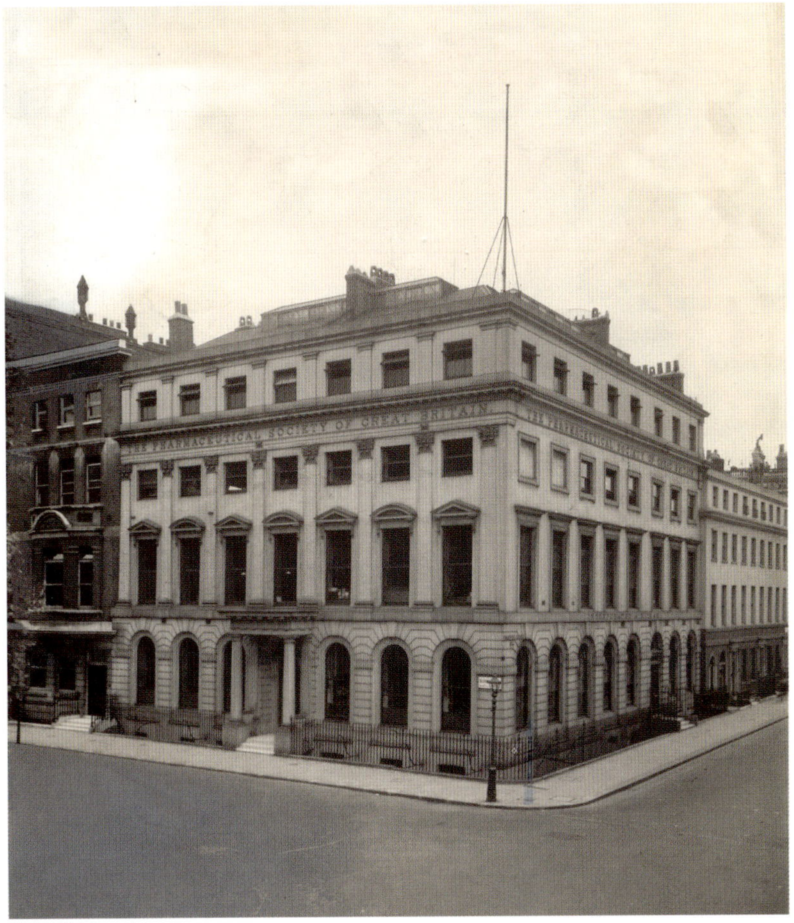

Taken in the 1930s, this photograph shows the main entrance to 17 Bloomsbury Square under the pillared porch, the secondary entrance on Great Russell Street, and number 16 Bloomsbury Square to the far left, that the Society had re-built in 1890.

Royal Pharmaceutical Society Museum

taking over areas of the building such as the library and various corridors. From the date of this announcement onwards, the changes made to the building were only minimal, such as a flagstaff to enable the Society to celebrate King George V's jubilee in 1935, the installation of a microphone and amplifying equipment in the hall in the same year and, as the *Square Chronicle* put it, "the installation of fans in certain of the Laboratories – but not in the Council Chamber – to let out the hot air."

The Society's 1930 Annual Report showed that the freehold of a block of houses on the north side of Brunswick Square had been purchased for demolition and this was to be the site for a new headquarters and School of Pharmacy. The houses were currently let to tenants, but the Council stated that they were prepared to wait for the leases to expire before taking over the block and demolishing it. They also expressed regret that they would have to leave Bloomsbury Square, but explained that as they were unable to buy the property, they were unable to stay. The space issue was the key factor. As the Society's president, Mr L. Moreton Parry, reported at the AGM:

> The Society is at the moment struggling to carry on its work with efficiency in a group of antiquated buildings providing inadequate accommodation, and in many respects ill adapted to the Society's purposes. Such buildings, moreover, are held on leases which commence to fall in a few years' time, and can only be renewed on much less favourable terms than those on which they are now held. The Society's future responsibilities are likely to entail more and not less accommodation, so that this problem of accommodation is becoming a most urgent one; and its solution turns on the question of finance. There are the expenses inseparable from the termination of a lease to provide for, but more important still is the question of raising the funds necessary to equip the Society with a modern building of a size adequate to provide for its present and, so far as can be foreseen, its future requirements, of a design specially suited to its needs, and placed on its own freehold site.

	was first published in 1936. The Act also introduced a Fourth Schedule of poisons which could only be sold with a prescription
1937	PAGB Code of Standards of Advertising Practice launched
1938	Food and Drugs Act prohibited the adulteration and mislabelling of drugs
1939	Cancer Act restricted the advertisement of products claiming to treat cancer
1940	under the Finance (No. 2) Act, purchase tax was imposed on a range of goods including most drugs and medicines at 33%
1941	Pharmacy and Medicines Act repealed the old medicine stamp duty. It forbade the general advertisement of products claiming to treat a number of specific illnesses, or to be effective in procuring an abortion. For the first time manufacturers were required to list the active ingredients of products on their packaging
1941	Statement upon Matters of Professional Conduct, the first simple code of ethics, published; the idea had been proposed in 1866
1947	Mrs Jean Irvine elected as the Pharmaceutical Society's first female president
1947	Penicillin Act

He explained that, in 1929, the Society had moved an additional £7,500 to its building fund, bringing the current total to £26,300. However, he also pointed out that they would need significantly more capital than this to embark on a new building.

BRUNSWICK SQUARE

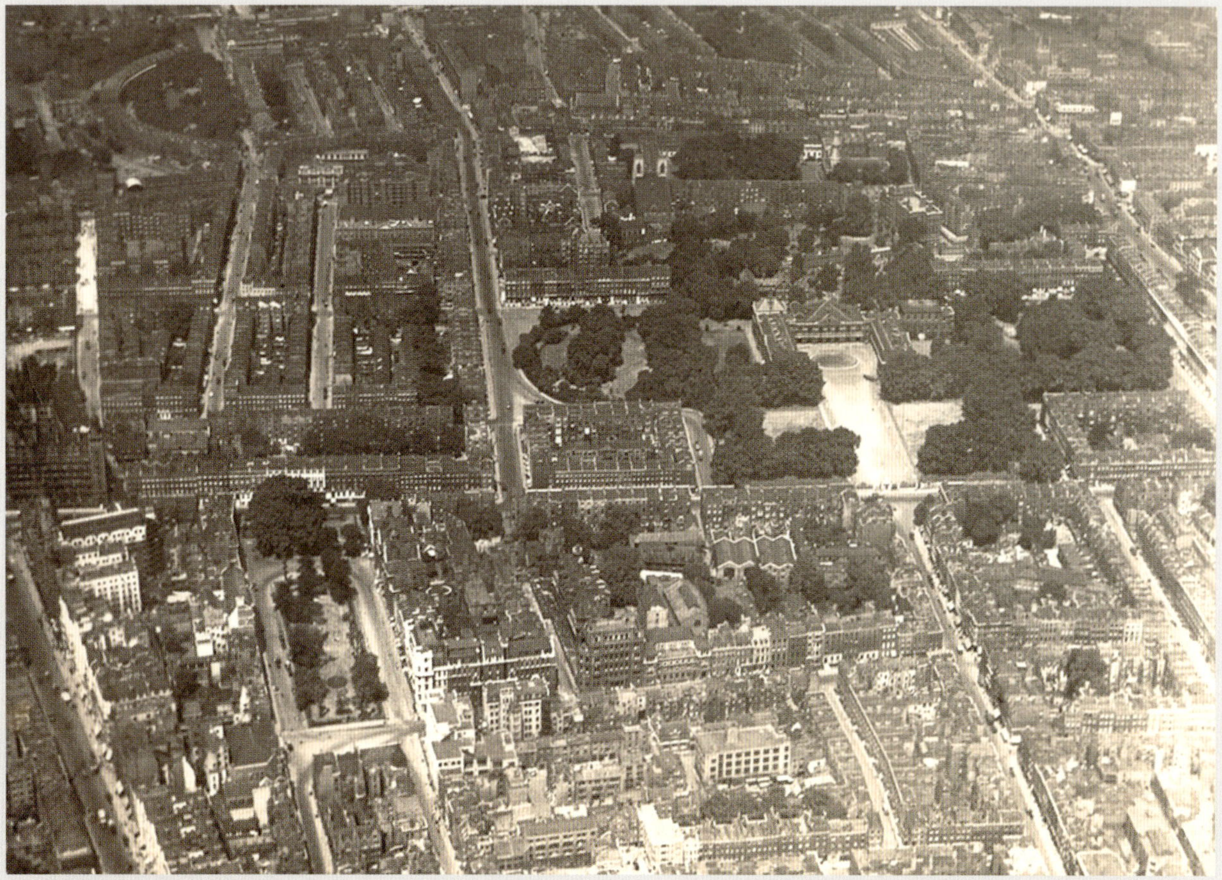

This aerial photograph was taken in 1938. You can see Brunswick Square with its Georgian terrace where the School was to stand, and the enormous Foundling Hospital complex to its right.

Royal Pharmaceutical Society Museum

Brunswick Square, along with Mecklenburgh Square, was built in part of the recreation grounds of the Foundling Hospital, an orphanage founded by the distinguished seaman Captain Thomas Coram, in 1739. In 1790, when the Hospital needed additional income, it leased the land to have houses built on it. Brunswick Square was finished by 1802. It was named after Caroline of Brunswick, wife of the Prince Regent, and later (briefly and controversially) Queen Caroline on his accession as George IV in 1820.

In the early nineteenth century, the Square had a reputation for being respectable rather than fashionable; it was also a convenient home for officers of the Foundling Hospital itself. John Hunter, vice-president of the Foundling Hospital (not the famous surgeon/anatomist), lived in the Square from 1803 to 1816.

Thomas Burgon, a Levant Company merchant who also worked in the nearby coin room of the British Museum, lived at number 11 from 1814 until the 1830s with his wife Catherine and their six children. According to the *Oxford Dictionary of National Biography*, they were part of a social circle that included the architect Thomas Leverton Donaldson, the painter Charles Robert Leslie and the poet Samuel Rogers.

In 1815, Jane Austen's novel *Emma* mentions the Square as the London residence of the Knightley family. Isabella Knightley boasts: "Our part of London is very superior to most others! You must not confound us with London in general, my dear sir. The neighbourhood of Brunswick Square is very different from almost all the rest. We are so very airy! I should be unwilling, I own, to live in any other part of the town – there is hardly any other that I could be satisfied to have my children in."

Other residents in the nineteenth century included the writer and editor William Maginn; the evangelical physician Thomas Harrison Burder; the surgeon and philanthropist Thomas Phillips; John Leech, caricaturist and illustrator of Dickens; the lawyer, and one of the founders of the Law Society, Bryan Holme; and the writer and campaigner for volunteer troops Alfred Bate Richards.

The Square's genteel reputation must have been damaged in the 1840s, when residents were recorded complaining of prostitutes working there at night. In 1878, another possibly unsavoury activity was centred here with Thomas Cooke's School of Anatomy, the last private anatomy school, providing Brunswick Square as its address. In the following year, the public benefactor Angela Burdett-Coutts and her friend Louisa Twining founded a home for female art students here, the first in London.

From 20th November 1911 to 29th October 1912, Virginia Stephen (later Woolf) lived at 38 Brunswick Square, part of the School's site. She shared the house with four young men, one of whom was her future husband, Leonard Woolf. He proposed to her whilst they were living in the house. In 1920, large premises on the west side were the first home of the progressive Minerva Club, a social centre for members of the Women's Freedom League. After the removal of the Foundling Hospital to the country in 1926, a new building was built as the headquarters of the Thomas Coram Foundation, which is still part of the complex neighbouring the School.

The Square's freeholds were later acquired by a subsidiary of McAlpine, which demolished the eighteenth-century terraces on the west side of the Square and replaced them with the Brunswick Centre, completed in 1972. It was a controversial development, described by Shirley Green in 1986 as "a residential-cum-shopping complex that looks like a 5-storey machine-gun emplacement." It achieved Grade II listed status in 2000.

Near the centre of the Square's garden is an extremely fine example of a London plane tree. It was officially awarded "Great Tree Status" in 1988.

In 1935, the Society felt confident enough to appoint an architect for the new building. The Council's Sub-Committee on Premises had visited buildings by eight architects before shortlisting three. At the Council meeting in February 1935, they recommended their choice to be approved by the Council. He was Herbert J. Rowse from Liverpool. He appears to have been a bold choice, with purely Liverpool buildings to his name

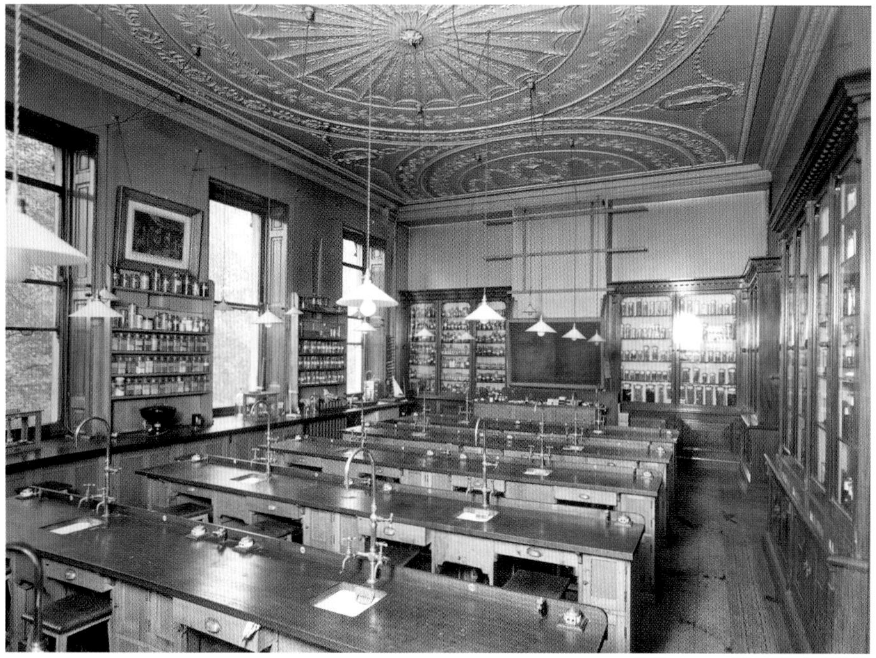

The Histology laboratory was refitted in 1926 with electric lighting, and a sink, water and gas supplies on each bench. However, the ornate ceiling was retained. Hanging between the windows is a framed image of the laboratory at John Bell and Co, shown on page 13.

Royal Pharmaceutical Society Museum

by the time of his appointment. However, they were extremely striking buildings: the India Buildings, Martins Bank, and the Liverpool tunnel entrances, toll booth and ventilation building exteriors for the Queensway Tunnel, completed in 1934. Rowse's plans were approved by the Council on 3rd February 1937. Meanwhile, the Society completed negotiations for a loan of £100,000 to meet half of the balance of the project that the Society was not able to pay in cash. The loan was to be repayable over 30 years at an interest rate of 3.5%.

The editor of the *Square Chronicle* expressed his delight in June 1936 that the School and the Society were to have a new building:

> Square students learn from their own experience the disadvantages resulting from the adaptation of an early eighteenth century mansion to the requirements of a modern school of pharmacy ... It is to be hoped that the new headquarters will in appearance be more worthy of Pharmacy, and will be sufficiently large to house adequately, both a School of increased size and scope, and an administration sufficiently extensive to allow the Society to play a more active part, not only in the advancement of the Science of Pharmacy, but also in prosecuting the welfare of Pharmacy in general.

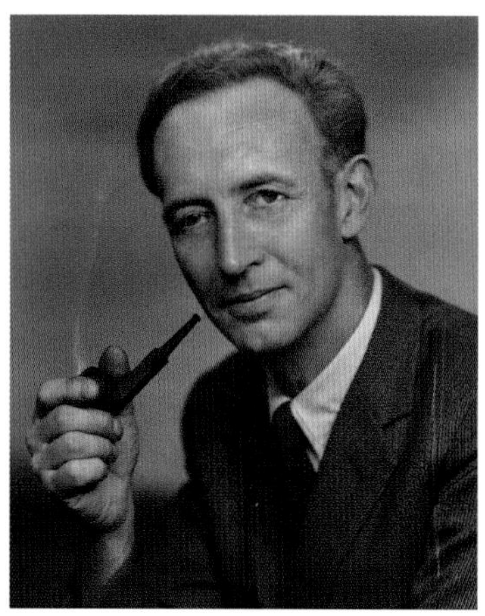

LEONARD GOODWIN (1915–2008)

© National Portrait Gallery, London

LEONARD GOODWIN (1915–2008)

Len Goodwin gained his BPharm at the Square in 1935, and then worked as a demonstrator for four years at UCL before approaching the Wellcome Laboratories to enquire about vacancies. Having gained a post there, he stayed for 24 years. He is best known for his discovery of pyrimethamine, one of the most valuable of the antimalarial drugs, which he developed alongside Ian Rollo at the Wellcome Laboratories. Whilst working in Kenya in 1951, he tested the new drug by infecting himself with malaria and taking the medicine until his return to London in February 1952. He also played a leading part in the evolution of sodium stibogluconate in the treatment of leishmaniasis, a disfiguring disease that is caused by protozoan parasites carried by certain types of sandfly.

When the Wellcome Laboratories closed in 1963, Goodwin became director of the Nuffield Institute of Comparative Medicine at London Zoo, then director of science to the Zoological Society. He was awarded the Galen gold medal of the Society of Apothecaries in 1975, elected a Fellow of the Royal Society in 1976 and appointed CMG in 1977. From 1984 to 1985 he was honorary director of the Wellcome Museum for Medical Science. He received an honorary doctorate from Brunel University in 1986.

A detailed illustrated article entitled "The Society's New Home" was produced in *The Pharmaceutical Journal* on 29th May 1937. It reproduced the architect's plans that had already been approved by the Council, and it was explained that working drawings and competitive estimates of costs were being prepared. The article also included illustrations of the building in Brunswick Square, and floor plans of all five floors. As for an aesthetic concept, the article stated:

> In the matter of form and architectural design, it has always been the Society's wish that their new home should be a building authentically belonging to its time, yet in its formal expression free from the eccentricities of fashionable experiments. It should have a general association with the collegiate tradition, and at the same time exhibit the character of a home for a professional body. The architect, Mr Rowse, has endeavoured to produce a building having its roots in a sound English tradition, at the same time utilising the diverse elements of the programme of requirements to produce an original scheme.

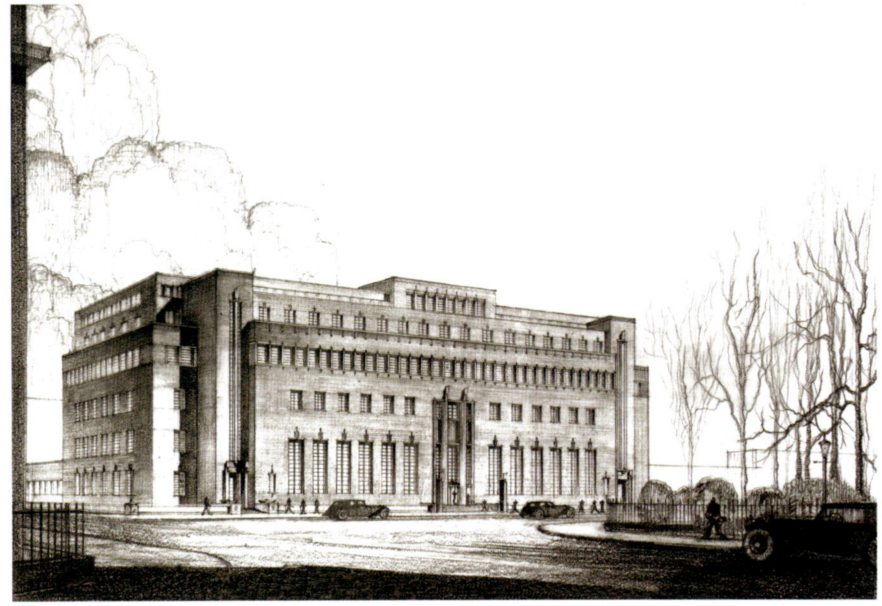

This perspective drawing of the new school building in Brunswick Square was included in an article titled 'The Society's New Home' in *The Pharmaceutical Journal* on 29 May 1937.

The Pharmaceutical Journal

The article went on to explain that brick had been chosen to fit in with the rest of the Square, and also because of its traditional associations. It chimed with their overall concept as it had an aesthetic appeal, and was not an experimental material.

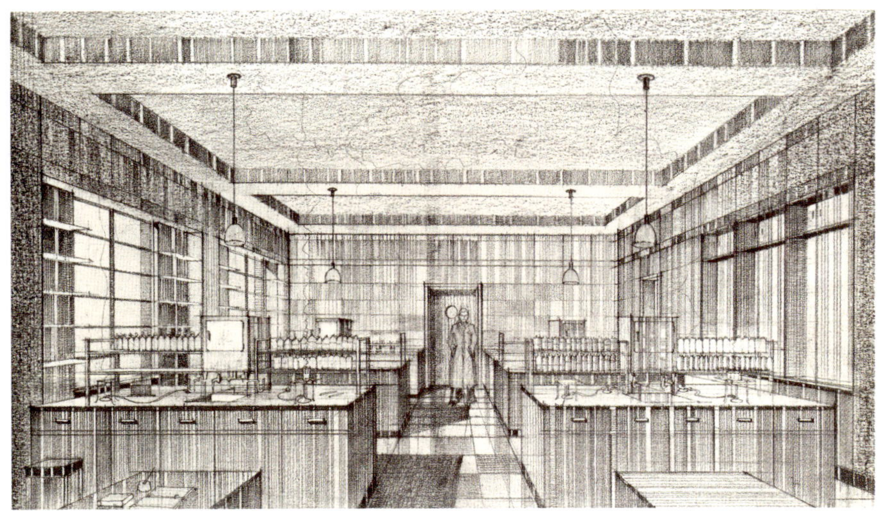

One of a series of perspective drawings prepared by architect Herbert Rowse to accompany his plans and elevations for the School's new building in 1938. This one shows a view of a proposed laboratory.

Royal Pharmaceutical Society Museum

The Council had established a Premises Sub-Committee to work with the architect. It was made clear that there could be extensions to the building in the future. Another key element for consideration was the lighting, presumably in stark contrast with Bloomsbury Square. The Committee was very keen to make the new building as light as possible, and the design included courts for cross-lighting. In terms of space allocation, three-eighths of the space was for the Society's domestic requirements: the library, council room, lecture theatre and offices. Five-eighths was intended for the School, which meant that it occupied the whole of the third and fourth floors, for pharmacy and chemistry, respectively, plus the east wing of the ground, first and second floors. The library would be on the ground floor with a mezzanine level available for expansion, although the reference museum displays were planned to be initially situated there. Examination rooms were located next to each department throughout the School.

Tenders for construction of the new building were invited in May 1938, and the lowest tender was accepted. Building work started later in 1938, and several scale models of the new building were taken to that year's British Pharmaceutical Conference for delegates to view. There was a growing belief that the move from Bloomsbury Square was actually going to happen imminently. In the *Square Chronicle* of March 1939, the Society's president, Hugh Linstead, remarked that the Square "spirit" "will stand the College in good stead when, in 1940, it crosses

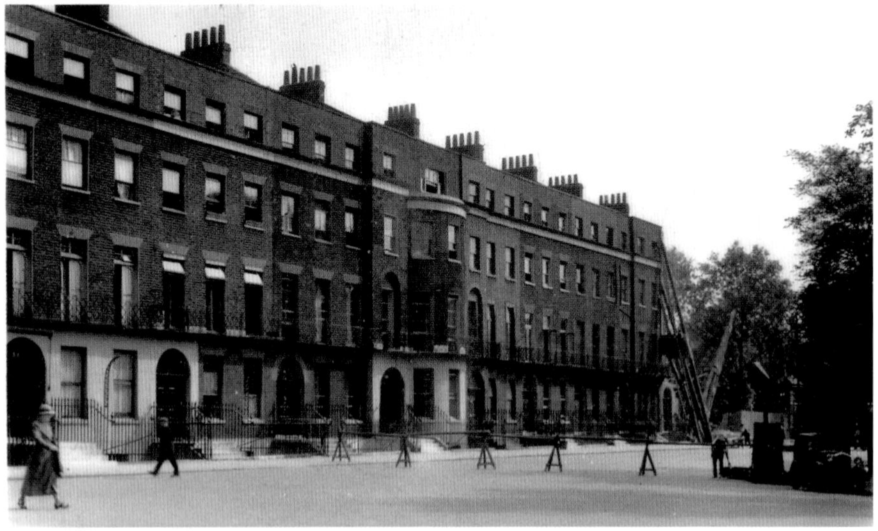

Work began to demolish the existing terrace of Georgian houses on the Brunswick Square site in 1938.

UCL School of Pharmacy Library

Southampton Row to Brunswick Square, and starts to accommodate itself to the emptiness of the new building. The immense gains of the move will be accompanied by certain very distinct losses, which perhaps only those who have worked in the building can fully feel." The Students' Union president, T. Eric Barker, added in the same edition of the *Chronicle*, "It is a happy thought that our arrival at Brunswick Square will approximately coincide with the opening of the new £100,000 ULU [University of London Union] Premises ..."

The leading article in *The Pharmaceutical Journal* on 11th February 1939 revealed that the original cost of the Brunswick Square site was £57,000. It suggested that the area was very suitable because of its proximity to the National Pharmaceutical Union, the Proprietary Articles Trade Association, the Wholesale Drug Trade Association, the British Medical Association and the University of London. It also explained that Rowse had been chosen as the architect as "one of the most prominent architects of the younger school." His relationship with the Society was very good, and staff and officers were very impressed with how he had understood the various needs of a school, research departments, a library and administration offices. However, the project was currently being challenged as rearmament across Europe in response to the threat of war had caused a rapid rise in the cost of building materials. The total cost of the new building was now estimated at £350,000, of which £275,000 had been found. The article concluded by calling for members and organisations to contribute to the fund for the building in order to secure its future.

Britain declared war on Germany on 3rd September 1939. At the Council meeting in December 1939, it was announced that construction work would have to be stopped. A report from the committee explained that the contractors would continue to complete the external structure of the building "and to postpone indefinitely work upon the interior apart from the installation of floors and certain services." In reality, the construction halted at the point where the shell was completed up to the third floor and much of the remaining steel structure was in place. A temporary roof was provided and during the war, the building used as depository for bombed-out furniture.

THE SECOND WORLD WAR

When war broke out, the School was advised by the University of London to evacuate immediately. It was decided to move the majority of its operations to Cardiff, a plan that had been formulated a year earlier in response to Hitler's aggression towards Czechoslovakia and the subsequent Munich crisis. Seeing that they needed to make plans for evacuation of all of the University of London colleges, staff from the university met with vice-chancellors from other universities across the country to work out potential arrangements. The School of Pharmacy would be partly accommodated in the University College building in Cathays Park, and partly in the botanical department in Newport Road, about 15 minutes away. The pharmacology laboratories moved to the National Institute for Research in Dairying at Shinfield, near Reading. As Rees

Vernon Lloyd, head of school at the Welsh School of Pharmacy, put it: "the College has been forced to tear up its roots in Bloomsbury and transplant them in the far distant City of Cardiff … the College equipment is not the only thing that had been brought from London. The members of the Association present must be congratulated on their successful transport of a very large quantity of the Square Spirit …"

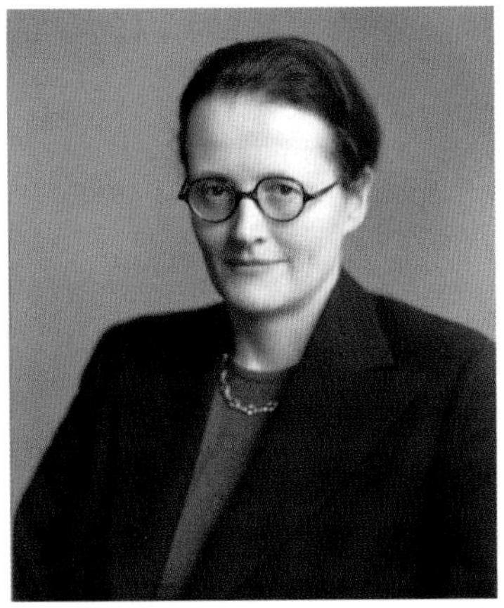

MARTHE LOUISE VOGT (1903–2003)

©Godfrey Argent Studio

MARTHE LOUISE VOGT (1903–2003)

Marthe Vogt was born in Berlin, the daughter of leading neuroanatomists. She studied chemistry and medicine at Berlin University from 1922, and achieved a PhD in 1929. Following neuroscience research in Germany, she won a Rockefeller Travelling Fellowship for one year and worked in Sir Henry Dale's laboratory in Hampstead, and in the pharmacology department at Cambridge University. She gained subsequent scholarships to enable her to continue her research in Britain. However, in 1939 she was categorised at a tribunal as an "enemy alien". She avoided internment through a campaign of letters of support which resulted in her recategorisation as a "friendly alien" in early 1940.

In June 1941, she joined the pharmacological laboratories at the Square, temporarily housed in the Agricultural Research Council facilities in Reading. She began work on the adrenal and its relation to stress, an area that she stayed in for the rest of her career. In 1947, she moved to the department of pharmacology at Edinburgh University. In 1952, she was elected a Fellow of the Royal Society, only the eighth woman to receive this distinction. In 1960, she became head of the pharmacology unit at the Agricultural Research Council's Institute of Animal Physiology, until her retirement in 1968. She continued to publish papers and to receive visiting workers into the 1980s. In fact, one-third of her publications appeared after her retirement. She has been described as "one of the leading neuroscientists of the twentieth century … Marthe's legacy cannot be judged only by what she was able to accomplish herself but by the impetus she gave to all those who followed to revolutionize the treatment of mental illness."

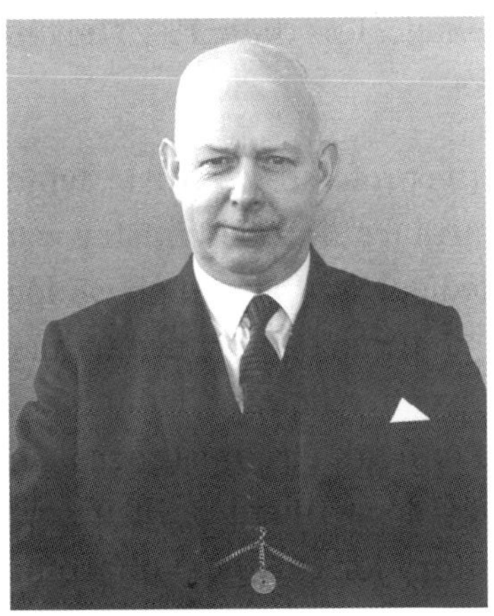

REES VERNON LLOYD (1902–1988)

Welsh School of Pharmacy and Pharmaceutical Sciences, Cardiff University

REES VERNON LLOYD (1902–1988)

Rees Vernon Lloyd studied at the Square as a Jacob Bell Scholar in 1924. In 1930, he was appointed head of the Welsh College of Pharmacy, part of the Cardiff Technical College. His main task on appointment was to instigate an internal degree within the remit of the University of Wales. Vernon Lloyd hosted staff and students from the Square during their evacuation from London to Cardiff during the Second World War, and served as president as the Students' Union in this period.

When the Technical College became the Welsh College of Advanced Technology (CAT) in 1957, the Welsh College of Pharmacy was renamed the Welsh School of Pharmacy. In 1959, Vernon Lloyd was appointed vice-principal of the Welsh CAT, and remained head of the Welsh School of Pharmacy. He retired in 1967, after 37 years in charge of the School. In 2010, the lecture theatre on the ground floor of the School was renamed the Vernon Lloyd Lecture Theatre in his memory.

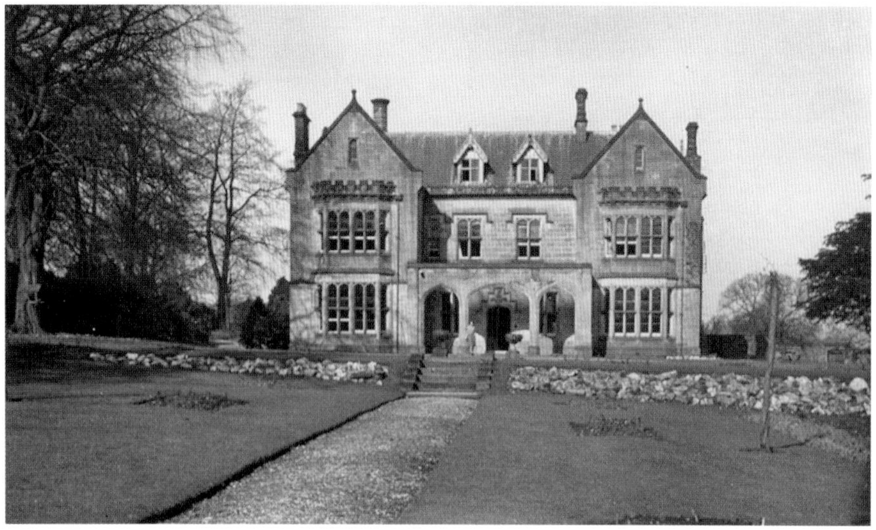

Birdsgrove House in Derbyshire was bought by the Pharmaceutical Society as a convalescent home for its members, but proved invaluable as a wartime headquarters during World War Two, when this photograph was taken.

Royal Pharmaceutical Society Museum

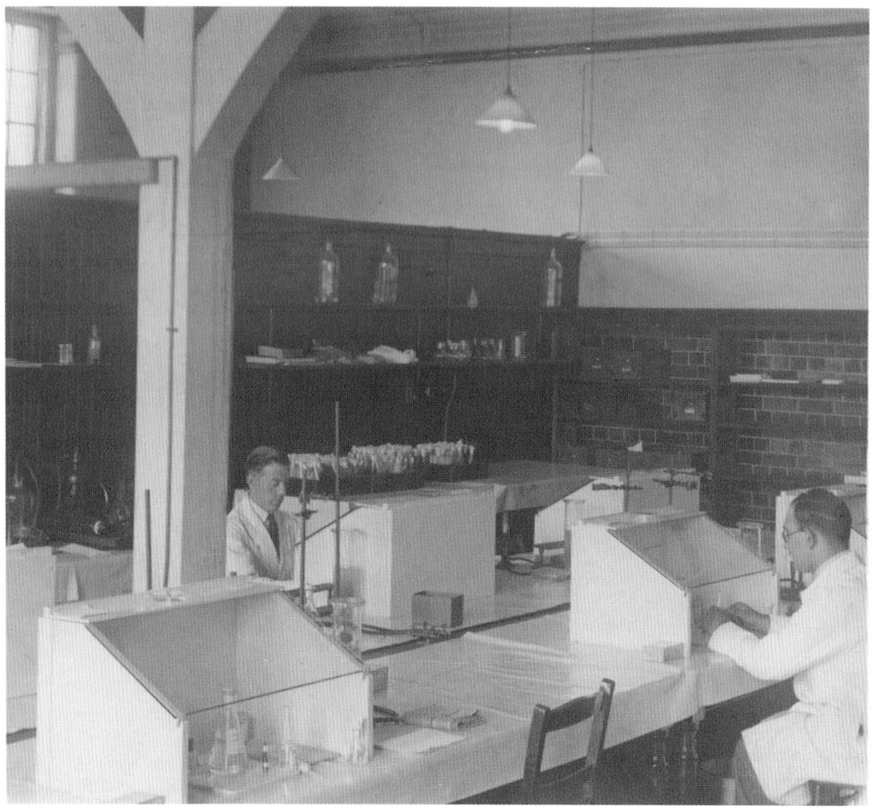

I. Michaels was a demonstrator and J. Mackay was a lab steward during the School's time in Cardiff. They are shown here in the Aseptic Lab.

UCL School of Pharmacy Library

The practicalities of the move, although planned, were not without issues, as a detailed article describing the evacuation in the *Square Chronicle* related. At end of August 1939, most of the staff were on holiday. The dean, Harry Berry, was about to head off to an International Pharmaceutical Federation (FIP) meeting in Berlin, but he received a message from the Foreign Office which made him change his arrangements. Plans for packing up the equipment and furniture had been made in advance. Vans usually used for transporting horses were used, as all racing fixtures were cancelled. Three vans arrived at Bloomsbury Square on Friday 8th September, and were loaded by 11am with 12 tons of the most important equipment from chemistry, pharmacy and physiology. As the article put it, "The musk deer [in the museum collection] gazed with sorrowful eyes at the departure of his friends, and the ancient rubbish they were leaving behind."

The Pharmaceutical Society evacuated its core functions, meanwhile, to Birdsgrove House in Derbyshire, which it had purchased in May 1939 as a convalescent home for pharmacists.

The journey to Cardiff seemed quite upbeat. As a wartime measure, lorries were not supposed to exceed 30 mph, but the School's vans apparently reached 60 mph when on the open road and away from the police. During the journey, those travelling on the vans learnt from the drivers that the lorries had carried several Derby winners. They took a route through Cheltenham and Gloucester "after a glorious run through the Cotswolds, where the rolling downs bared their green and brown splendour to the blue sky." Although the plan was to arrive in Cardiff at about 5pm, their actual arrival time was 6pm after a military traffic diversion. Students and staff helped to unload about half the equipment, and the rest of the unloading was finished the following morning. The vans then returned to London and a second convoy arrived on 14th September. The article reports very little breakage, less than 1%. The final trip was a lorry containing the dean's carpet and desks.

In Cardiff, the dean was allotted a room belonging to the professor of music, which still contained a grand piano. Pharmaceutics and pharmaceutical chemistry were taught at University College, pharmacology at the Medical School and physiology at the medical unit of Cardiff Royal Infirmary. The pharmacognosy department was housed in large wooden huts at the Cardiff University botany department. Both teaching and research continued in spite of the difficult circumstances, and the Welsh staff were very welcoming. The pharmacy department built its own laboratories, one dispensary and one practical laboratory for galenical pharmacy and bacteriology. The Welsh physiology department moved into the biochemistry laboratory in the Royal Infirmary in Cardiff to make space. There was initially some difficulty in finding accommodation for the chemistry department, as Cardiff University College had lost half of its laboratory space to government departments, but the London and Cardiff students ended up sharing a laboratory. In practical terms, this meant that they had to put their equipment in lockers at the end of each class as lots of different students were using the same benches, and it was impossible to run experiments over any period of time. Seven pharmacy research students had to find room in the chemistry department at the technical college as there was no room at University College. However, they did not seem to mind: "Some little time is wasted in many journeys to and from, through a very delightful park."

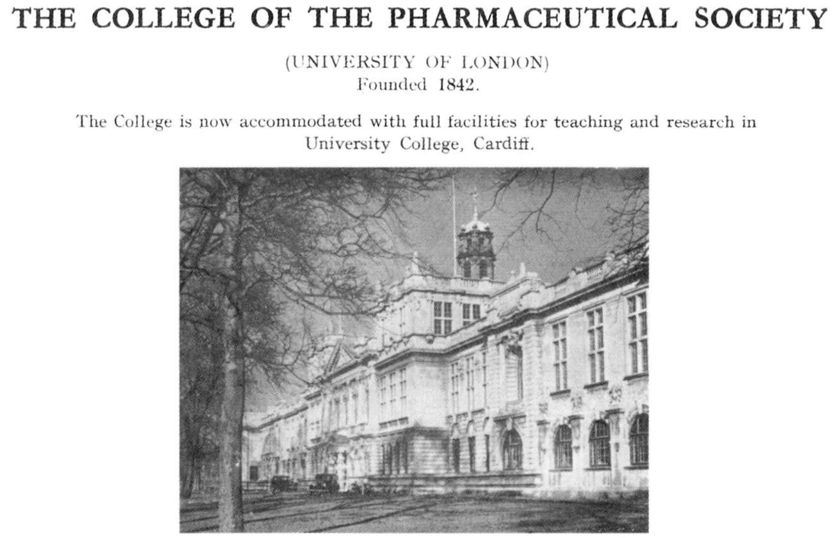
THE COLLEGE OF THE PHARMACEUTICAL SOCIETY

(UNIVERSITY OF LONDON)
Founded 1842.

The College is now accommodated with full facilities for teaching and research in University College, Cardiff.

UCL School of Pharmacy Library

Within three weeks of the first vans arriving, all the necessary equipment had been moved to Cardiff and the allocated laboratories had been adapted. Nearly all of the students who had been accepted for the session were able to come to Cardiff. Dr Linnell had arrived early to deputise for the dean and sort out rooms and student admissions. In fact, the session opened on time in October with the maximum number of students that could be accommodated. As the *Chronicle*'s "Special Correspondent" expressed it: "Although all of us are very comfortable in Cardiff, none of us will be sorry to return to Bloomsbury Square, where we may have difficulty in settling down again after the vastness of University College, the magnificent Civic Centre, and the chiming of the city clock to which we are gradually growing accustomed."

The School attempted to return to London after one year, but a bomb landed in Gower Street at the same time as a consignment of returning pharmaceutical apparatus, and so the return was abandoned. In 1940, the museum specimens, which were still in Bloomsbury Square, were packed in specially made wooden cases and taken care of by the Natural History Museum in South Kensington. Unbeknownst to the staff at the time, that was the end of their central presence in the building, as the museum room became a lecture room on the School's return after the war.

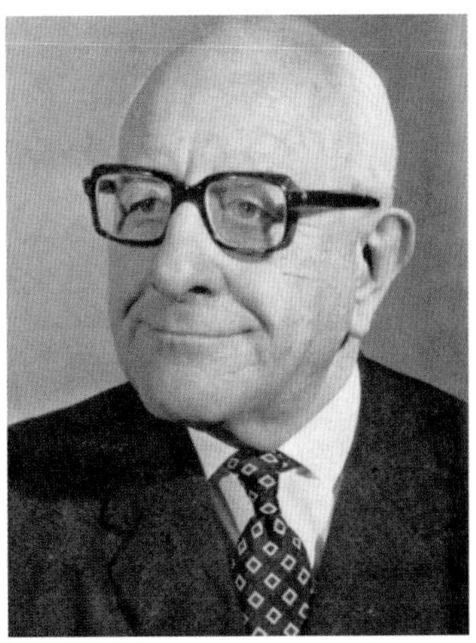

FRANK HARTLEY (1911–1997)

UCL School of Pharmacy Library

FRANK HARTLEY (1911–1997)

Frank Hartley served his apprenticeship in his native Lancashire, and became a chemist & druggist by studying at evening classes. He entered the School as a Bell Scholar in 1930, and registered as a pharmaceutical chemist in 1932. He worked as a demonstrator while studying at Birkbeck College for his BSc, which he gained in 1936. He continued his research under Professor Linnell, and achieved his PhD in 1940 for work on gamma fructose. He was appointed lecturer in pharmaceutical chemistry, and whilst teaching in Cardiff during the School's evacuation, he earned the nickname "8.58" for his punctuality in giving the 9am lectures. He became chief chemist at Organon Laboratories in 1940, aged 29.

During the war, he served as secretary to the Therapeutic Research Council, which was working on the development of penicillin and other antibiotics. He also acted as secretary of the Ministry of Supply's penicillin committee. In 1946, he joined British Drug Houses (BDH) as director of research and scientific services. He was involved in the development of early oral contraceptives, including dimethisterone and megestrol acetate.

He returned to the Square in 1962 as dean. He was co-opted on to the Senate of the University in 1968 and was elected deputy vice-chancellor in 1973 and vice-chancellor in 1976. He was made CBE in 1970, awarded the Pharmaceutical Society's Charter gold medal in 1974, and was knighted in 1977 for services to pharmacy. He was made an honorary Fellow of the Royal College of Physicians in 1979, and of the Royal College of Surgeons in 1980.

Hartley served as a Society examiner for eight years, and was chairman of the British Pharmaceutical Conference in 1957. In 1974, he was appointed chairman of the University Grants Committee. He served on the *British Pharmacopoeia* Commission from 1953 to 1980, and was its first pharmacist chairman. He was also the UK delegate to the *European Pharmacopeia* Commission from 1964 to 1980. He was a member of the Poisons Board, the Committee on Safety of Drugs and the Committee on Safety of Medicines, alongside a number of other government, pharmacy and education bodies and commissions. He was also president of the Royal Institute of Chemistry from 1965 to 1967. His successor as dean, James Swarbrick, commented: "Frank Hartley is a man who leaves large footprints – so large that it is really not possible to fill them. One is therefore forced to walk a somewhat different path."

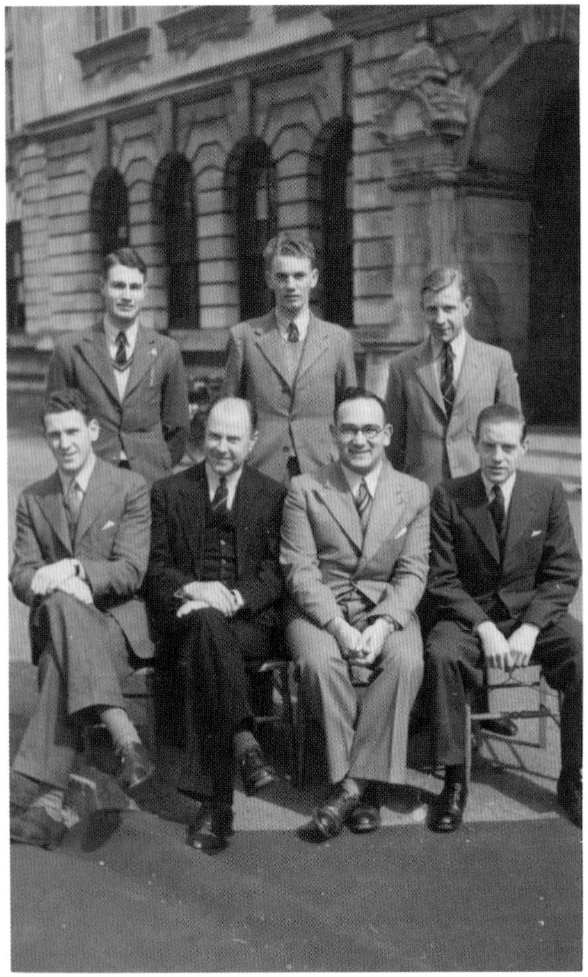

Staff pictured in Cardiff: J. Stenlake, J. Hindle and H. Bean in the back row, with J. Oakley, H. Berry, I. Michaels and J. Mackay in front.

UCL School of Pharmacy Library

The School was based in the Welsh capital for about three years. Their neighbours were the Ministry of Supply (Chemical Inspection) on one side and King's College of Household and Domestic Science on the other, both institutions also evacuated from their London bases. As the School had brought a big still with them, they ended up supplying their own distilled water, and also supplies for the government departments and the King's College of Household Science. The expertise of the staff was also appreciated in their temporary homes. Professor Berry, for example, was appointed Pharmaceutical Adviser to the Welsh Board of Health for South Wales.

The students' social life continued with the Pharmaceutical Students' Society as part of Cardiff University Students' Union. This meant that they were able to use the Students' Union building in Park Place, Cathays Park. Both staff and students felt that they benefited greatly from mixing with students from across the university during their time in Cardiff, something they did not manage to do as easily at Bloomsbury Square. In addition, the students were exposed to a different cultural influence when a group of "Czecho-Slovakian" pharmacists, forced to flee their homes when the Nazis invaded, attended a course at the College in 1941–42. Pharmacy students also took on fire-watching and home-guard duties in Cardiff during their time there.

The pharmacy students admitted that the standard of sport in the University teams was too high for them, but they were able to obtain help from the technical college students to arrange fixtures. However, the table tennis club was curtailed in Cardiff as they had no room or table. The pharmacy students also had to take it in turns to play soccer and rugby as they were unable to field teams for both sports on the same Saturday. They ran practice sessions for hockey, but did not hold any matches. A cycling club was formed. The students took advantage of the Cardiff rowing club facilities to form a boat club, and continued the rambling club, although an article in the *Chronicle* confessed that "Occasional difficulties were encountered because members of the Club did not know where they were going or how to pronounce the name when they arrived." The rambling club also decided not to continue with their traditional midnight ramble in case they were mistaken for enemy parachutists.

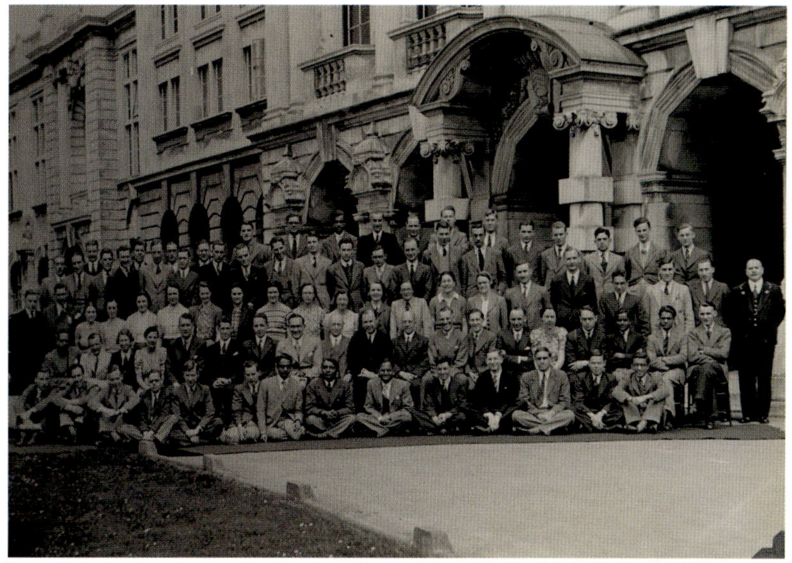

The School year group photograph for the first year in Cardiff, 1939-40, taken outside the impressive university buildings.

UCL School of Pharmacy Library

One of the key issues (at least for the male students) was a shortage of women pharmacy students, so students from the Welsh College of Domestic Arts were invited to the Christmas parties, alongside students from the Welsh College of Pharmacy. The annual college dinner was also continued, the first being held at the Carlton Restaurant in Cardiff on 24th January 1940.

The more formal elements of the Association also continued, such as maintaining its employment bureau from Cardiff. The *Square Chronicle* was produced throughout this period, although the type size was reduced greatly to maximise the amount of content that could be produced on limited paper supplies. By 1943, the thicker coloured cover had also disappeared and the editions were annual rather than twice a year. Although the minute book had been left in London, the Association's AGMs were held in Cardiff, with R.V. Lloyd, head of the Welsh School of Pharmacy, as the Association's president. However, the *Chronicle* of June 1943 explained that the Association had not celebrated the centenary of the School as they would have done "in more tranquil times".

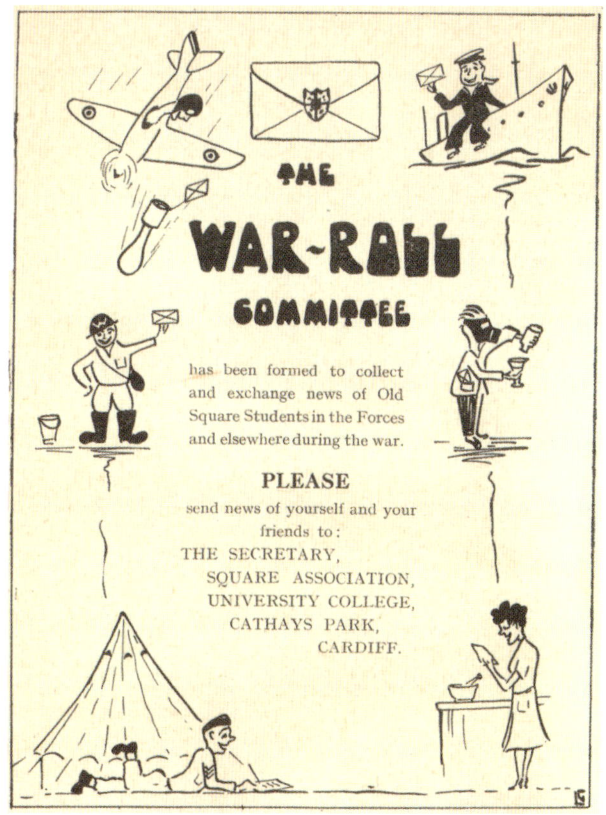

Square Chronicle, **October 1941.**

UCL School of Pharmacy Library

While Rees Lloyd took over as president of the Students' Association and its committee was restricted to those living in Cardiff, Hugh Linstead took up the responsibility to try to continue social events in London. On 6th March 1940, the Association held a dinner dance in place of old boys' and old girls' dinners. The following year, on 19th April 1941, a London lunch was held at the Holborn Restaurant, even though all of the windows had been blown out the night before. In 1942, a London Committee was formed to keep the Association going in the capital, and Miss M. Neal started a rambling club based in London. In the same year, the old boys' and old girls' dinners were reinstated and an entertainment evening was held at the Square.

However, the obituaries pages in the *Chronicle* showed that past students were not immune to the obvious dangers of staying in London. One edition reported that Mary Helen Whayman, who had qualified from the Square in 1934, was killed during an air raid in May 1941 when her house received a direct hit. She had been the chief pharmacist at Croydon General Hospital.

Sadly, the evacuated students were not safe in Cardiff, as the city, renowned for its ports, was heavily bombed throughout the war. K.M.N. MacClaren ("Mac"), social secretary of the Association in London and Cardiff, was killed during an air raid on Cardiff in February 1941. The *Chronicle* commented that

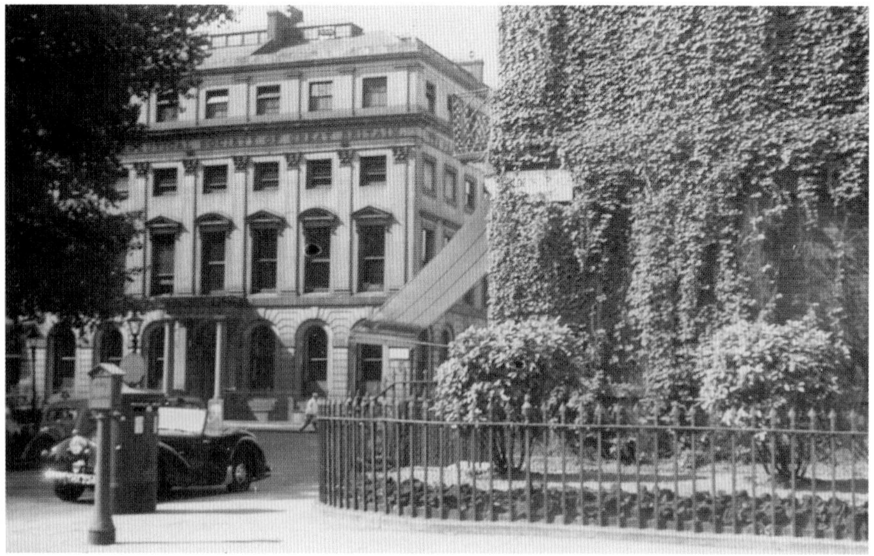

This unusual view of 17 Bloomsbury Square, taken from Bedford Place, was used for a Society greetings card in 1941.

Royal Pharmaceutical Society Museum

**“Paint is peeling from the ceiling
And the wall in the hall
But it will last, if used with care
Until we move to Brunswick Square!”**

E.M. Dickinson, Square Chronicle, March 1944

“Social activity during the Autumn Term has been maintained, despite the interruptions of the siren.” During the Cardiff Blitz, the University's student building was also damaged.

The decision to return to London was finally made in 1944, and the job of “Packing and unpacking”, as an article in the *Chronicle* titled it, had to be done. The article, written by a student who helped with the effort, explained that “Everything to be packed was either ‘Fragile’, ‘Exceedingly Fragile’, or ‘Irreplaceable’.” Everything was double-wrapped in corrugated card and then packed in straw. However, “Hell hath no fury like a demonstrator finding the 10,001st eight ounce bottle when 10,000 have already been packed.”

The scene at Bloomsbury Square on their arrival to unpack the equipment was mixed, to say the least. The main lecture theatre was still being decorated. The pharmacy laboratory looked like a “dark and dirty dungeon … Our eyes wandered round the wilderness and our hearts sank … The Dispensaries – still grubby after four scrubbings by the cleaners and Mary and Jo, were soon looking more business-like as mortars and pill machines piled up.” Their efforts to unpack and clean had quick effects: “The dungeon began to look a little more like a lab – but Oh! for the airyness [*sic*] of Cardiff!” The effect of the war years on the house was clearly quite shocking: “The common rooms (common rubbish dumps they seem to have been during the time we were away) – were straightened up, but still looked bare and empty”, but the team work to get it back into use was evident from the article: “The tale of how the large refrigerator was taken upstairs by so few was recounted with obvious pride … At last, with the Lecture Theatre cleaned up after the decorators, all was ready (at least to an uncritical eye) for the Inaugural Meeting.”

The School's dean who had to reinvigorate the organisation after the war was Harry Berry. His secretary, Margaret Fleming (“Flem”), had been injured by a V1 bomb and was unable to work.

He called back staff and students from war service early, including Jack Oakley, John Stenlake, Arnold Beckett and David Train. By October 1944, he had enough staff in place to reopen the School. Sixty per cent of the students were ex-service men and 50% of the applicants were women. Berry fixed a quota of 30% female students. Berry and Wilfred Linnell had been confirmed as professors of London University in 1943, and when Gladwin Buttle was appointed head of pharmacology in 1945, he also received recognition from the University. Jim Fairbairn took over as head of pharmacognosy from T.E. Wallis, to allow him to reduce his work commitments, although he still continued in the department, aged 69.

Louis Sharpe, working as one of the demonstrators in the first session back in Bloomsbury Square from October 1944, recalled that there were 28 first year students in two sections, and 10 second year students

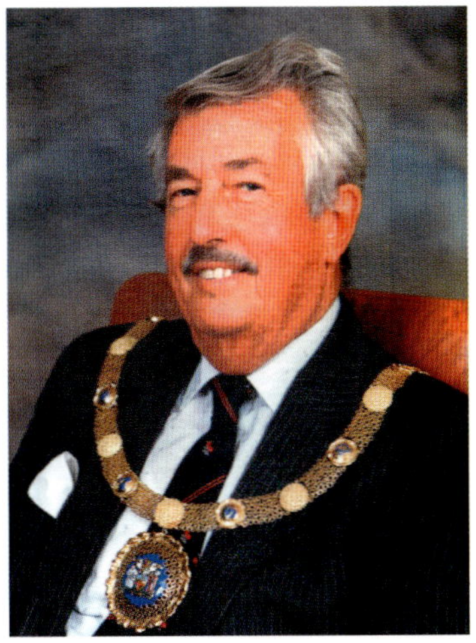

ARNOLD HEYWORTH BECKETT (1920–2010)

Royal Pharmaceutical Society Museum

ARNOLD HEYWORTH BECKETT (1920–2010)

Arnold Beckett finished his doctorate at the Square in 1950, having registered as a pharmaceutical chemist in 1941. In 1958, he was appointed co-editor of the *Journal of Medicinal and Pharmaceutical Chemistry*. His textbooks, written with John Stenlake, and his publications on drug metabolism, the chemistry of natural products and the relationship between stereochemistry and analgesic action were all extremely influential, and he published over 460 scientific papers and supervised 95 PhD students during his career. He became head of the Chelsea School of Pharmacy in 1959, and remained there for more than 30 years.

In 1965, the International Cycling Union asked him to carry out drug tests on competitors in the Milk Race. In 1966, Beckett supervised drugs testing at the football World Cup in England, which led to an invitation from the Olympics Committee to be involved in this area of work when they set up a medical commission in 1967. Beckett gained an international reputation as an expert on drugs in sport. He subsequently served on the medical commissions of various Commonwealth Games and on the British and International Olympic Committees. He was also a member of the medical panel of the International Federation of Football Associations. However, from the 1990s onwards, he worked on the side of accused athletes, such as skier Alain Baxter, to advise them in their defence against the official boards. He served as a non-executive chairman of the nutraceutical company Vitabiotics for 18 years.

Professor Beckett was president of the Pharmaceutical Society in 1981, and served continuously on the Council from 1965 to 1990. He received the Society's Hanbury memorial medal in 1974, its Charter gold medal in 1977, and a number of awards from foreign pharmacy organisations. He was president of the Board of Pharmaceutical Sciences at the FIP in the 1970s, and was awarded their highest pharmaceutical sciences award in 1982.

in the year. Although there was a research laboratory for each department, there were very few research students because of the war, and most of the research was carried out by staff. The total number of academic staff was 12, consisting of heads of department and full-time demonstrators. The course at this point was a full five-day week, including nine or 10 hours each week in both the chemistry and pharmaceutics laboratories. The principal of the University of London reflected in 1944 that, with the colleges back in London, academic life was returning to normal. He remarked that the examinations that year were carried out "without casualties, other than those normally caused by these exacting but essential tests."

VE (Victory in Europe) Day, 8th May 1945, was a momentous occasion, not least for those students at the Square. They organised food in the lecture theatre, and then walked down Kingsway to Trafalgar Square to join the thousands crowded into the London landmark, seeing themselves later in a photograph in the *Daily Sketch* newspaper. The students reported that they did the "Conger" [*sic*] through the Mall and sat

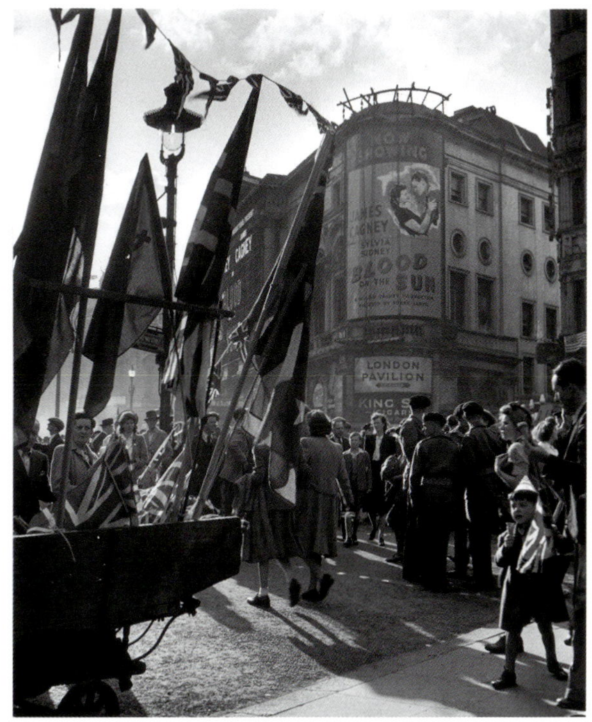

Photographer Wolf Suschitzky captured the atmosphere of VE Day in Piccadilly Circus.

© Museum of London

in St James's Park, and then came back to the Square and had a scented foot bath in the women's common room. They went back out into Holborn in the early hours of the morning, and then came back to sleep in the common room.

Although the war was now over, the impact on pharmacy was significant. Pharmacists and pharmacy students had been a reserved occupation, but they had served an important function on the home front. As R.V. Lloyd put it, "In peace time the man in the street has always looked upon the chemist in his shop as a friend in need. In war time, this relationship can become a very valuable aid in preserving the morale of the general public." The impact of the war on the profession was particularly significant for women pharmacists. During the war, the Ministry of Labour and National Service issued instructions that women pharmacists and dispensers were not to be called up. Miss Islip, the National Association of Women Pharmacist's employment secretary, asked in *The Pharmaceutical Journal* of 18th April 1942 that "married and retired women who could return to pharmacy during the present emergency should do so as soon as possible." The shortages that the war had produced also affected pharmacy supplies. The editor of the *Chronicle* in October 1941 commented: "It is somewhat baffling to peruse a Pharmacopoeia, which consists of a nightmare collection of everything T.E.W. [T.E. Wallis] so recently taught us to shun. We hopefully await the day when olive oil, glycerine and syrup of orange reappear on the shelves, and when eggs and tinned fruit cease to be merely pleasant recollections." The *National War Formulary* and amendments to the *British Pharmaceutical Codex* specified substitutes to be used in case of shortages. Wartime rationing did not fully end until 1954, and the austerity that such a long period of conflict inevitably produced had both physical and psychological impact for many years to come.

However, as is well documented, the impact of the war on drug development was nothing short of revolutionary. The most famous story is that of penicillin, with the war providing Howard Florey's existing team in Oxford with increased urgency to produce effective antibacterials. Mass production of penicillin in the United States allowed supplies in sufficient quantities in time for the D-Day landings in 1944. After the war, the search for other antibacterial drugs launched "the antibiotic era." Another key wartime development was in the field of antimalarials. It had been anticipated that German supplies of existing drugs, such as mepacrine, would be interrupted, and so projects to produce alternatives began in the early war years. The successes were proguanil for ICI in 1945 and chloroquine for Winthrop in 1946. These developments were the first of many and, alongside the launch of the National Health Service in 1948, marked a new age for pharmacy in the postwar period. Cyril Maplethorpe, chairman of the Society's Education Committee, identified the consequences of these developments for pharmacy: "if the pharmacist of to-day hopes to take his proper place in the new health service his pharmacy must be so equipped that he can handle any of the specialised products [penicillin] which are being called for by the medical practitioner."

EXAMINATIONS

The first candidate for the newly instituted BPharm degree took the examination in 1927, and was successful. She was Phyllis Sully from Chelsea Polytechnic, not a student from the Square. She went on to achieve the BSc (Lond) in Botany in 1935.

In 1928, the exam regulations were reviewed, and in the following year, the teaching of organic chemistry was transferred back from University College London (UCL) to the Square. The regulations were amended again in 1932 to include recognition of apprenticeships in manufacturing pharmaceutical laboratories. However, this appreciation of the reality of the breadth of the profession was at odds with a 1930 report from a Council committee, which suggested that retail pharmacists should remain at the lower chemist & druggist level and hospital pharmacists should qualify as pharmaceutical chemists. The proposal was that the two types of pharmacists should follow different educational routes. It was rejected, not because of any apparent concerns about restricting the academic achievements of individuals in any particular sector of pharmacy, but because it was seen to be impractical to run two parallel courses at most schools of pharmacy.

In the context of increasing drug development, the Society introduced postgraduate diplomas in Pharmaceutical Analysis and Biochemical Analysis in 1932. The research laboratories had established themselves in the prewar period as a strong centre for pharmacological science. Their first success was to set up a standard for tincture of *Strophanthus*, working with Dr J.W. Trevan of Wellcome Physiological Research Laboratories. Their reputation grew internationally, and in the first 11 years of their existence, Professor Burn later recalled that research students came from Australia, Belgium, China, Denmark, France, Hungary, Iceland, India, South Africa, Spain, Thailand and the United States.

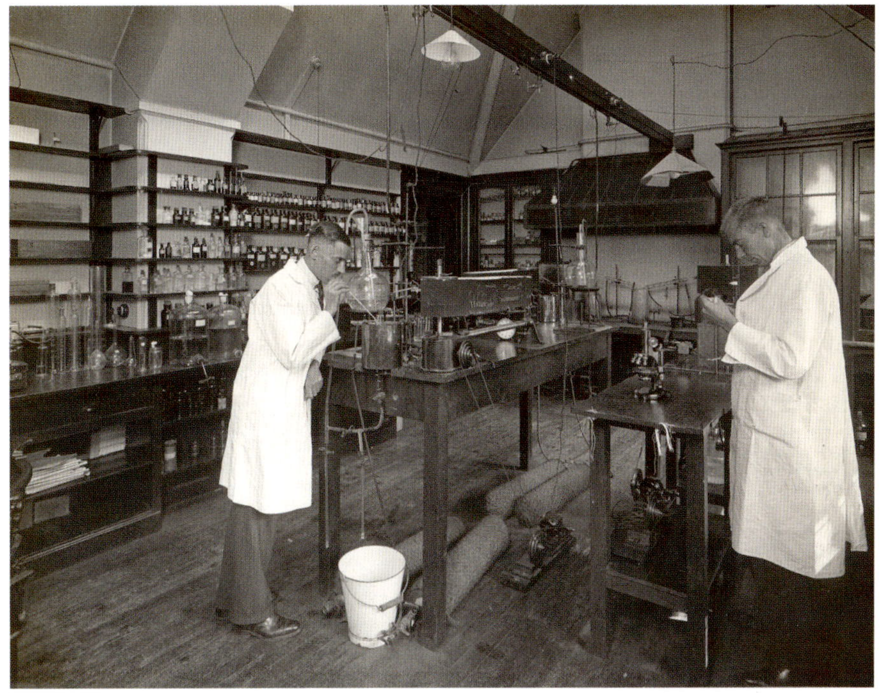

By the late 1920s, this research laboratory in the Galen Place extension which had been first established for galenical pharmacy, was being used for pharmacology work.

Royal Pharmaceutical Society Museum

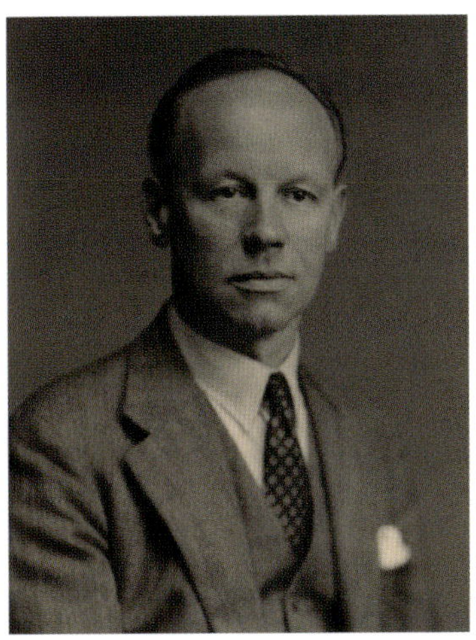

JOSHUA HAROLD BURN (1892–1981)

© National Portrait Gallery, London

JOSHUA HAROLD BURN (1892–1981)

J.H. Burn studied natural sciences at Emmanuel College, Cambridge, before working as a pharmacologist at the Wellcome Physiological Research Laboratory. When the First World War broke out, he joined the Royal Engineers (Signals). In 1918, he qualified in Medicine at Guy's Hospital, London, and then joined the Medical Research Council. He was appointed in 1926 as the director of the Pharmaceutical Society's new Pharmacological Laboratory, and continued his research on pharmacological assays of material such as ergot, digitalis and vitamin A. In 1933, he was appointed professor of pharmacology and dean of the College of Pharmacy. He resigned in 1937 to move to the post of professor of pharmacology at the University of Oxford.

He was a founder member of the British Pharmacological Society in 1931, and a member of the *British Pharmacopoeia* Commission for the 1932 edition. In 1940, he was nominated as a member of the General Council of Medical Education and Registration of the United Kingdom. In 1942, he was elected a Fellow of the Royal Society, and served on its Council in 1944–5. He was the author of numerous papers and the books *Methods of Biological Assay* (1928), *Recent Advances in Materia Medica* (1931) and *Biological Standardisation* (1937).

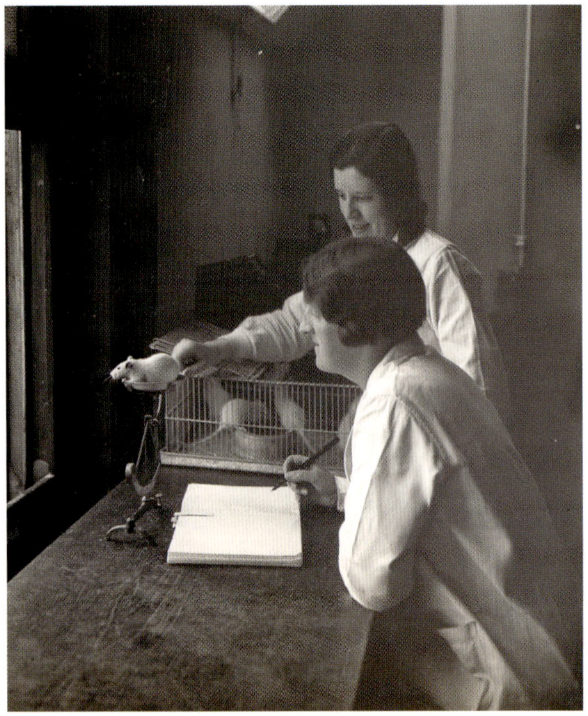

Experiments involving animals were an accepted part of pharmacy teaching when this photograph was taken in about 1928.

Royal Pharmaceutical Society Museum

J.H. Burn, head of the Society's pharmacology laboratories since their opening in 1926, was in a perfect position to influence the emphasis of the courses to meet the challenges of the new therapeutic environment. In an article in *The Pharmaceutical Journal* in August 1933, he suggested that physiology and pharmacology should be introduced into the curriculum as long as this did not have a negative impact on the standard of the existing subjects. He argued that it was only interesting to prepare a medicine if you understood how it might be used, and that these new subjects would "illuminate and inform" a pharmacy student's work. He suggested that a knowledge of physiology and pharmacology would enable the pharmacist to provide a much better service, to advise the doctor who was unable to keep up to speed with the rapid increase in the number of drugs, and to serve a wider audience, for example by carrying out chemical tests. In fact, this was a long-standing argument. As early as 1859, Dr George Wilson of Edinburgh had proposed that physiology should be added to the pharmacy course as one of the three essential areas of knowledge for pharmacists. He argued that a pharmacist needed an understanding of the physiological action or influence of medicines on the body in order to be "a safe dispenser of drugs".

On Greenish's retirement in 1933, Burn took on the role of dean and was therefore in a good position to carry these changes through. From 1934, physiology, later changed to pharmacology, was taught in the School by the laboratories' staff. Burn was joined in 1934 by Harry Berry as vice-dean and reader in pharmaceutics, with a special interest in bacteriology.

In the 1933 *Journal* article, Burn also defended the educational standards for pharmacy, stating that it was a "sad fact" that pharmacists have to rely on trading for income, but this did not decrease the amount of training that a retail pharmacist required. On the contrary, criticism from other professionals could only be met if the educational standard of pharmacists was increased. In addition, the likelihood of the welfare state being extended to wives and families, rather than just the wage-earner as in the existing National Health Insurance Scheme, would require at least a maintenance of the current educational standard. Burn felt strongly that all pharmacy students should aim to take the BPharm to give them the best opportunities for the future, and to provide time in the course to do more than just learn what was needed for the examinations.

> **"The age of the older chemist is passing, the age of the Biochemist, the Biophysicist and the Biopharmacist is dawning, despite the fact that some may not welcome the dawn."**
>
> *Square Chronicle, November 1933*

The major update to the exam regulations came in 1935, following a report of the Society's Syllabus Committee in the previous year. The ability to continue directly from qualifying as a chemist & druggist to a pharmaceutical chemist was confirmed. The syllabus of the Qualifying exam was changed to include physiology, and a practical exam in pharmacognosy. Physiology was also introduced into the chemist & druggist and pharmaceutical chemist exams, botany was discontinued and pharmacognosy was reduced. The subjects for both the London BPharm degree and the pharmaceutical chemist qualification were therefore altered to be pharmaceutical chemistry, pharmacy, physiology, pharmacognosy and forensic pharmacy, which meant a more vocational content. It also allowed the first year of the higher course to be assimilated into the chemist & druggist course. London University matriculation was adopted as the preliminary standard. The subject of biology, meaning zoology combined with botany, was added to the preliminary scientific exam. The Society's Council was also given the power by the Privy Council to lay down the conditions under which apprenticeships should be served.

The inclusion of more biology content and physiology finally provided students with some understanding of recent therapeutic developments including vaccines and sera. Combined with a higher standard of knowledge of the chemistry of drugs, students were better trained to understand the action of drugs. In 1935, Ernest Saville Peck reported that "These advances tend to a closer approximation of pharmacy to the altered conditions due to the progress made in medical science and should be conducive to the fuller recognition of the important place which pharmacy occupies in the health service of the Nation." The students at the Square fully engaged with the changes to the syllabus, including holding a debate in 1935 with the motion "In the opinion of this House the introduction of Physiology into Pharmacy is unnecessary." The motion was proposed by Mr Fitch, editor of *The Pharmaceutical Journal*, and opposed by Mr Berry, then reader in pharmaceutics. Although the motion was lost by a large majority, the author of the report in the *Chronicle* teased, "We wonder if the opinion of the meeting was still the same after the first Physiology test." The facts that most pharmacy students had studied no biology at school and that there were no biologists on the staffs of most schools of pharmacy definitely presented a challenge.

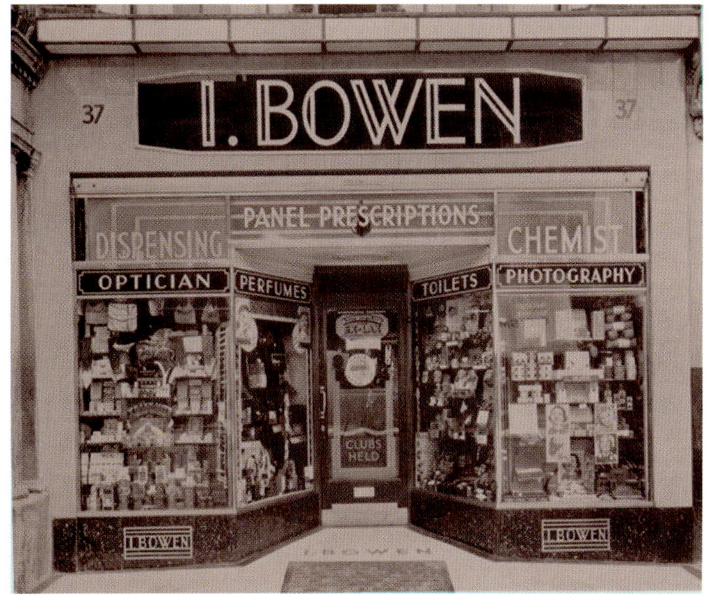

I. Bowen's pharmacy with its distinctive Art Deco styling of the 1930s, advertised above the door that it dispensed "panel prescriptions" for those who were eligible under the National Health Insurance scheme, first launched in 1912.

Royal Pharmaceutical Society Museum

From 1935, all teaching for BPharm courses was transferred to the Square. The editor of the *Square Chronicle* recognised how difficult the situation had been with subjects split between the School and UCL, not least the distance between the buildings and the different methods of teaching. However, there had also been the impact on the social life at the Square, as the second years had split loyalties between School and University clubs and events. The current session would be "memorable as the year in which the Square once more becomes a unity." In 1937, the School stopped teaching for the Major exam, and only ran courses for the new chemist & druggist Qualifying exam, the pharmaceutical chemist diploma exam accredited by the Society and for the final exams of the new pharmacy degree. As such, through the 1940s, the School was the major national pharmacy examination centre for Society exams and for the internal and external BPharm degree courses of the University.

"The growth of pseudo-scientific knowledge among laymen, due, in part, to a smattering of science taught in schools, and also the craze for articles on popular science in the daily press written in an elementary manner – occasionally by scientists but more often by ill-informed journalists – has largely dispersed the mysterious halo enveloping our craft. The pharmacist is no longer regarded in the same light as the alchemist of old."

Square Chronicle, November 1934

During the war, the University of London had decided that all degrees should require three years' study from Intermediate or Higher School Certificate level, rather than two. For the School of Pharmacy, this meant a rethink of the proposed layout of the new building and a reduction of the number of students that could be accepted each year. Of course, this meant less income through fees. The three-year BPharm honours degree course was first introduced in 1946. From 1950, it was the only course on offer at the Square. Until the 1960s, the BPharm syllabus served as a model for newer courses in the United Kingdom and throughout the world.

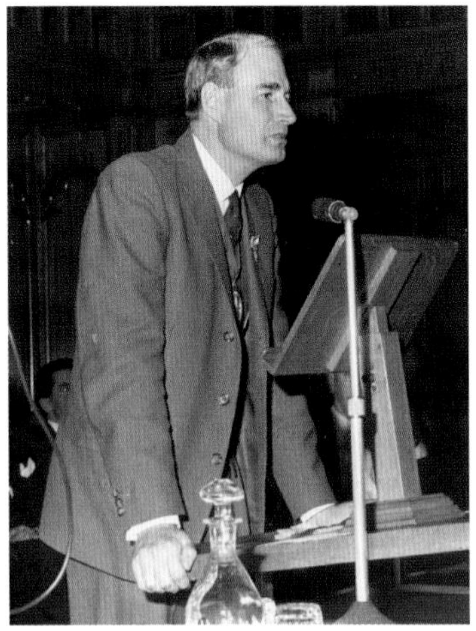

JOHN BEDFORD STENLAKE (1920–2006)

Royal Pharmaceutical Society Museum

JOHN BEDFORD STENLAKE (1920–2006)

After an apprenticeship with Boots, John Stenlake entered the Square as a Jacob Bell Scholar in 1939. He served in the Royal Air Force during the Second World War, and returned to the School as a demonstrator and then as an assistant lecturer. Meanwhile, he gained a BSc from Birkbeck College, and then his doctorate in 1950. He was promoted to lecturer in pharmaceutical chemistry at the same time.

In 1952, he took a post as senior lecturer in pharmaceutical chemistry at the Royal College of Science and Technology in Glasgow. In 1962, he became professor and head of the pharmacy department at the College, where he oversaw the transition of the college to the University of Strathclyde, and became dean of the university's School of Pharmaceutical Sciences from 1967 to 1975.

He was a member of the *British Pharmacopoeia* Commission from 1963 and leader of the UK delegation to the *European Pharmacopoeia* Commission. He was a member of the Committee on Safety of Medicines from 1970 to 1979, and a member of the Medicines Commission.

His most influential achievement was his contribution to the discovery of atracurium besylate, the first short-acting and readily reversible skeletal muscle relaxant for use in surgery. The drug was developed by a research team led by Professor Stenlake in the pharmacy department of Strathclyde University in collaboration with the Wellcome Foundation.

Professor Stenlake was made a CBE in 1985. He was awarded the Society's Charter gold medal in 1990. He also received the Society's Harrison memorial medal in 1974.

The postwar education policy at the Society was primarily based on the findings of a Committee of Enquiry set up after the 1933 Pharmacy and Poisons Act. One of the major developments was the ultimate phasing out of the chemist & druggist course, with the aspiration that pharmacy should be an all-graduate profession. One of the more immediate discussions in the 1940s was whether pharmacognosy was still relevant for students. The argument for its retention was not helped by the fact that most students were not enthusiastic. Of course, this could be blamed on the existing syllabus, which had not kept up with recent research, and relied mainly on a passive ability to memorise plants. As the editor of the *Chronicle* put it, "the facts, which he [the pharmacy student] would have been expected to remember in Botany, he will now be required to be acquainted with under the synonym of Pharmacognosy." Derrick Dunlop, acting as the Privy Council Visitor in 1947, sympathised with the students' lack of enthusiasm: "While a knowledge of plant anatomy may be of some slight importance for a candidate's future studies in pharmacognosy, a combined broad course in the biology of living things would be of much more fundamental and stimulating educational value than the learning of the details of the morphology of fruits, stems, leaves and dogfish." Dunlop also recognised that the pharmacy students were stuck with some outdated aspects of their course because of wider issues within the medical profession: "it is unfortunate that young pharmacists should have to pass a special examination in the deciphering of prescriptions written by members of a learned profession. It seems, however, that as long as medical men prescribe old-fashioned remedies in undecipherable Latin, pharmaceutical students will have to suffer."

"What is the future to be – are we merely to be vendors of packed products, ethical or otherwise, or are we to be highly skilled professional people who, with doctors, dentists and others fit into a fully co-ordinated health service? Much depends on us – we must move forward in education."

C.W. Maplethorpe, February 1946

The 1944 Education Act set up a grant system for the first time to encourage school leavers to go straight into higher education. For pharmacy students to take advantage of this, apprenticeships and pupilages had to take place after the Qualifying exam, and so the development of today's preregistration period was set in train.

In 1946, the student body at the Square was markedly different from its prewar make-up. In 1933, there had been 60 students on the chemist & druggist course, 14 studying for the pharmaceutical chemist exam, eight aiming for the BPharm degree and six research students. In 1946, the biggest group was the 37 students for the degree course, followed by 19 aspiring pharmaceutical chemists. There were 18 research students, and only 16 on the chemist & druggist course. Students were finally leaving behind the Victorian educational structure, ready to face the challenges ahead.

OTHER SCHOOLS

The external London BPharm degree, established in 1925, was slow to catch on outside London. It seemed that most pharmacy students purely wanted to gain the basic level of qualification, and not anything more academic. For example, at Nottingham School of Pharmacy, the normal intake in the 1930s was up to 80 students, but nearly all took the chemist & druggist qualification. In 1932, only two students took the BPharm and three took the pharmaceutical chemist course. In 1939, this was still only four BPharms and two pharmaceutical chemists.

In 1932, the Society's Council reviewed the position of various schools other than its own, particularly private ones. They took the new policy direction that there was no longer a place for private pharmacy schools, and decided not to recognise new ones. Their intention was that the old ones would gradually fade away owing to their inability to keep up with the new standards, and the increasing number of public teaching institutions for pharmacy. During the 1930s, the University of Manchester absorbed the private schools in its area, the private schools in Bath were taken over by Merchant Venturers College in Bristol, and the private schools in Leeds were taken over by the University of Leeds. By 1938, only three private schools survived: the London College, the South of England College and the Liverpool School of Pharmacy. Liverpool was the last to close, in 1949, when it was taken over by the technical college.

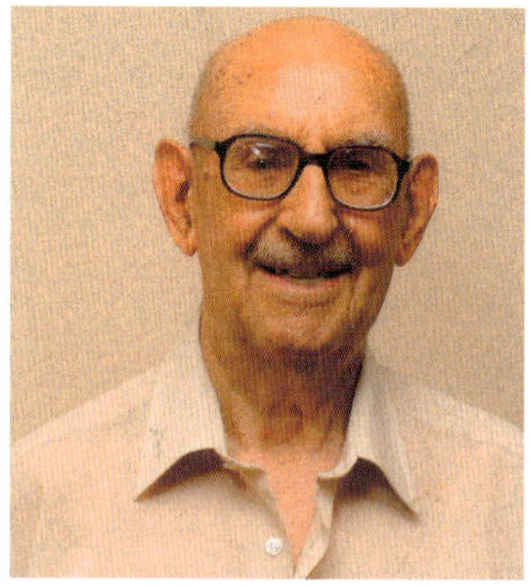

EDWARD JOSEPH SHELLARD (1914–2010)

© Richard Harper

EDWARD JOSEPH SHELLARD (1914–2010)

Joe Shellard registered as a pharmaceutical chemist in 1937. He spent some time working as a research pharmacist in industry before taking a post teaching pharmacognosy at the Merchant Venturers' Technical College in Bristol. He moved to Chelsea College in 1957, where he built up a pharmacognosy research group in the department of pharmacy. He gained his PhD on *Ipomoea* and jalap resins in the late 1950s. He was made professor of pharmacognosy in 1969. He was a pioneer in the use of chromatographic techniques for the separation of complex plant product mixtures. He published many scientific papers, but was also an expert in the history of pharmacognosy, and wrote a series of papers in his retirement on "A History of British Pharmacognosy, 1842–1980", published in *The Pharmaceutical Journal.* He also carried out a number of oral history interviews, including with his teacher, T.E. Wallis, for the Pharmaceutical Society.

He served on the Society's Adjudicating Committee. He was president of the Medicinal Plants Section of FIP from 1980 to 1984, having been an active member of the section since the 1950s. He wrote two textbooks, *Practical Plant Chemistry for Pharmacy Students* (1957) and *Quantitative Paper and Thin-Layer Chromatography* (1968).

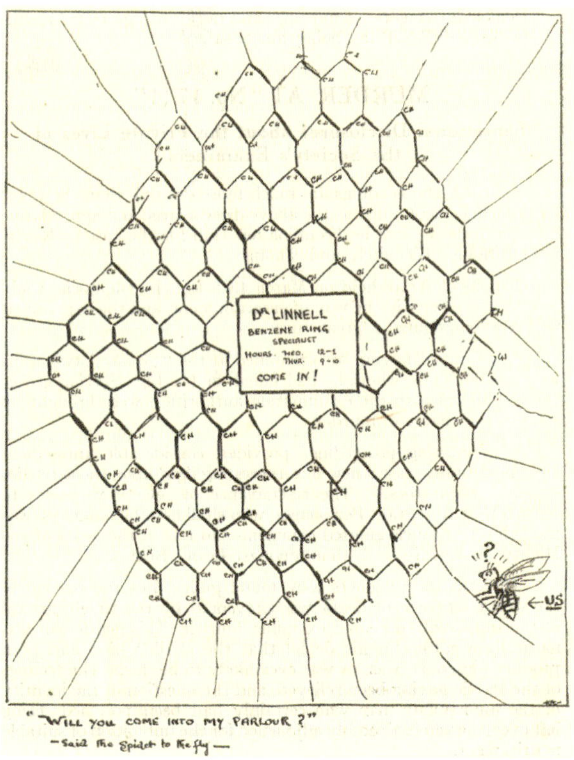

Dr Linnell, "Benzene Ring Specialist", is depicted as a spider inviting the student flies into his web in this cartoon published in the *Square Chronicle* in August 1930. The ring form of benzene had been discovered in 1865, but details of its hexagonal flat structure had only recently been published by Kathleen Lonsdale in the *Proceedings of the Royal Society* in 1929.

UCL School of Pharmacy Library

TEACHING

Throughout this period, pharmacy teaching struggled to keep up with the new developments in drugs and testing. An article in the *Square Chronicle* in July 1927 called for more training for pharmacists in laboratory methods such as diagnosis and bacteriology. It also recognised that the pharmacist's role within the public health team should not be overlooked, and that pharmacists needed to work hard to earn their place alongside other professionals: "it may well be that nothing short of a reformed public health service will give them a status and remuneration to justify the effort involved."

A new course in bacteriology for second year students had been introduced in the 1932–3 session, run for two weeks before the usual term start date. The newly created bacteriology laboratory was also used for microscopy for pharmacognosy and by biochemical analysts in a new course. A fire in the new laboratory on 28th December 1932 resulted in the attendance of three or four fire engines, but very little damage to the facilities. In 1933, the small lecture theatre was renovated to act as a sterile dispensing area.

As for the more established subjects, the place for materia medica, or pharmacognosy, in the course was under threat. Having had informal charge of the museum in his role as lecturer in botany from 1925, Dr Wallis accepted a post as its part-time curator in 1927. His condition was that he could personally report directly to Council. Wallis kept Holmes's set-up of a separate collection for the School, and actively encouraged funded scholars to work on museum specimens. However, changes in the syllabus from about 1926 meant that small samples of drugs were supplied to the students in the laboratories, rather than using the museum as a teaching and study room. From 1934, it became more difficult to develop the museum's activities as expansion of the School and Society administration offices meant that space available for a museum was reduced.

However, tongue-in-cheek, the *Square Chronicle*'s editor suggested that interest in materia medica was increasing: "I wonder, Mr Editor, whether you have ever noticed how eagerly students are devoting themselves to the study of drugs now that the subject that we used to know as Materia Medica has been rechristened Pharmacognosy. There is a positively weird magic in the name."

An article in the *Chronicle*, written as a fictional letter home from a new student in 1930, illustrated the comic difficulties that he was facing: "For six hours a week we pull flowers and leaves to pieces and draw sketches of what they would look like if we hadn't pulled them to pieces. This is called Pharmacognosy. Chemistry is a subject I find difficult because there are often two samples of stuff for analysis and I sometimes get the result for the sample I haven't used."

The *Square Chronicle* reported in January 1930, "During August [1929], the chemical laboratories were redecorated, stains and other remnants of bygone days being removed or covered over. A journey up several spiral staircases is now suitably rewarded by brighter surroundings." However, a piece in the *Chronicle* in February 1933 called for a new chemistry textbook. It gives a fictional title and author, and then leaves a large space on the page with the caption: "This space was reserved for a review of this long-awaited text book. Unfortunately, it appears to have become lost in the press, no news of it having been received for some considerable time."

In 1937, Burn left to become professor of pharmacology at the University of Oxford. His vice-dean, Berry, took over as dean, and John (Jack) Gaddum joined as the director of the pharmacological laboratories and professor of pharmacology.

After the war, the developments of the 1930s to bring the course and facilities up to date continued. In 1944, Harry Berry was appointed professor of pharmaceutics by the University of London. Under his guidance, facilities were set up for work on aseptic techniques, bacteriology and sterilisation, and a teaching room was established for biochemistry. Dr Linnell, who had held the post of lecturer of chemistry since 1926, was awarded a DSc by the University of London in 1939, a recognition of his research in chemotherapy. In 1946, he was appointed professor of pharmaceutical chemistry.

Also in 1946, the Wellcome Trustees endowed a chair of pharmacology in the School of Pharmacy by transferring to the University of London £66,666 redemption 3% stock. The first Wellcome professor of pharmacology was Professor G.A.H. Buttle, who also benefited from Wellcome funding for research in pharmacology in its application to pharmacy.

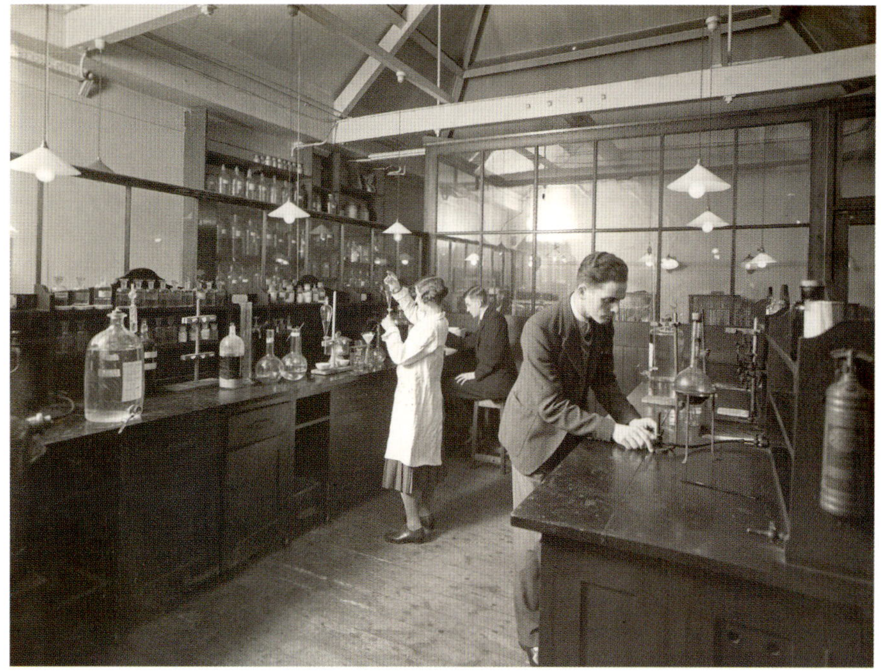

Miss Tickle and Mr Glyn (in the foreground) pose for the photographer in this shot of the chemistry laboratory in 1931.

Royal Pharmaceutical Society Museum

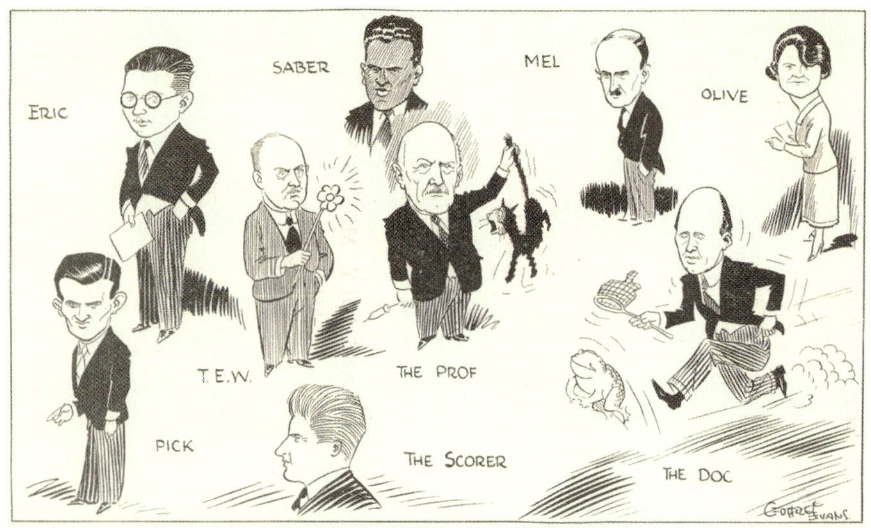

Mr Saber, a visiting researcher from Cairo, joins Melhuish, Wallis, Greenish and Linnell, alongside other School staff in this cartoon from the *Square Chronicle* in February 1933.

UCL School of Pharmacy Library

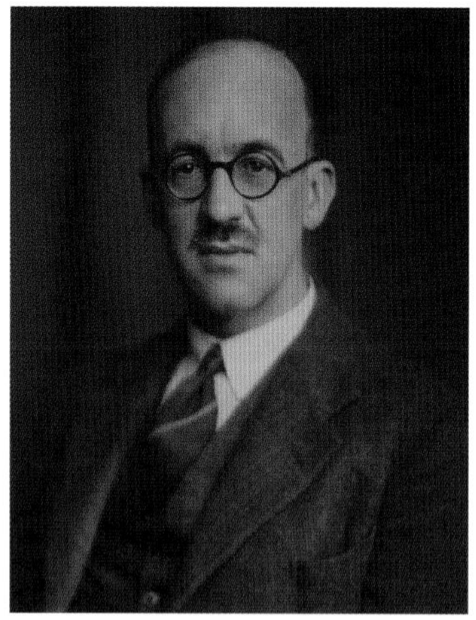

JOHN HENRY GADDUM (1900–1965)

JOHN HENRY GADDUM (1900–1965)

Jack Gaddum won a scholarship to Trinity College, Cambridge, where he studied Medicine from 1919. In 1922, he became a medical student at University College Hospital, and in 1925 he took a post at the Wellcome Research Laboratories. From 1925, he worked at the National Institute for Medical Research in the laboratory of Sir Henry Hallett Dale. Working with Ulf von Euler, he discovered a previously unknown vasodepressor substance in the brain and intestine (substance P). He was also able to establish the role of acetylcholine in sympathetic nerve transmission. His later research focused on the mode of action of drugs, and his studies on the effects of lysergic acid diethylamide (LSD) led to a better understanding of serotonin. In 1934, he became professor of pharmacology at the University of Cairo, but he returned to London in the following year to take the same role at UCL. In 1937, he joined the School of Pharmacy as director of the pharmacological laboratories and professor of pharmacology.

During the war, he worked at the Chemical Defence Research Station, Porton Down, studying the toxicity of gases. In 1942, he moved to become professor of materia medica at the University of Edinburgh. His final post was as director of the Institute of Animal Physiology in Cambridge, which he took in 1958. He was knighted in 1964, and received an honorary degree from the University of Edinburgh in the same year.

UNIVERSITY OF LONDON

Although the School had become a school of the University of London in 1925, most of its funding continued to be provided by the Society until after the war. In 1932, the pharmacological laboratories under Burn were recognised as part of the University, and the title of the School was changed to the College of the Pharmaceutical Society (University of London) so both School and laboratories were under one title.

In 1931, it was explained in the *Square Chronicle* that all students at the Square would be full subscribing members of the University of London Union of Students (ULUS) from the coming session. ULUS had been established on 28th May 1929. The closer ties between the School and the University were also shown with a full account in the *Chronicle* of the laying of the foundation stone of the new Senate House University building by King George V on 26th June 1933. At 209 feet high, it was the tallest secular building in London.

However, the role of the School within the Society's remit continued to be questioned, as it had been at critical points throughout the nineteenth century. At the British Pharmaceutical Conference in 1938, the Society's Birmingham branch put forward a radical proposal that the Society should no longer run a school of pharmacy, and should instead be concentrating on other core functions. Its motion read:

> That it is the opinion of this Conference that the Pharmaceutical Society should confine itself to its proper functions, examining, legislative and administrative, there being no longer any reason why the School of Pharmacy should continue to be conducted by subsidy from the Society's funds.

The motivation behind the proposal was the long-standing sense that Society funds going towards a central school disadvantaged provincial students, and also that the membership should not be subsidising the education of an elite few who could afford to study at the Square. The motion was heavily defeated. Speakers from the floor supported the London school as a model school for others around the country, as a centre for research, and because overcentralisation was "the danger of our age".

An article in the *Square Chronicle* in May 1944 also questioned the future of the College. The author wondered whether the Society should keep funding the School, particularly now that there were good technical colleges and the University of London BPharm course. Members were paying for public colleges in their taxes, and for the Square with their fees. One possibility that might be revived was that the Society could spread its funds over a number of colleges through grants, scholarships and professorships. Another possibility was that the School could merge with a medical school to improve relationships between pharmacists and doctors in the future. A final option presented was that the School could be more independent with its own finances and charter, and keep links with the Society via annual funding, and representatives on the governing body. The article concluded that the Students' Association should set up a subcommittee to consider the School's future.

The Society's financial situation forced the decision before the past students could debate it further. By 1945, the escalating costs meant that the Society's building project would need to be modified. In 1939, the total cost of running the College had been nearly £8,800, of which the University contributed £640. The steep rise in postwar costs finally tipped the balance for the School entirely towards the University. The Society was unable to meet the capital costs needed to complete the new building, and would certainly not be able to afford the running costs afterwards. In 1946, the Society detailed its case in a memorandum to the University, appealing for it to take over the funding and the accommodation for the School. After providing a brief history of the subjects taught and the importance of its research role, the memo proposed that Articles of Association were obtained to establish the School's independence. An agreement was reached that the University would purchase the partially completed building. The Society transferred its funding responsibility to the University, and handed over the School's assets, its equipment, benches and stores, to the University without payment, and provided a £10,000 grant for the first 10 years.

From 1948, the School's title reverted to the School of Pharmacy (University of London). Meanwhile, the plan for the Pharmaceutical Society to move into the Brunswick Square building with the School was cancelled, and when the School moved into the new building, the Society would remain at 17 Bloomsbury Square.

The editor of the *Square Chronicle* in 1944 expressed the nostalgia for the old School building that he was sure he shared with other former students:

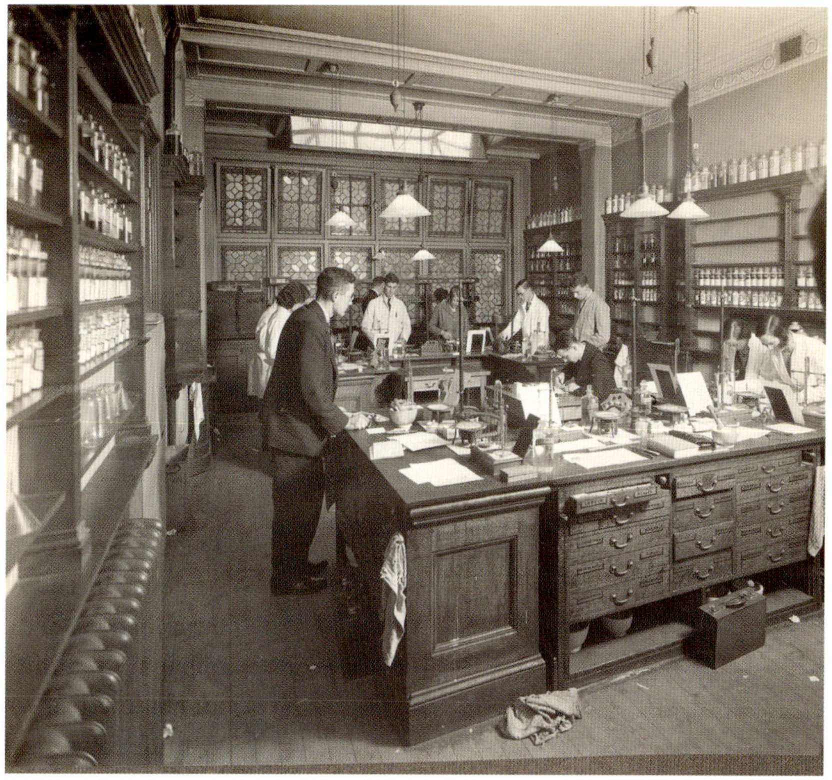

The large examination dispensary in the basement was set up to test students' dispensing skills. It was created in the 1880s to house 12 students, and was still in use when this photograph was taken in around 1928.

Royal Pharmaceutical Society Museum

> No. 17 Bloomsbury Square has a very pronounced character of its own. Upon a foundation of gentlemanly aloofness acquired in the service of the Sardinian Ambassador, the building has become saturated with the atmosphere produced by generations of youthful high spirits. The air is aromatic with an indescribable mixture of the essences distilled from old leather bindings and Council Room upholstery, the volatile metabolites of moulds and beetles in the herbarium collection, the pot-pourri of a thousand substances used in pharmacy, together with the cruder chemical odours and stale tobacco smoke from above, and a residuum of fried eggs and bacon from below. Just such a smell can be found nowhere else in the world. To a newcomer, the air of dingy aloofness and the lack of so-called modern conveniences are apt to be oppressive, but most of our readers will have personal experience of the hold that the wretched old place can get upon the heart, when a year or two have been spent in it.

THE STUDENT EXPERIENCE

In spite of changes to teaching and courses, the students continued to make the most of their time at the Square, probably more so as the year groups were now firmly established as mixed male and female. In 1935, the *Chronicle* contained an announcement from the social club that "It is our belief that too great adherence to academic work is a disease, its chief effect being to produce persons who are 'mentally muscle bound.' To attain the happy medium should be the aim of all Square students ..."

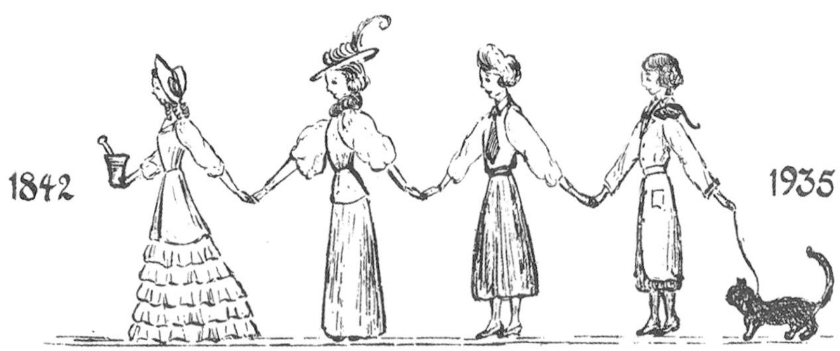

The progression of women students was shown in cartoon form in the *Square Chronicle* throughout the 1930s.

UCL School of Pharmacy Library

A report of the new use of the exam hall for social functions in the *Chronicle* of March 1927 commented that "It is an excellent idea from the exam point of view, since a candidate is less likely to be awed in a room where he or she has danced (or is it performed?) the Charleston." The Charleston, originally dating from 1923 when a tune of the same name was published by James P. Johnson in America, reached the height of its popularity in London in 1926 and 1927, so the pharmacy students were clearly up with the times. In 1933, the dance of choice appeared to be the "military Paul Jones", a mixer dance to ensure that you changed partners. In November 1933, the mixing seemed to be working well. The hall was apparently very full for a dance. "However, numbers of couples unselfishly distributed themselves all over the building, and, according to some reports, the crowding was greatest in the Sterile Dispensary."

The presence of so many female students also led to a humorous article providing guidance for the male students in the *Chronicle*, entitled "A Short Introduction to the Study of Ornithognosy", which is later described as "bird fancying". It included a section on preservation ("this is accomplished by the scientific application of divers creams, powders, lotions, and other secret cosmetics") and on types of birds (blondes and brunettes, with subdivisions, bobbed, shingled, eton cropped, full-fledged). It is not recorded how this attitude towards the women was met by the women, not least Ella Caird, now Mrs Corfield, who became the Association's first female president in 1930.

The male students also seemed to be following current clothing fashions. For example, after a lecture by Hugh Linstead, reported in the *Chronicle* of February 1933, it was stated that Mr Desmond proposed a vote of thanks. "We should like to know why the proposer found it necessary to stand on a lecture bench to make his speech, his badly-creased flannel 'bags' being already well-known."

It seems that nothing changes as far as student behaviour is concerned. The comment from the *Chronicle* on the new seating in the lecture theatre installed in 1928 after 70 years with the previous furniture was that "The new benches are much more comfortable than the old ones. By leaning against the desk, the sleep which follows comes sooner and is more restful than before." A social club report in February 1933 explained that refreshments had been provided before a lecture by the dean: "Apparently having had nothing to eat since they last ate, the students made the sumptuously laid refreshment table look as though a tornado had passed through the Lecture Theatre." If they had money in their pockets, it seems that they headed for the New Oxford Street Lyons' Café, on the corner of Tottenham Court Road, as there is a poem singing its virtues in the same edition of the *Chronicle*. On 6th May 1935, Jubilee Day, the Association held a dance: "The morning after, many were the dreary shapes which dragged themselves round the School, tottered into the dispensaries, dispensed overdoses by the score, and cracked emulsions with ease. We can sympathise with them, but all will agree that it is better to have had a morning after, than never to have had a night before."

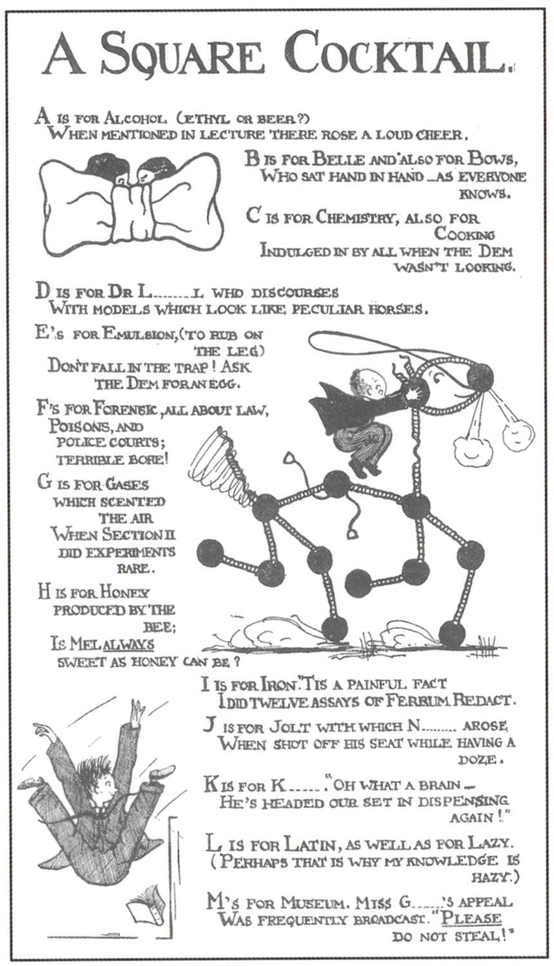

Published in the *Square Chronicle* in May 1934, this cartoon gives a fascinating insight into all aspects of life at the Square.

UCL School of Pharmacy Library

The attitude of the students towards the staff also seems perennial. The *Square Chronicle* of June 1937 included a series of mock monographs from the *British Pharmacopoeia*. One is headed "Demonstratorium": "Demonstrator is an overgrown student which has been collected in the first week in October and injected with an enormous superiority complex ... Manner, extremely sarcastic and suspicious ... Storage. – In a cool place, protected from light, in underground caverns at 17 Bloomsbury Square."

> **"The new benches [in the lecture theatre] are much more comfortable than the old ones. By leaning against the desk, the sleep which follows comes sooner and is more restful than before."**
>
> *Square Chronicle, May 1929*

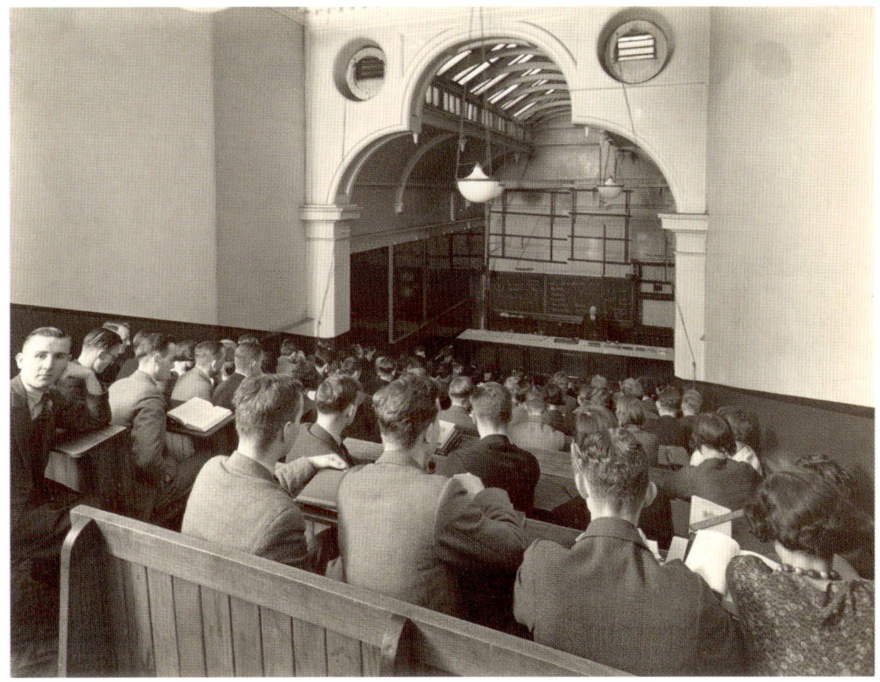

A full house in the Bloomsbury Square lecture theatre for Professor Greenish in 1931.

Royal Pharmaceutical Society Museum

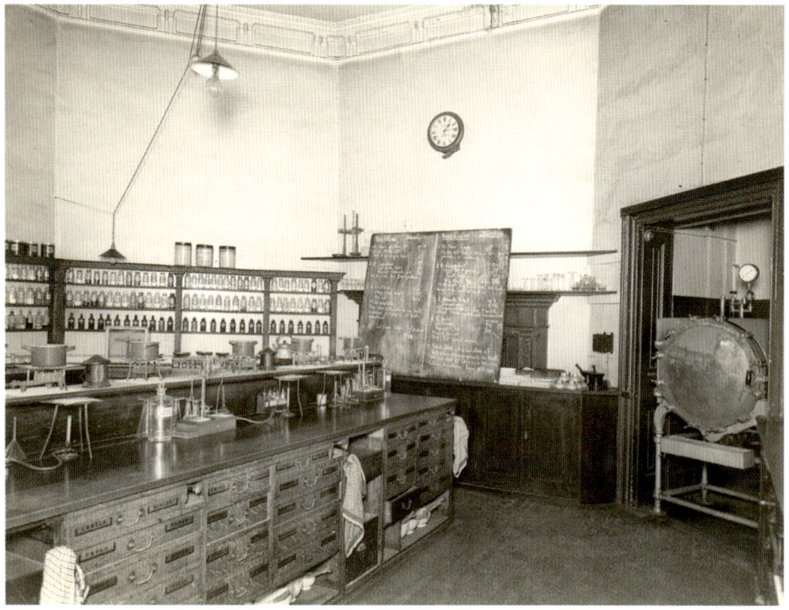

The Octagon was still used as a teaching dispensary in the 1930s. The benches' drawers have traditional gilt labels showing that they held scales, paper, stirrers, silver leaf, knives and other supplies for making and dispensing medicines. The blackboard, leaned against an ornate fireplace, shows four prescriptions to be completed in the morning and five in the afternoon, including pills and mixtures.

Royal Pharmaceutical Society Museum

The next is "Lecturorum": "Lecturer is an overgrown Demonstrator, collected some years ago, carefully preserved and becoming dry. Contains not less than 217 soporific units and considerably less than 1 per cent of dry humour."

Another way to pass time was in rivalry with other schools of pharmacy, and not on the sports field. In the *Square Chronicle* for September 1932 there is a detailed account of the "Battle of Bloomsbury", a precursor to long-running disputes in later decades, most notably with Chelsea College. In this instance, the rivals were the London College of Pharmacy. Students from the Square had taken an empty barrel painted with the Square's colours for use as a mascot by the soccer club. It was stolen by London College of Pharmacy supporters at a match. When two Square students went to the College to try to retrieve it, they returned with the College mascot instead. The College retaliated by using an open-top motor car to race around Bloomsbury Square and throw eggs at number 17. The Square students used eggs and water in response. The next day, the Square students took overripe grapefruit from Covent Garden, with soot, flour and eggs to Clapham Road by barrow after lunch. The College students had got wind of what was coming their way and had eggs and soot ready. However, when the students arrived at Stockwell Tube Station, they were met by police, marking the end of the battle. It is not reported how the mascots were repatriated, but the barrel was back at the Square by the next edition of the *Chronicle*.

In the *Chronicle* of May 1944, the barrel was allowed to tell its full history to date in an article entitled "The Barrel Speaks". Having been bought from a stall in Caledonian Market for 15 shillings, and painted red, yellow and blue, it was first taken to Northolt for a football match against the London College of Pharmacy. The Battle of Bloomsbury incident had been sparked when, in retaliation for stealing the barrel, Square students stole the London College's mascots, a wheel and a fire bell. In 1936, after a match, the barrel was taken to St Pancras by Nottingham students, wrapped as a parcel and left at the lost luggage office. In 1938, the barrel was lost outside the Princess Louise pub after a soccer match with Nottingham. It was successfully taken back to Nottingham. Although Squarites telegraphed for its return, no one arrived to meet the parcel, so it was taken back to Nottingham and stayed in its pharmacognosy department until 1941. In the spring of that year, Mr West, a Square student, was at University College Nottingham, saw the barrel and put it in his car. He returned it to the School, now evacuated to Cardiff, and eventually after the war it was returned to Bloomsbury Square.

In March 1928, it was announced in the *Chronicle* that a new anthem would be adopted for the School, as many other University departments had their own song. Set to the tune of "Marching thro' Georgia", an American marching song by Henry Clay Work, dating from 1865, it had its own pharmacy-related words set to it by the students. The new anthem was introduced at that year's school dinner where it was given its first public airing, but by August 1928 it had been abandoned, and the *Chronicle* was running a competition for a new one. In 1934, a Choral Society was formed, conducted by Dr W.H. Linnell: "The Pharmacological Laboratories report that the singing had a very definite effect on the rats, and rendered

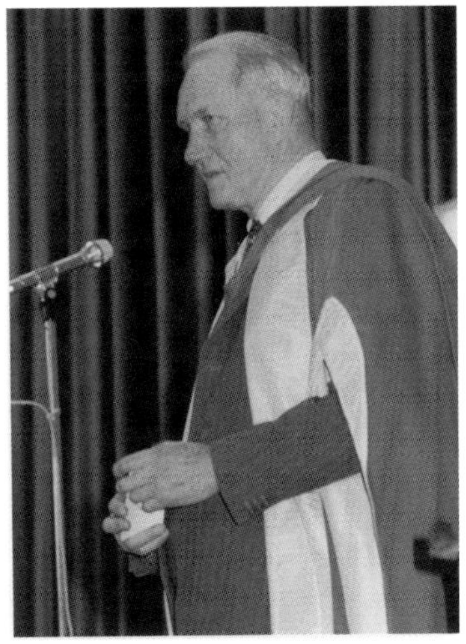

GEOFFREY BUCKLE WEST (1916–1990)

With kind permission from Springer Science and Business Media

GEOFFREY BUCKLE WEST (1916–1990)

Geoff West graduated with a BPharm from the Square in 1938 and gained his doctorate on work associated with adrenaline in 1942. He worked with Jack Gaddum to establish physiological pharmacology at the School and beyond. In 1950, he left to take up a post in the department of pharmacology at the University of St Andrews in Dundee, where, in 1952, his work with J.F. Riley localised histamine in mast cells, a significant milestone for the understanding and treatment of allergies and inflammation. He was awarded the DSc by the University of London in 1954. He then returned to the Square as reader in pharmacology, continuing his research on histamine. In 1965, he took the post of head of information at the British Industrial Biological Research Association, and in 1970 he became reader in pharmacology at the North East London Polytechnic. He was secretary-general of the European Histamine Research Society for more than 10 years.

them unfit for any further experiments." The fashion at the Square for singing even produced a publication, *The Square Students' Song Book*, published by the School of Pharmacy Students' Association, in 1938. In the foreword, E.R. Withell explained that it had been put together for sing-songs held regularly at the Square, and had been printed in a small enough format so that it could also fit in a pocket for rambles and bus journeys. In addition, the small green hardback book with the School badge embossed on the front provided a permanent record of one aspect of life at the Square. The book's contents are 84 songs, starting with "Waltzing Matilda" and ending with "Rose, Rose". Other well-known tunes included were "Campdown Races", "Loch Lomond", "Polly Wolly Doodle", "The Bear Went Over the Mountain" and "One Man Went to Mow".

Whether it was intended that the School anthem or the tunes in the song book should be sung at sports events is unclear, but these events carried on successfully through this period. In August 1928, there was the report of a new swimming club, and the rugby club seemed to be experiencing a new lease of life. Perhaps the most fashionable new sporting addition was in 1931, when a ping-pong table was bought by the Association for the Women's Common Room. The following edition of the *Chronicle* reported a table tennis knockout tournament. The rambling club was also revived. In 1930, they went out on two "charas" to Devil's Punch Bowl at Hindhead, and ran other trips closer into London monthly. The *Chronicle* had an easy explanation for the club's success: "it is very easy for two persons, so willed, to get lost – and what more does one want than to get lost in congenial company!"

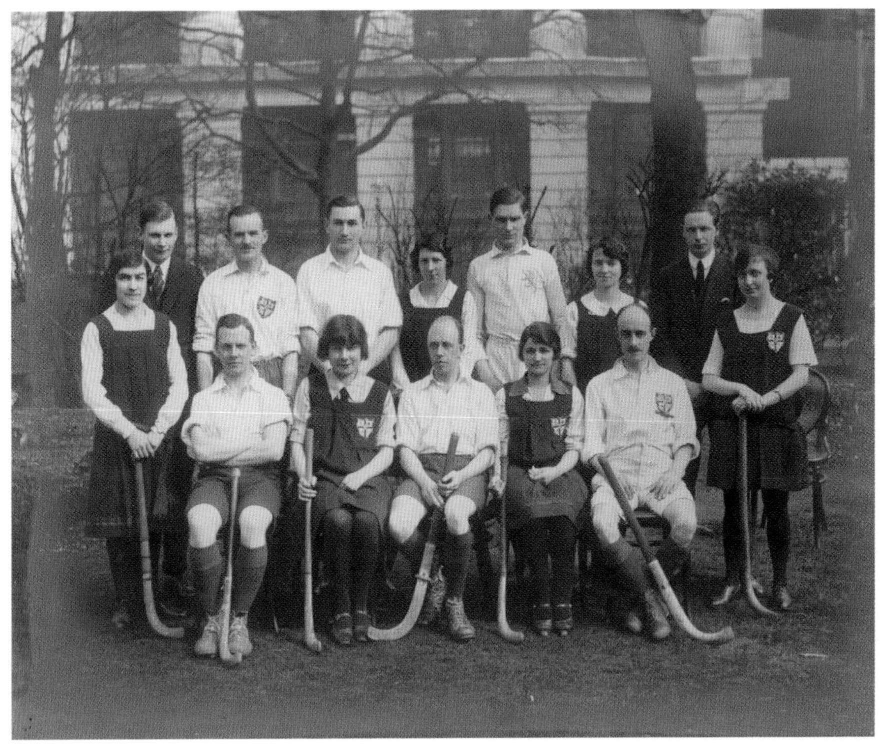

The 1926-7 hockey team went on to produce a professor and dean at the School, W.H. Linnell, and two people who became Pharmaceutical Society Secretary and Registrar, F.W. Adams and H.N. Linstead.

UCL School of Pharmacy Library

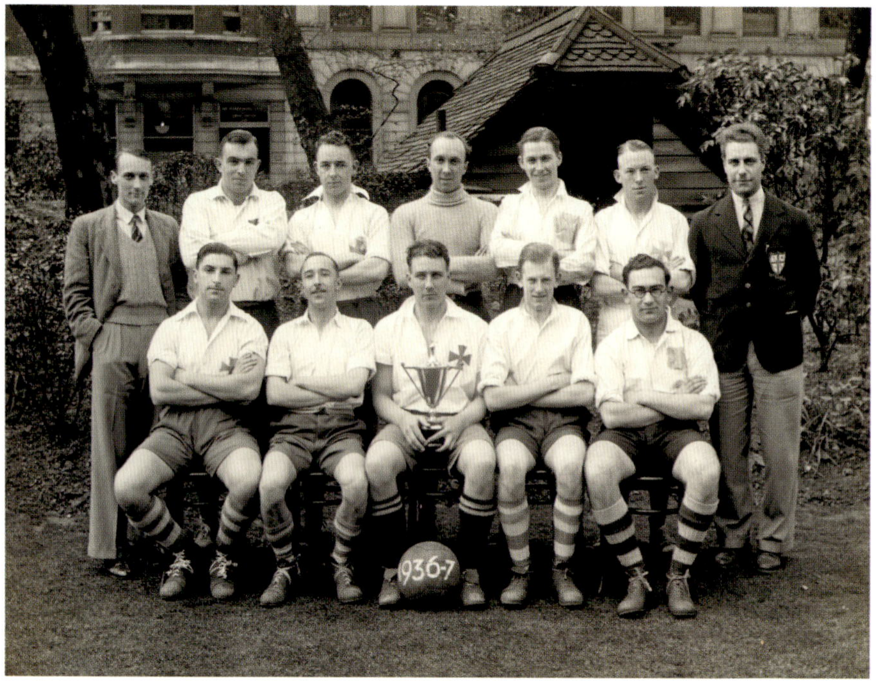

The football team seem to have been less successful in the 1930s, but no less popular.

UCL School of Pharmacy Library

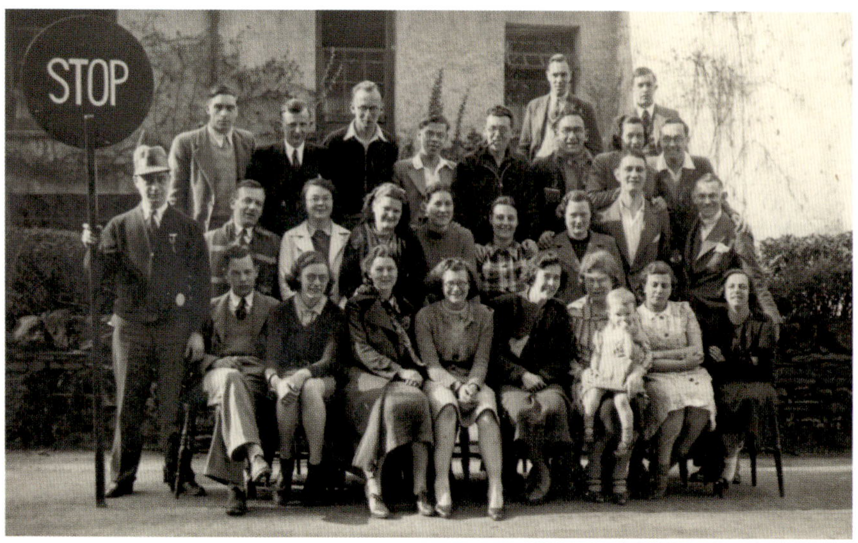

What part the man with a stop sign had to play in the annual trip to the Lake District in 1938 is lost in history. The older lady with a toddler in the front row may have been involved in hosting the trip.

UCL School of Pharmacy Library

And in 1934, the students set up a cross-country running club, the Square Harriers. In the 1930s, football and hockey matches were played at Allen and Hanburys' sports ground at Chadwell Heath, a long trek from Bloomsbury Square to what was then still Essex rather than Greater London. This arrangement ended in 1939. In the same year, the students formed a badminton club, and permission was given by Council for the exam hall to be marked out as a court.

Over Easter 1935, the Association organised the first of many annual trips to the Lake District. Most participants travelled by train from Euston, and the detailed reports in the *Chronicles* show how much fun was had and how many friendships were cemented. From 1935, the formal annual dinner was held at Grosvenor House with a greater focus on socialising, consisting of a dance, shorter speeches and no entertainment.

A milestone in the make-up of the student body was reached in the late 1930s with the first Indian student to achieve the BPharm degree. Mr Shantilal H. Merchant achieved his degree in 1940 and went back to forge a successful career in India, initially as the first hospital pharmacist at King Edward VII Memorial Hospital in Mumbai, and later as deputy drugs controller for India.

In 1938, the Students' Association adopted a new constitution and rules including allowing honorary members. At the same time, the Association changed its name to The Square Association, and became a group for past and present students, staff and honorary members. A new group, the "Students' Union", was established just for present students. The *Square Chronicle* of March 1939 explained that the delay since the last publication was because of these changes to the Association. In an article detailing the new set-up, it reports that the changes arose because current students wanted to run their own affairs. The Association would continue to cater for past students through the *Chronicle*, the annual dinner and past students' day. However, the new arrangements would help students to learn management and financial skills. In addition, the Association set up an Association Employment Bureau to help past students to find work.

The Square students also initiated a national students' group, the British Pharmaceutical Students' Association (BPSA). It started in 1942 as an initiative of the Square's Students' Union, when a delegation of pharmacy students from 11 schools of pharmacy attended a meeting of the National Union of Students (NUS). At the meeting, they argued the case to set up a national pharmacy student association, originally named the Pharmacy Faculty of the National Union of Students. In August 1942, representatives from Brighton, Bristol, Chelsea, Dundee, Portsmouth and the Square all met with Council. The Square agreed to take the initiative to form a permanent group. According to BPSA records, many of their initial meetings were held beneath the Square in 1942 while on air-raid duty with F.W. Adams, secretary and registrar of the Society. BPSA held its first conference in 1943 at the Square, at which they adopted their current name. John Shinner, president of the Square Students' Union, was elected first BPSA president. A piece by Shinner in the *Chronicle* of that year expressed his aspirations: "If well organized, it will be a valuable and powerful mouthpiece for the pharmaceutical youth of the future, and be a means by which Pharmacy can play its full part, as other faculties do, in the student life of the community." A temporary committee, set up with the support of 19 pharmacy student bodies from Aberdeen to Plymouth and the Society, expressed the group's broad policy objectives as:

- To foster the furtherance of Pharmacy as a scientific subject, and to secure adequate recognition for it.
- To co-ordinate the services of Pharmacy with medicine and the social sciences in securing an adequate health service as envisaged by the Beveridge Report.
- To co-ordinate the various branches of pharmacy and pharmaceutical study.

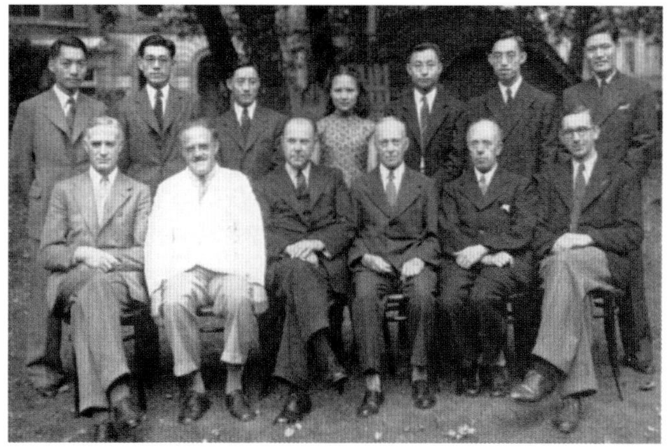

Seven Chinese students attended the School to study for the BPharm in 1947. They are shown in the back row here. In the front row are F.W. Adams, Deputy Secretary to the Pharmaceutical Society and past student at the School, Professor Buttle, Professor Berry, Dr Wallis, Professor Linnell and Dr Fairbairn.

Royal Pharmaceutical Society Museum

In 1944, it was announced that the Pharmacy Faculty Committee of the NUS would continue to function as the British Pharmaceutical Students' Association in order to include Scotland. The BPSA held its annual conference over Easter 1944 in Nottingham.

After the war, the Square students' social scene gathered momentum. Although it was reported in 1944 that the cycling club was not as popular in London as it had been in Cardiff, the table tennis club was back up and running. Louis Sharpe, one of the demonstrators working in 1944, remembered that the men's common room was almost completely filled by a table tennis table. Meanwhile, the women's common room had a three-piece suite, but with rats living in the sofa, as the whole house was infested. Sharpe also remembered that there was no refectory, and so they used to take in sandwiches, or go out for lunch to the "Express" or the "Montrose", or to the Museum Tavern if they wanted to go to a pub. The girls made tea each morning and afternoon on a gas ring in their common room, organised with a rota and a weekly sub.

Other social functions were held in The Hut, belonging to the ULU, after the Square's exam hall was turned into an aseptic laboratory. The ULU building was a huge prefab with a primitive stage, which is where the staff/student pantomime took place during this period. The dramatic club was now a recognised club of the Association, having started with a burlesque pantomime for the small number of London members in 1942. In 1945, the Association ran its trip to the Lake District for the first time since 1940. A debating society was founded in 1945. And in 1946, a new Square music society was established for regular record recitals, listening to recorded music in the physiology laboratory after hours, plus visits to concerts at the Royal Albert Hall. Unfortunately, the record recitals had to be postponed as the Society no longer had a suitable radiogram.

During the war, the dramatic section of the Association raised money for the Society's War Aid Fund. In 1946, it suggested to the Committee that a separate charity be set up, the Square Educational Trust Fund, to provide grants for equipment, courses or materials, or entry fees for Society, University and other exam bodies, with past and present students eligible to apply.

CHAPTER 5

THE "OLDEST NEW BUILDING" IN LONDON: 1949–1960

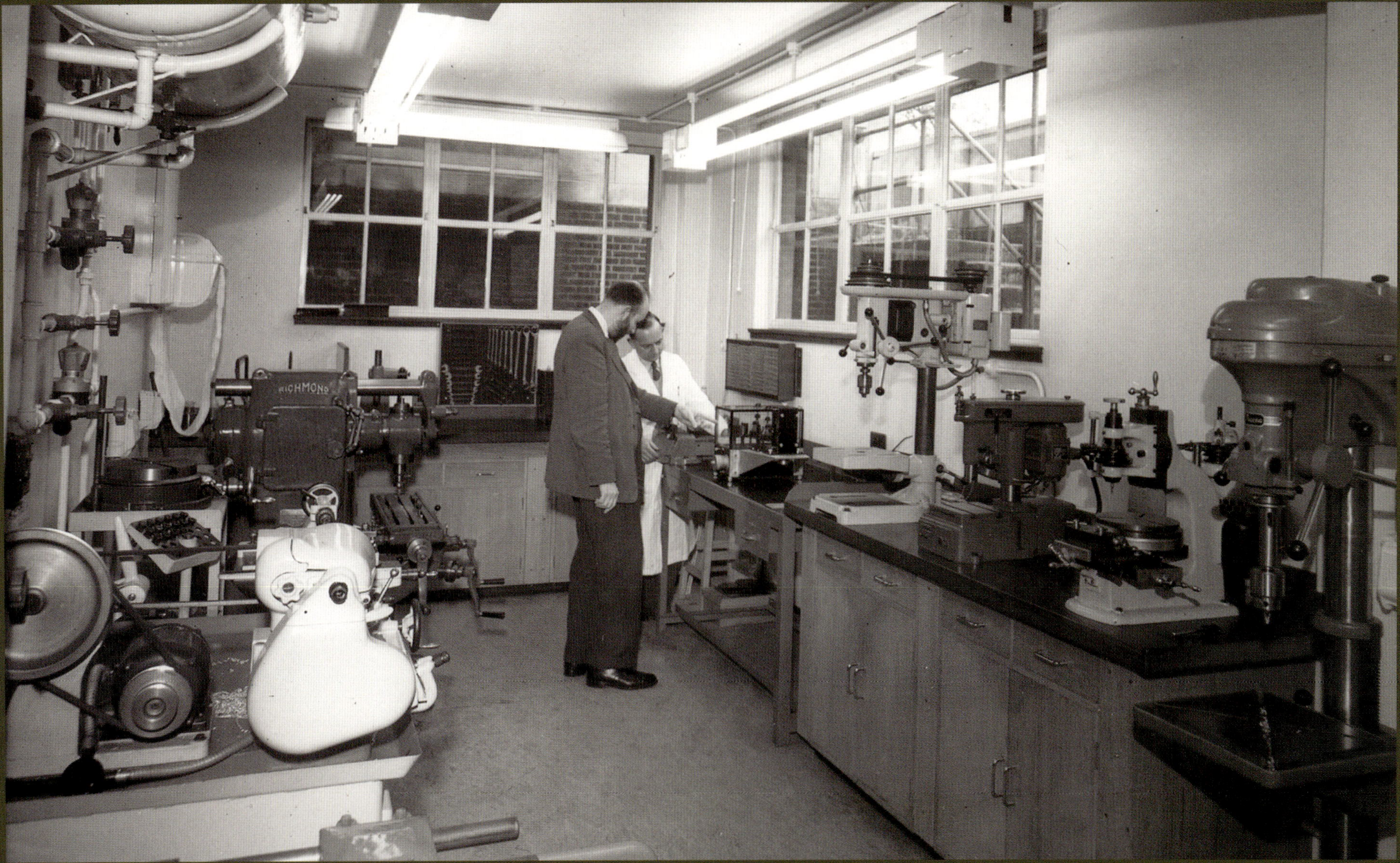

Dr Glenn with a technician in the Physical Chemistry Instrument Room in the basement, 1960. This facility was where special apparatus, including most of the equipment for the microchemical laboratory, was made.

Reproduced with permission from the Royal Pharmaceutical Society Museum

MILESTONES

London Life

1951	Festival of Britain
1952	a four-day fog in December caused an estimated 4,000 deaths
1955	Heathrow airport opened

National News

1952	death of King George VI
1953	coronation of Queen Elizabeth II
1954	end of food rationing

The Wider World

1949	formation of NATO
1950–1953	Korean War
1950–1954	McCarthyism in the USA
1950s	civil rights movement in the USA
1953	structure of DNA discovered
1953	heart–lung machine developed
1954	first successful kidney transplant
1954	CERN, the European Organization for Nuclear Research, established
1955	start of Vietnam War
1956	disarmament movement began
1957	USSR launched Sputnik I
1957	EEC established

Drug Developments

1950	Largactil (chlorpromazine) synthesised, for schizophrenia
1952	Rimifon (isoniazid), for tuberculosis
1952	Salk polio vaccine developed
1955	first oral treatment for diabetes
1957	interferon first isolated and named
1957	Tofranil (imipramine), for depression
1957	halothane anaesthetic gas
1959	first semi-synthetic penicillin marketed
1960	Celbenin (methicillin), active against many resistant bacteria
1960	Flagyl (metronidazole), for parasitic and anaerobic bacterial infections

Pharmacy Milestones

1952	prescription charge introduced
1953	PSGB Supplemental Charter granted: primary focus was to widen the Society's objectives to cover all pharmacists, and to bring more of its actions under the control of its own by-laws
1956	Therapeutic Substances Act
1957	first *British National Formulary* published

The postwar period was one of austerity. However, for the School and pharmacy more widely it was also an exciting time. The establishment of the National Health Service (NHS) in 1948 put pharmacists at the centre of the provision of medicines for the public, and provided a catalyst for increased professionalism and status. Coupled with this was an explosion of new drug developments, starting with antibiotics, followed quickly by steroids to treat rheumatoid arthritis, polio vaccination, and the first medicinal treatments for mental health conditions. Simply taking the *Square Chronicle* as a historical source, the introduction of advertisements in this period points to the scale of the developments. In April 1947, the advertisements included Burroughs Wellcome products, Allen & Hanburys' penicillin, May & Baker sulphonamides, WB medical products, Parke Davis Euthymol toothpaste, Evans products, British Drug Houses supplies, and Flatters and Garnett microscopical preparations.

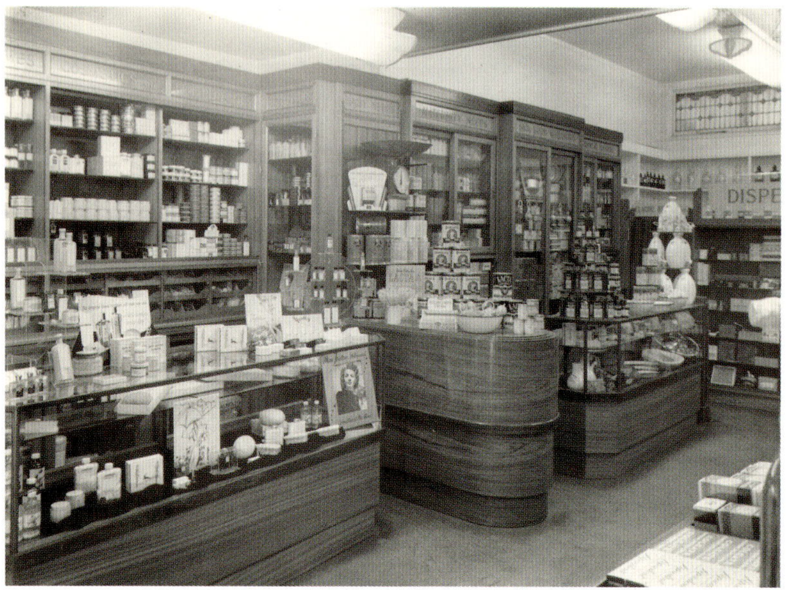

Claude Benton Ltd stocked a typical mix of cosmetics, including an advert for "Max Factor of Hollywood, Cosmetics of the Stars", alongside their "Baby Needs" at their shop in Norwich in around 1950. Note the baby weighing scales at the top of the display of milk formula, and an impressive display of ceramic bed warmers at the rear of the shop.

Royal Pharmaceutical Society Museum

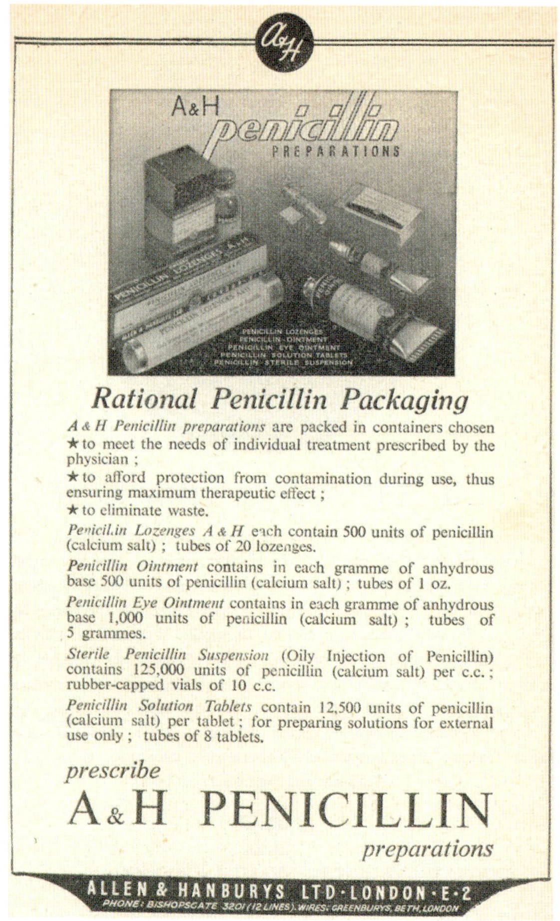

Penicillin was first advertised in the *Square Chronicle* in April 1947. The Penicillin Act of the same year controlled the supply of the "wonder drug".

UCL School of Pharmacy Library

THE BUILDING

The School's move to its new Brunswick Square building was already a project of more than 20 years' duration by the time that the University of London took over the financial and governance reins in 1949. Both the capital and recurrent costs of the School were assumed by the University. The deal was very favourable to the University, with the five-eighths of the accommodation intended for the School sold at 1939 actual costs, and the remaining three-eighths that had been intended for the Society's functions sold at estimated market value in 1949. At the Charter dinner and dance in 1952, the principal guest, Dr Douglas Logan, principal of the University, revealed that the estimated cost of completing the building was £600,000. The three-eighths of the building that were now not going to be used by the Society were allocated to the University examinations department, which changed some of the internal planning. The fact that the Society was not moving from Bloomsbury Square with the School also meant that the School would need its own library, and as a result, new floor loadings had to be calculated. Once the Brunswick Square building had been transferred to the University, staff could not resist taking an unofficial look around the empty shell. They remembered lecturer Ken Wibberley crawling around in the darkness. There is even some tragic folklore that a university administration officer died after walking over an unprotected floor edge.

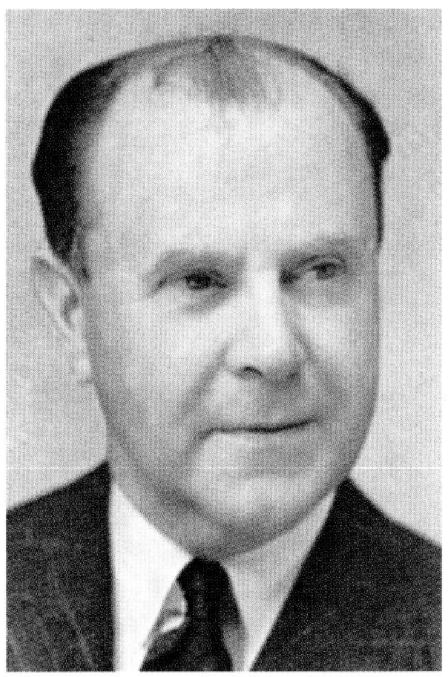

HAROLD BERRY (1890–1982)

HAROLD BERRY (1890–1982)

Harry Berry studied in his native North West, and passed the Minor and Major exams in 1912 at the Northern College of Pharmacy, Manchester. He joined the staff at the College before moving to the pharmacy department at UCL. He served in the Royal Fusiliers, then the Royal Engineers and then the Royal Garrison Artillery in the First World War. After the war, he worked as a lecturer in pharmacy at Robert Gordon College in Aberdeen, before transferring to the Birmingham Technical College. He gained his BSc in Chemistry in 1926, and in the following year was appointed head of the pharmacy department at Birmingham.

In 1933, he became reader in pharmaceutics at the University of London, and vice-dean of the College of the Pharmaceutical Society. He received the Diploma of Bacteriology of the University of London soon afterwards. In 1937, he became dean of the School, and was appointed professor of pharmaceutics in 1944, playing a key role in introducing microbiology into the pharmacy curriculum.

As dean, he was instrumental in the School's establishment as part of the University of London, and oversaw the acquisition of its Grant of Arms and its Charter. In addition to his academic role, Berry served as an examiner for the Society, and the universities of London, Manchester, Glasgow and Wales. He was a member of the *British Pharmacopeia* Commission and of the *Codex* Revision Committee. He was chairman of the British Pharmaceutical Conference in 1951. He was made an honorary fellow of the School in 1956. His successor as dean, Professor Linnell, commented: "It is doubtful if any other period in the life of the School has been so eventful, or so fruitful, as that during which Professor Berry shouldered the major responsibilities … No one has contributed more to the success and future progress of the School."

The move to the larger modern building could not come soon enough for the staff and students at Bloomsbury Square struggling within the confines of the mainly eighteenth century building with nineteenth century fixtures and fittings. As the *Square Chronicle* put it in April 1948, "The Pharmacognosy Lab is rather like a Victorian drawing room, lacking only the lace curtains and aspidistra." In fact, 17 Bloomsbury Square was listed as being of important historical value in 1952. But as Professor Berry explained in his report to the Charter Inaugural Meeting on 8th October 1952, "It is difficult to describe the congestion which obtains in the present building in Bloomsbury Square, or to describe our intense longing for some amelioration of the conditions under which we have to work." Space at Bloomsbury Square, even bursting at the seams, was limited to 88 students. To help the situation, Birkbeck College had provided two laboratories for use by pharmaceutical chemistry, and the Royal Veterinary College had provided two laboratories for pharmacology. The dean was playing a waiting game for the University to prioritise the building work within its busy postwar programme. In 1952, he reported, "it is a relief to be able to say that there is now reasonable ground to hope that it will be possible to fit into the current University building programme a part of the work necessary for the completion of the new building in Brunswick Square." A year later, he reported, "It is hardly possible to describe our relief when we learned from the University that at long last it was possible to make a start on the completion of the new building in Brunswick Square."

"It is difficult to describe the congestion which obtains in the present building in Bloomsbury Square, or to describe our intense longing for some amelioration of the conditions under which we have to work."

Professor Berry, October 1952

Building work restarted in 1954, but because of the large sums involved, grants were made in instalments by the University Court to finish self-contained elements of the building which could be brought into use on completion. This meant that various departments had to transfer into the building at different times. The space allocated to each department was worked out carefully. Pharmaceutics and pharmaceutical engineering science would have 12,600 square feet or 34% of the departmental space, pharmaceutical chemistry would take 30% or 11,100 square feet, pharmacognosy was given 4,500 square feet or 12% of the total, and pharmacology had 24% or 8,900 square feet. The students knew exactly what amenities were important to them, as outlined in a humorous article in the *Chronicle* in September 1954, entitled "The 'New Building' Policy or What the Students Should Have When They Go to the New Building." Their list of demands included efficient electric fires in the common room, daily lectures on permutations for those who did the football pools and, intriguingly, the establishment of a marriage guidance council.

The first department scheduled to move into the third floor of the building was Pharmaceutics, with a hope that they could get settled in to start the 1954–5 session, but it was not to be. Berry reported, "It was with considerable disappointment, tinged with a good deal of anxiety, that we learned that the scheme could not be completed during the session and that the third floor could not be occupied this October." David Train became the department's executive site representative for the School's contract, whilst Ted Shotton with Ken Wibberley and Cyril Ridout had responsibility for the move of both the undergraduate and research laboratories. Archie Cook planned the move of the microbiology and aseptic studies areas, and David Train was responsible for the recently established pharmaceutical engineering science course and its workshops. During 1954, funds were made available for equipping the new laboratories. Staff bought supplies direct from the makers to be most economical, such as spatulas by the gross from the manufacturers in Sheffield.

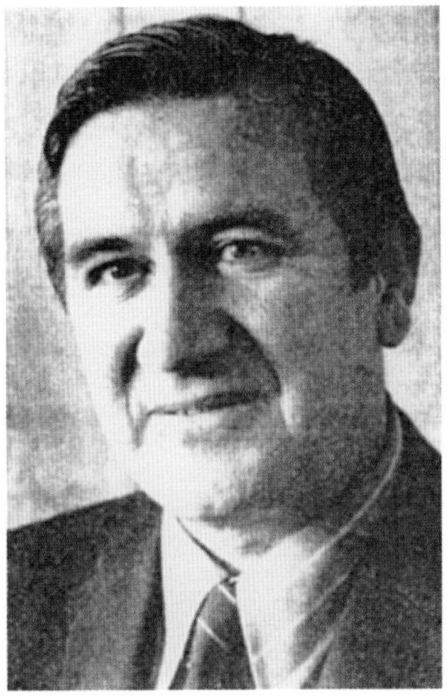

SIR DAVID JACK (1924–2011)

SIR DAVID JACK (1924–2011)

The son of a Scottish miner, David Jack served his apprenticeship at Boots, and then gained a degree in Pharmacy and Pharmacology at Glasgow University and the Royal Technical College. During the war, he taught at the Army School of Health. In 1951, he joined the research department at Glaxo, and then moved to work on product development at Menley and James. In the 1950s, he studied part time for a PhD at the Square, supervised by Professor Beckett. In 1961, he was appointed research director of Glaxo's subsidiary Allen & Hanburys. He stayed at Glaxo until his retirement, serving as director of research and development from 1978 to 1987.

He headed an extremely successful team of research scientists. In 1966, they achieved a major breakthrough with the development of the bronchodilator salbutamol, a new treatment for asthma. It was launched as Ventolin in 1969 and is still incredibly successful. In competition with James (later Sir James) Black at Smith Kline and French, he next turned his attention to duodenal and gastric ulcers. Black's paper on histamine H_2 antagonists prompted Jack to form a group to investigate them for Glaxo. In 1976, Black produced cimetidine (launched as Tagamet), but Jack's team developed a more effective drug, ranitidine hydrochloride, launched as Zantac in 1981. It became the first drug to achieve worldwide sales of more than $1 billion a year.

Jack's team also developed Becotide (beclomethasone) in 1972, Severent (salmeterol) in 1990 and fluticasone propionate, used as an inhalation to treat asthma and hayfever, and as a cream for eczema and psoriasis. They went on to launch Zofran (ondansetron) in 1991 and Imigran (sumatriptan) in the same year. Jack continued with research after his retirement from Glaxo.

He was appointed a CBE in 1982 and knighted in 1993. He also won several Queen's Awards for Industry and was elected a Fellow of the Royal Society of Edinburgh in 1978, and of the Royal Society in 1992.

By October 1954, the School had been given Easter 1955 as a moving date. With the amount of time that they then had for planning, staff were able to organise labelled packages that went straight into their new positions. Practical classes therefore began in the summer term of 1955. The *Chronicle* marked the occasion with an article devoted to the pharmaceutical engineers, no doubt written by one of their number: "The Cream of the Square, the Engineers, have at last left their foetid dungeon and gone to the airy chaos of Brunswick Square. Fifty-six days after Pancake Tuesday they emerged, blinking like pit ponies in the unaccustomed light, and disappeared towards their new home, dragging their Expresso [*sic*] machine behind them." It was reported that they had left the pharmaceutical engineering boiler, a "triumph of mediaeval engineering", behind at Bloomsbury Square. The light, space, airiness and facilities of the new building impressed everyone, staff and students, but working conditions were noisy, as the rest of the building was still a construction site. Berry was nevertheless pleased: "It is difficult to express adequately our feelings of relief from congestion, and our appreciation of the freshness and modernity of the new accommodation." During this period, with the departments at a distance from each other, Derek King, a pharmacology teaching technician from August 1950 onwards, remembered that the School bought a three-wheeled Reliant van to ferry goods and equipment around. Professor Buttle eventually bought the van for his own use.

The students were also pleased, not least for the hoped-for impact that the new building would have on their full university experience. In the *Square Chronicle* of September 1955, the editor explained that:

> For the last few years the walls of No. 17 have been visibly bulging to contain the large numbers of Staff and Students and the masses of equipment for which this building was never designed. Now this problem of crowding will be solved. In the airy, well set out rooms of Brunswick Square there should be no more complaints about space ... We are going to have a new degree in a new building, and with the increase of space for work let us have an increase in the spaciousness of the degree course. At present it is rather too crowded for all students to enjoy university life to the full, and for the weaker of them to keep up with their studies.

However, Berry explained in his Dean's Report of 1955 that there was still not enough funding to complete the building. Pharmacy was only a small school in a large University. Professor Berry retired as dean in 1956, so did not see the building finished whilst head of School. Professor Linnell took over as dean and as the manager of the building project. With pharmaceutics settled in, he concluded that "The move is proving a great success, and one can already recognise the effect of the freshness and modern equipment of the building on the attitude of both staff and students." The University confirmed that it would supply a grant for the completion of the building in the 1957 programme. This had an impact beyond the morale and performance of current students and staff, as it finally allowed an increase in the student intake to 48 per year. Linnell explained in 1956 that "A tentative move in this direction has been made this year as, greatly daring, 36 students have been accepted in the first year course."

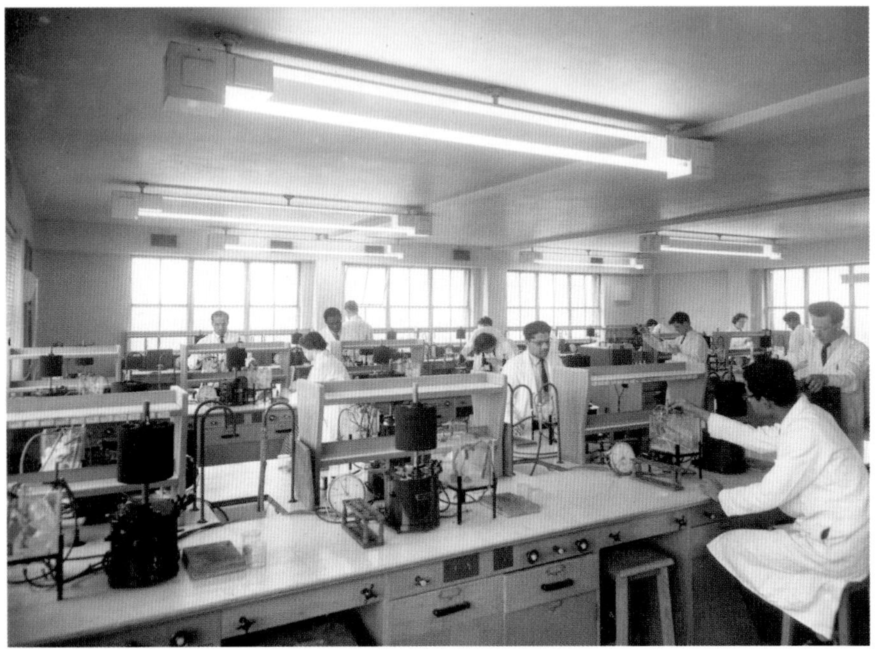

The pharmacology teaching laboratory for first and second year students on the fifth floor, 1960.
Royal Pharmaceutical Society Museum

The pharmaceutical chemistry department joined pharmaceutics in the new building, by taking up its place on the fourth floor in October 1956. Linnell felt that both the students and the staff felt the benefit, both practically and psychologically. He also reported that "Many foreign visitors have been entertained at Brunswick Square and they are unanimous in confirming our own impression that, on completion, our School will be the finest school of pharmacy in the world. This constitutes a great challenge to the staff in order to maintain this position – a challenge which I am sure will be well and truly met."

In the Easter vacation of 1957, the pharmacology department moved into the fifth and sixth floors. Although the new accommodation was fantastic, the Dean's Report of that year fended off any potential criticism that they would not be making the most of the new set-up: "the only handicap to full use of the excellent facilities is one of finance. Research in Pharmacology is extremely expensive owing to the high cost of animals, and lack of money will limit the number of workers who can be accepted."

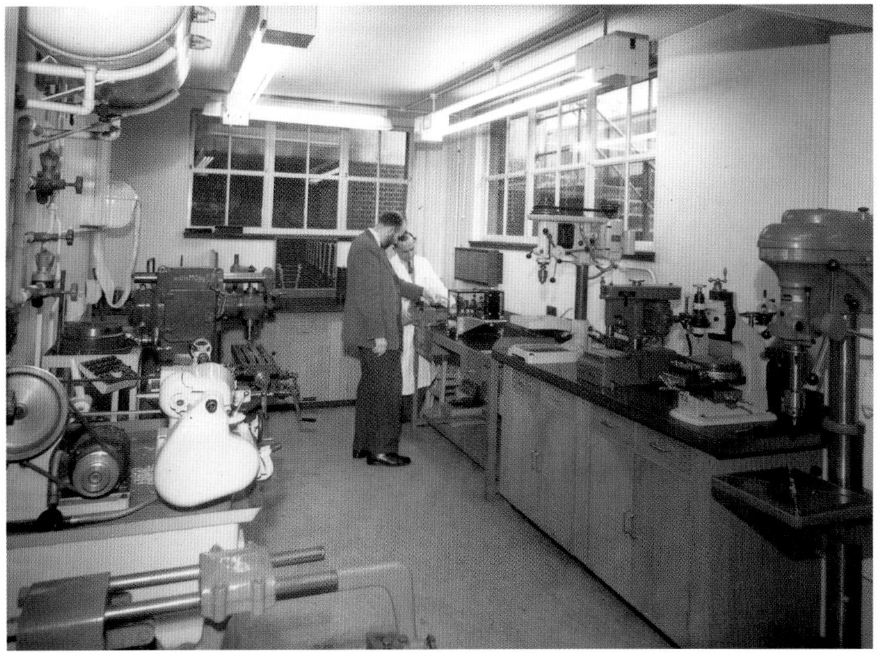

Dr Glenn with a technician in the Physical Chemistry Instrument Room in the basement, 1960. This facility was where special apparatus, including most of the equipment for the microchemical laboratory, was made.

Royal Pharmaceutical Society Museum

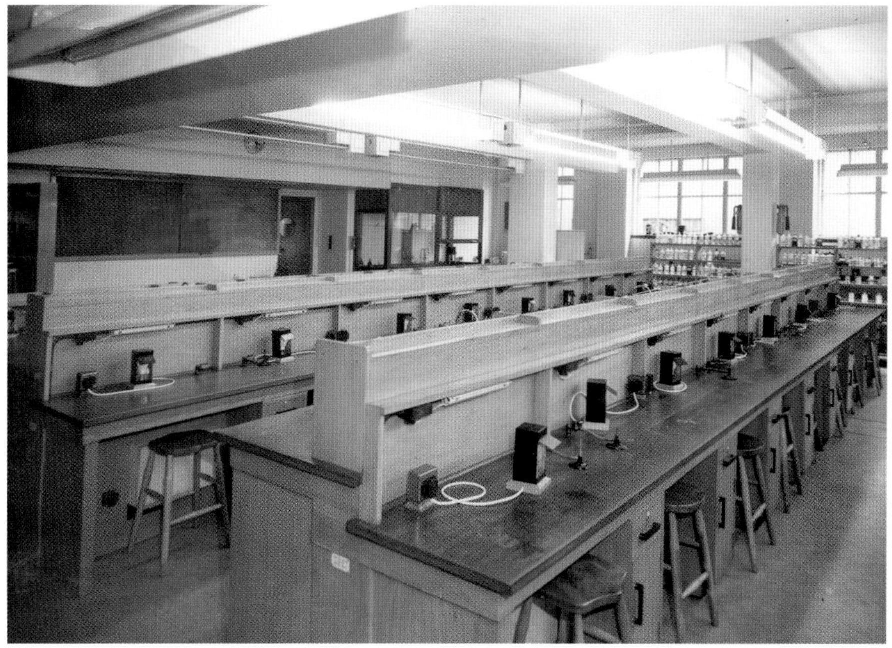

The practical pharmacognosy teaching laboratory in the basement, 1960.

Royal Pharmaceutical Society Museum

It had been hoped that all of the departments would have been moved in to start teaching in October 1958, but the physical chemistry section of pharmaceutical chemistry and the whole of the pharmacognosy department had to stay in Bloomsbury Square for another term. They moved to their new areas in the basement in 1959. The *Square Chronicle* reported that "The Pharmacognosy department, the last department of the School to remain in its entirety at No. 17, has been practically blasted out of the building by the workmen who have been converting the former Chemistry laboratories on the third floor into offices for the Society."

Finally, all teaching and research staff and facilities were in the building for the academic year starting October 1959. Linnell expressed the dean's customary annual sense of relief: "With the last removal from Bloomsbury Square taking place on August 5th, 117 years of high endeavour reap a just reward in the acquisition of premises suitable for a School of the University of London." The student body was also very relieved. The Students' Union president admitted that "For years now we have regarded the new Building

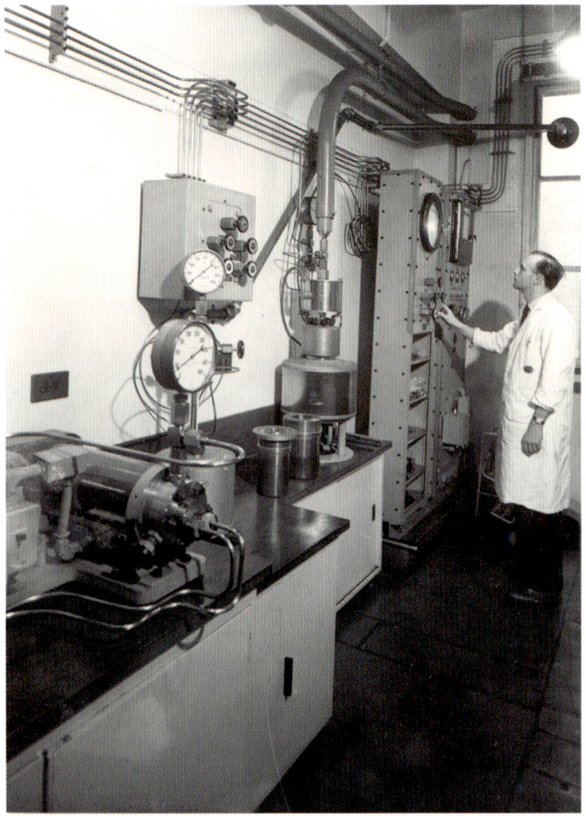

The pharmaceutical chemistry hydrogenation room on the fourth floor, 1960.

Royal Pharmaceutical Society Museum

at Brunswick Square as an empire upon which the concrete never sets ..." and the editor of the *Square Chronicle* summed up the contrast that they were experiencing: "the School of Pharmacy now may well represent the student's dream of a college, and the excellent facilities of the new building do not remotely resemble those of its predecessor 'way back' in Bloomsbury."

In parallel with the building's official opening, a significant illustrated article appeared in *The Pharmaceutical Journal* on 30th April 1960, particularly focused on the equipment and facilities in the new School. The pharmaceutics department could boast a multipurpose Erweka apparatus which, with attachments, covered triple roll milling, mixing, granulation and tablet coating. The department was also using a Ferranti–Shirley viscometer and a Dognon–Abribat surface tension balance to do research into the surface activity of emulsions. The School also had a refrigerated centrifuge for microbiology research. In the pharmaceutical engineering science department, a major emphasis was on research into the preparation of tablets, using equipment that included a 20 ton Apex hydraulic press. The pharmaceutical chemistry department was built to include a fireproof room so that volatile solvents could be left unattended and the room would be automatically flooded with carbon dioxide in the event of a fire. Microbalances were held in a separate room with temperature control to plus or minus one degree. Physical chemistry had use of an optical room with a Gouy diffusion apparatus, thought to be the largest in the world. The department also had a light-scatterer in a dust-controlled room, and a thermostatically controlled infrared room. The radiochemistry laboratory had been installed with a special one-piece floor so that it could be easily cleaned if radioactive material was spilled. A water purification plant was established that supplied deionised water on tap to the whole building. The pharmacology department's research included commercial biological testing for pyrogens, assay of pituitary extract, digitalis and steroids, and acute and chronic toxicity tests. The article also mentioned that the new dean's dining room was furnished and equipped as a gift from the Society.

" Many foreign visitors have been entertained at Brunswick Square and they are unanimous in confirming our own impression that, on completion, our School will be the finest school of pharmacy in the world. This constitutes a great challenge to the staff in order to maintain this position – a challenge which I am sure will be well and truly met. "

Professor Linnell, 1957

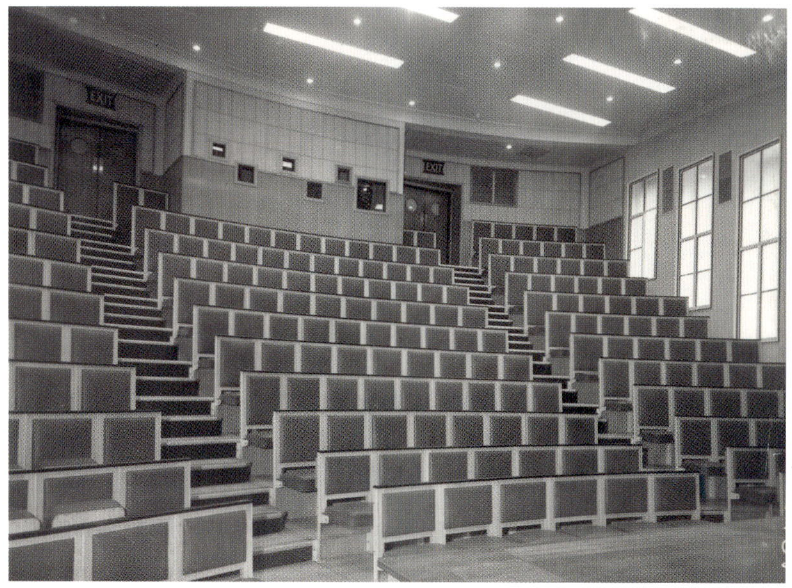

The Large Lecture Theatre (now the John Hanbury Lecture Theatre), 1960. The theatre was kitted out with electrically-controlled blinds, and a preparation room, working bench and fume cupboard which could be revealed by raising the blackboards.

Royal Pharmaceutical Society Museum

Her Majesty Queen Elizabeth, the Queen Mother, Chancellor of the University of London, opened the building officially on 27th April 1960. A section of the Welsh Guards band played a musical accompaniment, and students and invited guests filled the hall to capacity. At the opening ceremony, she remarked, amid laughter, that as its construction had started as early as 1938, it was the "oldest new building" in London. Her Majesty continued by saying:

> [the School] can be justly proud of the influence it has exercised on pharmaceutical education. In this century the education of the pharmacist has changed from a meagre academic course, followed by a long apprenticeship, to a full honours discipline in the University augmented by a brief period of practical training. This change was essential in order to keep pace with the metamorphosis of pharmacy itself from an art – or craft – tinctured with a soupçon of mystery to a profession firmly based on sound scientific principles.

She unveiled a commemorative plaque set into the Italian marble wall of the central entrance hall, saying, "And now, as Chancellor of the University, it gives me great pleasure to declare this building open. And to those who work in it I wish success and happiness in their labours." Her tour of the building and the many exhibits of work by staff and students was very popular. The *Chronicle* reported that the involvement of so many students on the day was very much appreciated, and that "Her Majesty won the hearts of the students by chatting to them about their exhibits and asking them various questions about themselves and their work."

"[the School] can be justly proud of the influence it has exercised on pharmaceutical education. In this century the education of the pharmacist has changed from a meagre academic course, followed by a long apprenticeship, to a full honours discipline in the University augmented by a brief period of practical training."

Her Majesty Queen Elizabeth, the Queen Mother, 1960

However, the move to the new building did not fully alleviate the challenges facing the School. Linnell had articulated one of the key issues before the building was finished. In his Dean's Report for 1958, he explained that "The anomaly presents itself that before the new building is completed it must be admitted that the accommodation is not sufficient to meet the need created by the modern trend of pharmaceutical education and policy." Even with the capacity for an annual intake of 48 students, the School was not meeting the demand for places. The Pharmaceutical Society's ambition for all pharmacists to be university educated had to depend on the support of the universities in terms of financing this capacity. In the following year, Linnell confessed that in spite of the massive development in pharmaceutical education in the last 50 years, the School was only able to keep up with the development of basic sciences. One of the key areas was the need to stimulate research, which was expensive and relied on the Government to provide additional grants to universities, with some passed on to the School as it had been that year. The other issue around space was that with all 144 undergraduates in residence for the first time from October 1959, the School was unable to accommodate any external students, other than a few that could not be accommodated by their own institution for Part II (third year).

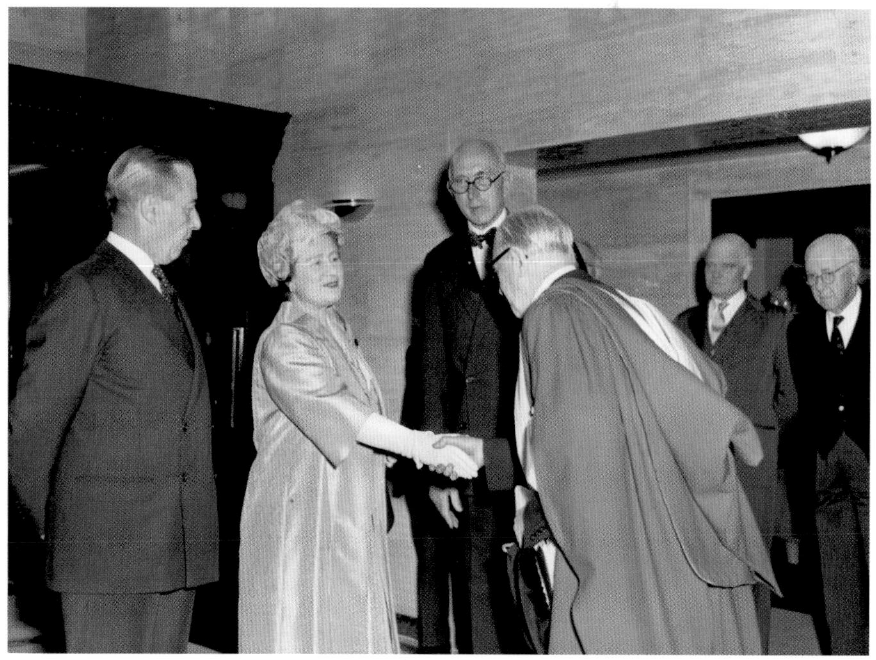

Her Majesty Queen Elizabeth, the Queen Mother, Chancellor of the University of London, being received, before opening the building officially on 27th April 1960.

UCL School of Pharmacy Library

“ The anomaly presents itself that before the new building is completed it must be admitted that the accommodation is not sufficient to meet the need created by the modern trend of pharmaceutical education and policy. ”

Professor Linnell, 1958

In its “Royal Opening Number” of December 1960, the *Square Chronicle* noted a possible solution to the capacity issue:

With the last nail barely banged in, the new school in Brunswick Square was ceremoniously opened by the Royal Chancellor. And so, more than a century after its inception, the School of Pharmacy has finally quitted 17 Bloomsbury Square, and the borough of Holborn, and now dominates the north side of Brunswick Square in the borough of St Pancras, although it still enjoys the most “U” postal district in London, WC1. In the same way as the latest fighter planes are out of date before they leave the ground, so is the New Building no longer adequate, although it has been longer than is customary in construction. Many of the requirements of the original plan are no longer wanted and many things that are required now were not then even conceived. The School is also too small and the higher powers are already thoughtfully casting their eyes hungrily on the building now occupied, but presently to be vacated, by the Royal Free Hospital School of Medicine.

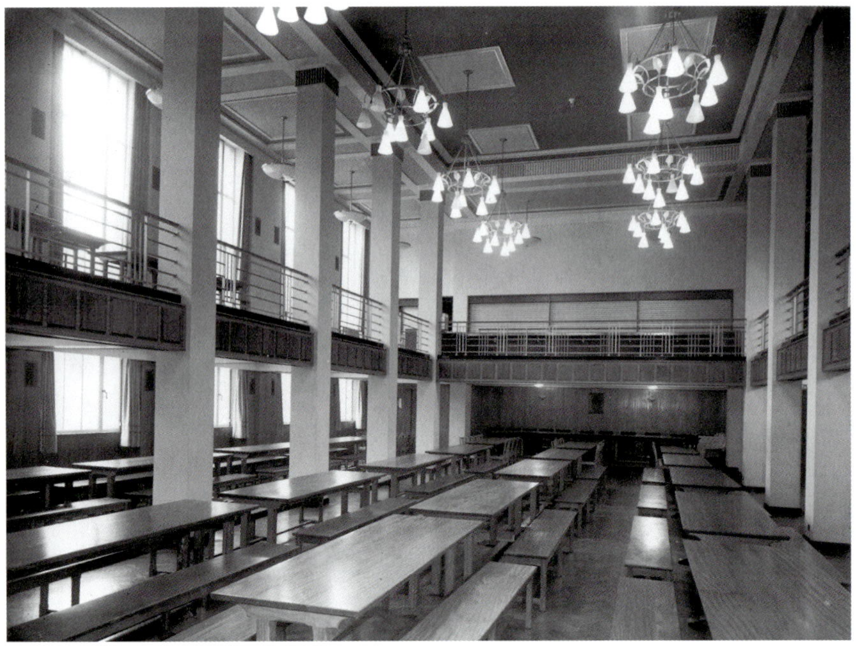

A strangely empty refectory with a snack bar on the gallery, 1960.
Royal Pharmaceutical Society Museum

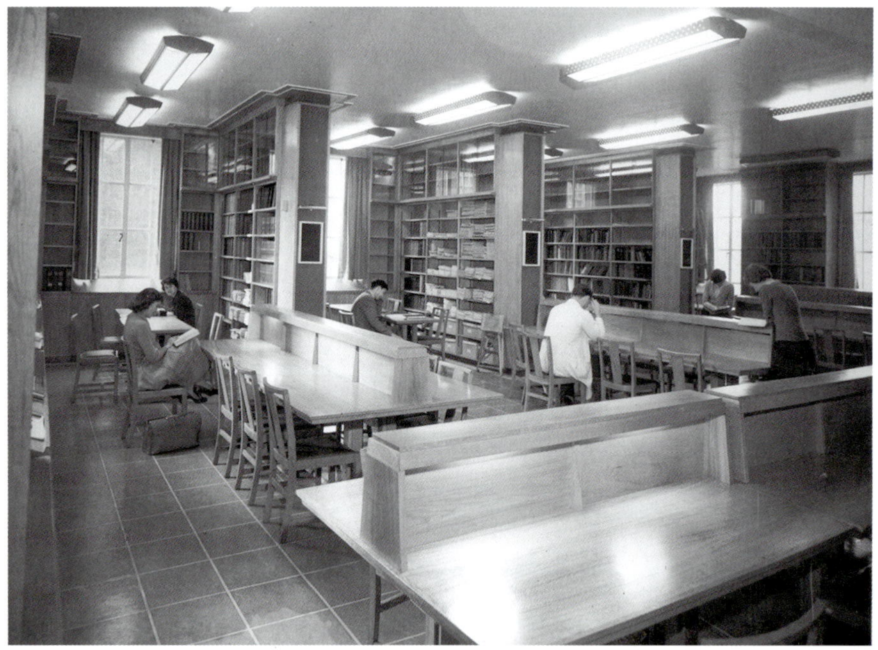

The main library, 1960.
Royal Pharmaceutical Society Museum

There were also inevitable teething problems with the new building. The refectory only just managed to open in January 1960, but was very popular. The library first opened in November 1959, under the first librarian at Brunswick Square, Anthony (Tony) John Evans. At Bloomsbury Square, students had used the Society’s library, with each department maintaining its own collection too. Professor Evans therefore started the Brunswick Square library from scratch. The original plans for it to be sited on the ground floor were altered and it was located on the first floor from the start, with the refectory in the library's original place. The library experienced difficulties due to staff shortages, particularly in opening the library in the evenings. However, having initially only opened until 5.30pm, it was soon able to open until 9pm. The refectory arranged to serve light meals until 6.30pm so that students could continue to study in the evening if their living accommodation was not suitable. A significant advantage of the new accommodation was that outside organisations could hire the facilities. Early examples included the School's neighbour, the Royal Free Hospital Medical School, the Pharmacological Society, and summer schools on a wide range of topics including "Art, Literature and Music in England, 1660–1780."

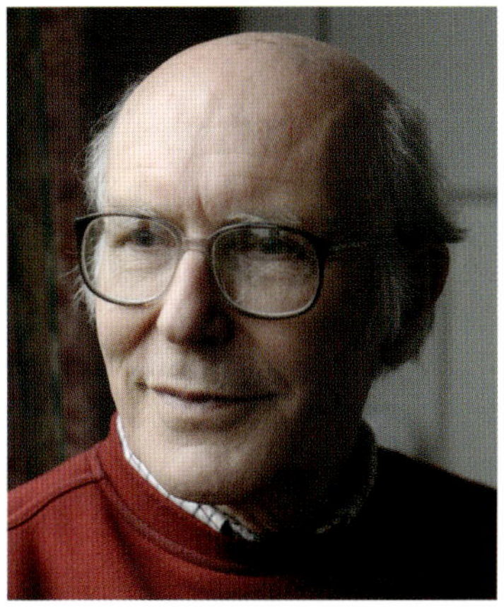

AINLEY WADE (1936–)

AINLEY WADE (1936–)

Following advice from Tony Evans, Ainley applied to the Square and took the BPharm (1954–1957). Although intending to be an analyst, he trained in pharmaceutical development at BDH Ltd in Islington and returned there for five years after two years of National Service. While studying part time for an MPhil at Chelsea, he was inspired by meeting editors from the Pharmaceutical Society and joined the department of pharmaceutical sciences on the staff of *Martindale: The Extra Pharmacopoeia* in 1965. From 1966 to 1968 he was fortunate to assist in the founding of the British Society for the History of Pharmacy. He was appointed assistant editor in 1970 and editor in 1972–1978 for the 27th edition of *Martindale*. He then became the general editor of the Pharmaceutical Society's scientific books and worked on the development and launch of the new *British National Formulary* from 1978 to 1981 and joint secretary of the Joint Formulary Committee with the British Medical Association and Department of Health. He was involved in the publication of three editions of the *Handbook of Pharmaceutical Excipients* with the American Pharmaceutical Association, *Pharmaceutical Codex* and *Herbal Medicine*. Before his retirement in 1996, electronic versions of *Martindale* and the *BNF* were launched. He is a fellow of the School and editor of *Pharmaceutical Historian*.

But what did the students think of their new school? In 1960, a piece in the *Guardian* had described the building as "the clumsy, dull, School of Pharmacy". The students had their own views. Beyond the universally positive reaction to the increased space, light and modernity, opinions of contributors to the *Square Chronicle* on the aesthetic appeal of the building were less than complimentary. One article in 1955 put it simply: "Brunswick Square from outside is red and tall, and the setting of its doors and windows too mathematically precise to be pleasing." Another article suggested that the new building looked like a prison camp, calling it "Stalag Brunswick". However, a cartoon perhaps summed it up best for a building that was designed in the 1930s but not completed until 1960, depicting the School as a cinema.

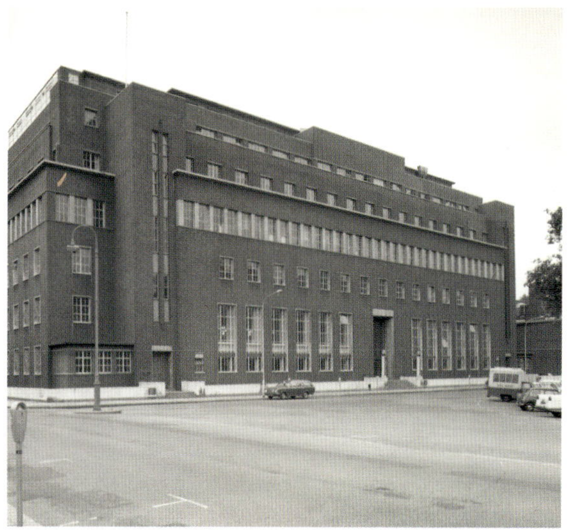

The new School of Pharmacy building, Brunswick Square, 1960.
UCL School of Pharmacy Library

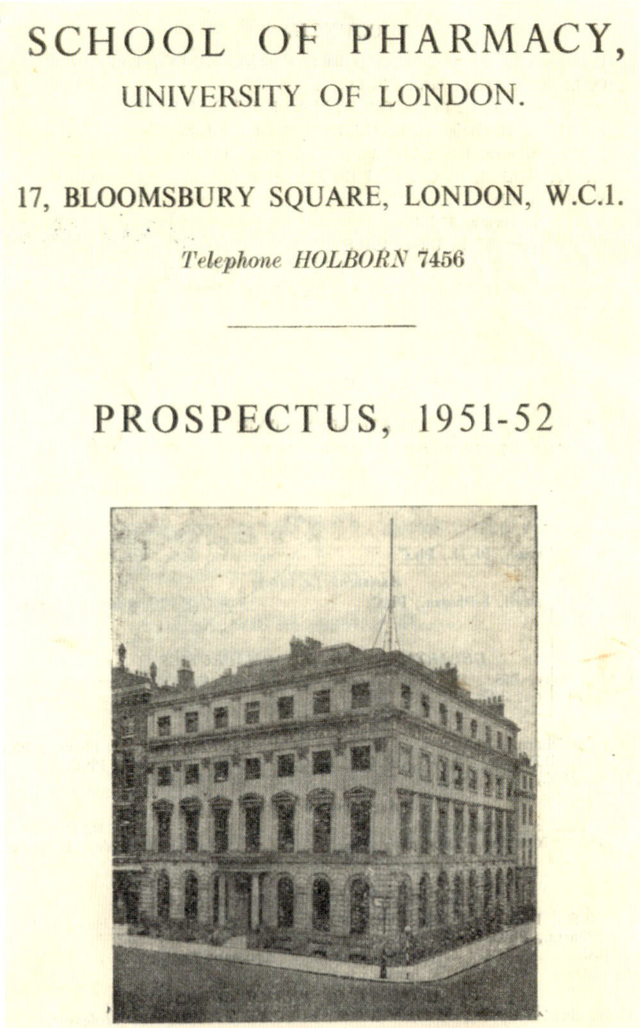

SCHOOL OF PHARMACY,
UNIVERSITY OF LONDON.

17, BLOOMSBURY SQUARE, LONDON, W.C.1.

Telephone HOLBORN 7456

PROSPECTUS, 1951-52

UCL School of Pharmacy Library

A UNIVERSITY SCHOOL

At the meeting of the Society's Council in March 1949, the president, Clement Shaw, officially reported that the Society had ceased to be responsible for the School. The School was incorporated as an independent entity with its own governing body upon which sat representatives of the University of London, the Pharmaceutical Society and the academic staff, together with a number of co-opted persons. Stanley Curtis was appointed as the first secretary of the School on 1st September 1948 and oversaw the development of the Society's administration of the School into an independent office organisation. Berry also registered the School as a company limited by guarantee in January 1949. The School benefited from a greatly increased budget of £50,000 in 1949–50.

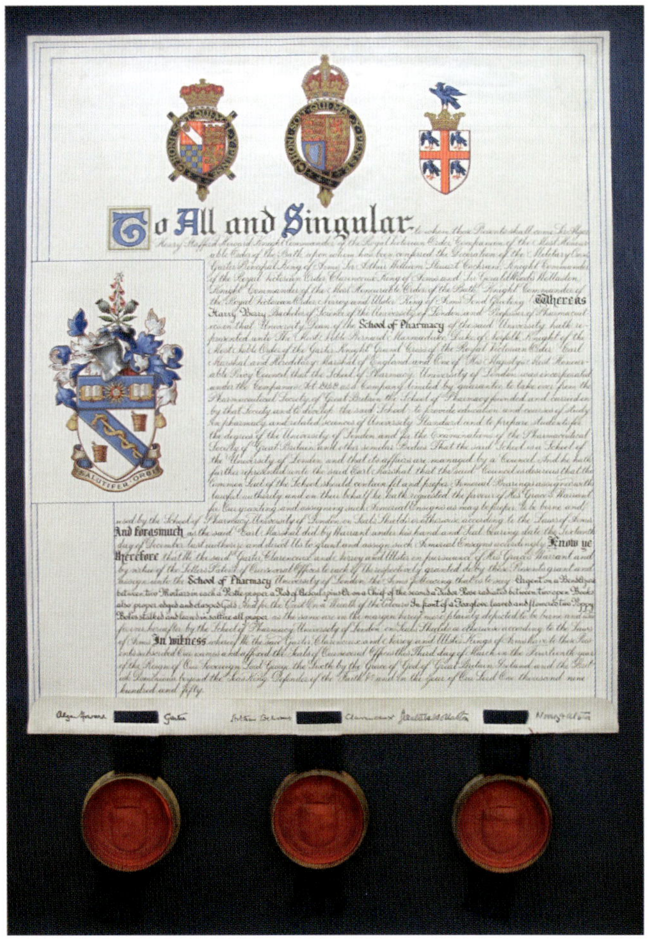

The School's coat of arms includes two mortars and pestles, the medicinal symbol of the staff of Aesculapius, two poppy heads and a foxglove. The inclusion of the Tudor rose and two open books are part of the arms of the University of London. The motto, 'Salutifer orbi', means "Bringing health to the world."

UCL School of Pharmacy

"I believe a sound foundation has now been laid for the School, which will enable it to develop satisfactorily along its own special lines, to take its proper place in the Faculty of Medicine, and to make its contribution to the advancement of medical science."

Professor Berry, October 1952

As a key development in the establishment of the School as an independent organisation, it received a grant of arms in March 1950. The coat of arms included the pharmaceutical symbols of the staff of Aesculapius, a mortar and pestle, and poppy heads and a foxglove. It also included the University of London symbols of open books and a Tudor rose. The motto, "Salutifer Orbi", translates as "Bringing health to the world".

In 1952, a Royal Charter of Incorporation was granted to the School. The signatories included the president and vice-president of the Pharmaceutical Society, the chancellor and vice-chancellor of the University, the chair and vice-chairman of the School Council, and the dean, Professor Berry. The petition for the Charter had been submitted to King George VI in October 1951 by the University of London's chancellor, the Earl of Athlone. The petition put forward the advantages for the School of holding a Royal Charter. It will:

> tend to the great advantage of the School and to the promotion of its interests, by giving it a higher status and more efficient form of government, thus ensuring its stability and the more effective performance of its duties by fostering public spirit, by instituting a greater pride in the School and its traditions, by encouraging measures for further development and improvement of the School, and by giving to the School additional dignity and influence which will enable it to hold that position among the Schools of the Kingdom to which its past history and its growing influence and sphere of importance would appear justly to entitle it.

However, the King's death on 6th February 1952 meant that it was Queen Elizabeth II who granted that Charter on 7th May 1952, only three months after her accession. Professor Berry was quite rightly very pleased:

> There is no doubt that the announcement of the granting of the Charter was received with great satisfaction by all pharmacists for they rightly deemed it an honour conferred upon Pharmacy. The School would appear now to have acquired its rightful and permanent status in the scientific world by the great generosity of the University of London, and to have realised the ambition of those early pioneers – Redwood, Attfield, Bentley, Reynolds, Green, Crossley and Greenish – who each in his way established the ideals of the School which can be summed up as the prosecution of research, the pioneering of new developments and the provision of a centre of pharmaceutical education where students can foregather and acquire a liberal and balanced outlook on Pharmacy.

From the point of view of the School's history, it is worthy of note that point 9 of the Charter put the battles over women students of the 1870s firmly into its history: "No religious test shall be imposed upon any officer or teacher or any student of the School, nor shall any disability be imposed on the grounds of sex."

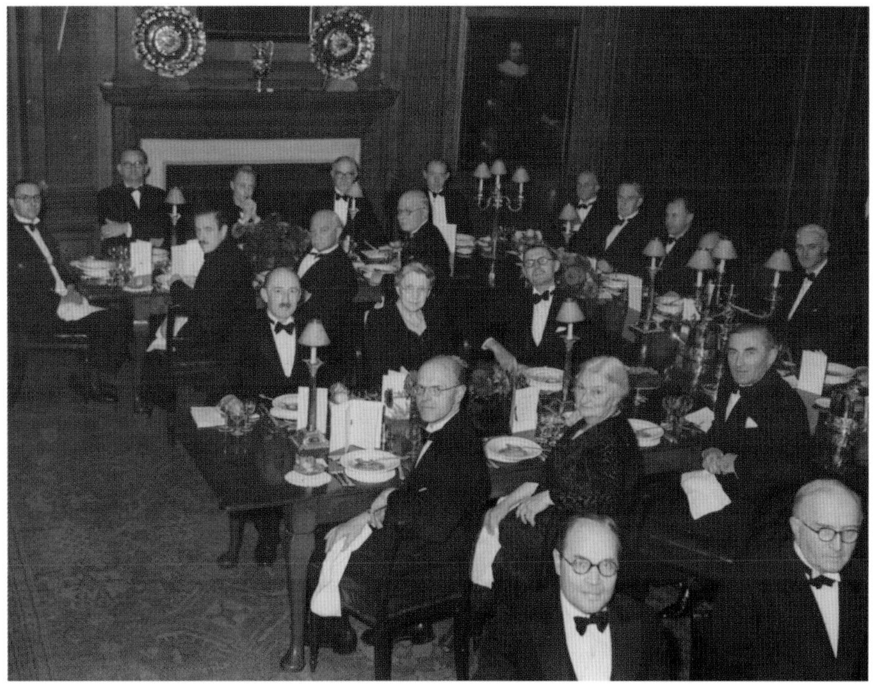

The School's annual dinner was renamed the Charter dinner, with the first being held at Mercers' Hall in November 1952.

Royal Pharmaceutical Society Museum

The granting of the Charter was commemorated each year by the School Council, by renaming the annual school dinner the Charter dinner. The first Charter dinner and dance in November 1952 was attended by Princess Alice and her husband, the Earl of Athlone, the chancellor of the University, as principal guests, alongside 400 other guests. The occasion was celebrated with saddles of roast lamb.

The Pharmaceutical Society Council marked the occasion with a gift of £2,000 to start a Charter Fund to fund research or any other activity. However, the financial situation was not comfortable. A University Grants Committee report for 1952–3 outlined the School's balance sheet. There were 32 teaching staff and 105 full-time students. The School's total income was £80,794, of which £70,000 was from government grants, £4,876 from tuition fees and £2,000 from endowments (the Charter Fund). Total expenditure was £82,066, of which £35,210 was teaching staff salaries. From this year onward, the School's calendars begin to show a growing emphasis on encouraging grants from pharmaceutical manufacturers in order to develop the facilities. In the calendar for the 1954–5 session, the donors are listed as Allen & Hanburys with £250 per annum for seven years, Boots with a grant of £15,000 spread over seven years, British Drug Houses giving £250 per annum for seven years, Distillers Company with £500 per annum for three years, Glaxo Laboratories donating £2,100 per annum for seven years, and the Pharmaceutical Society with £2,000 per annum for five years. This public recognition of external funding was only the beginning of a new financial environment for the School. In his Dean's Report of 1957, Linnell explained that although the University of London had been very sympathetic financially, the Government had restricted funding for universities such that no capital development could take place at the School over the next five years.

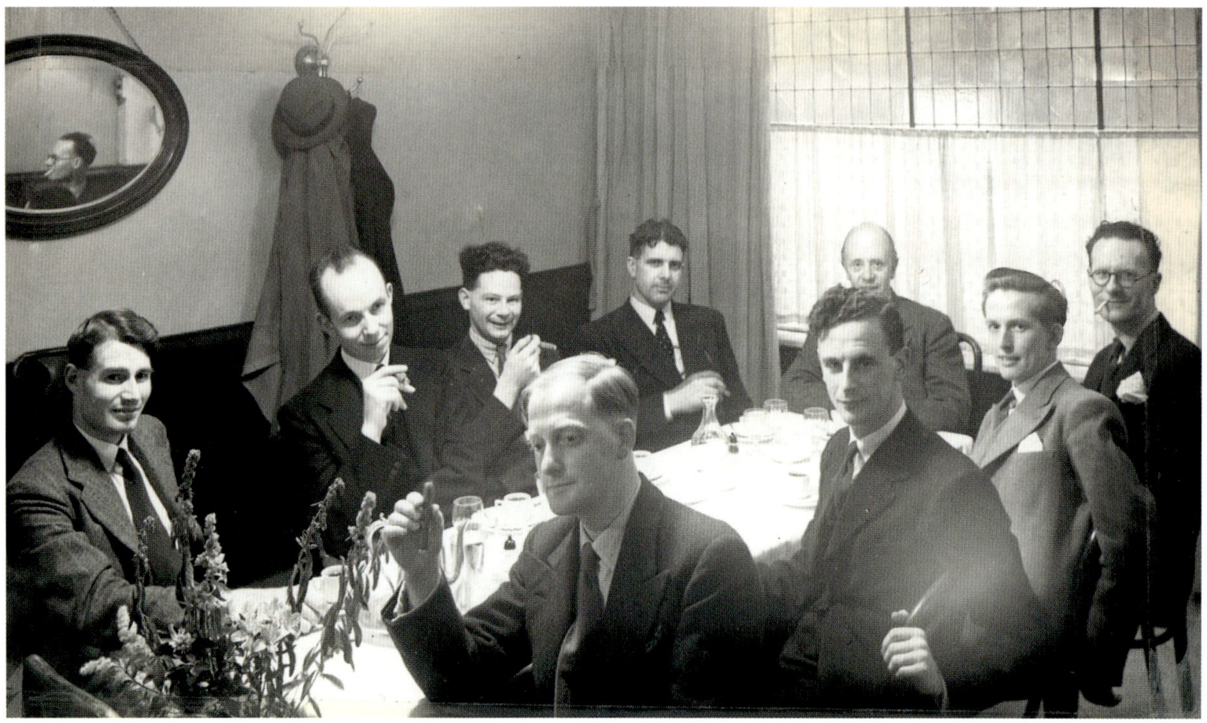

Professor Linnell, as head of department, heads the table in this informal photograph of a chemistry staff gathering in around 1949.

UCL School of Pharmacy Library

THE COURSE

In 1950, new syllabuses for the Society's Qualifying exam were published. All entrants for the exam from 1952 onwards had to take a new two-year course in Physiology and Pharmacology. After two decades, these modernising elements had finally become compulsory. The Pharmacy Act of 1953 was the catalyst for more long-term changes. The chemist & druggist register was finally abolished, and all existing chemists & druggists were transferred to the pharmaceutical chemists' register as Members of the Pharmaceutical Society (MPS). Those who were already pharmaceutical chemists were now designated Fellows of the Pharmaceutical Society (FPS), and a new Honorary Fellowship category was inaugurated to recognise exceptional service to the profession. In fact, the 1953 Act was a Transitional Act, and was replaced by the 1954 Pharmacy Act which repealed it, plus the 1852, 1868 and 1908 Pharmacy Acts. The old Victorian and Edwardian membership and educational order was swept away.

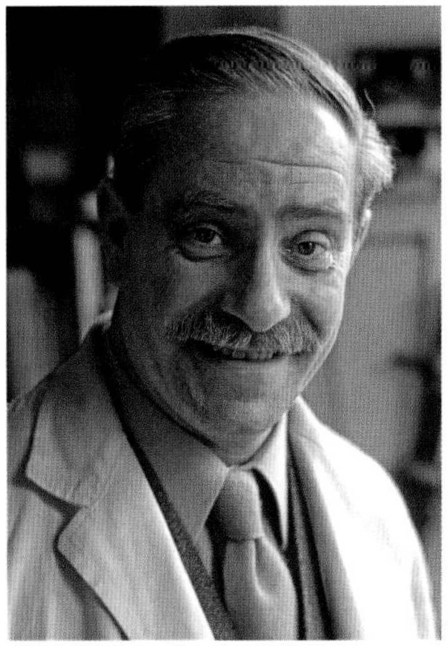

PATRICK D'ARCY (1928–2001)

Victor Patterson

PATRICK D'ARCY (1928–2001)

Patrick D'Arcy gained his BPharm at the School in 1952, and then lectured in pharmacology while studying for his PhD, which he gained in 1956. He joined Allen & Hanburys as head of the pharmacology department in 1958, but left in 1962 to go to Sudan, where he established pharmacy as an academic subject at the University of Khartoum and he became dean. In 1967, he moved to take up the post of technical director at Riker Laboratories. He then became the first head of the pharmacy department at Queen's University, Belfast, where he stayed for 16 years. He also became director of the International Pharmaceutical Federation's Third World Department.

He edited *Pharmacy International*, the *International Pharmacy Journal* and the *International Journal of Pharmaceutics*. Professor D'Arcy was science chairman for the British Pharmaceutical Conference in 1980. In 1981, he was awarded an OBE for services to pharmacy. In 1984, he received the Pharmaceutical Society's Harrison memorial medal and was made a fellow of the School of Pharmacy in 1993 for his contribution to pharmacy, both nationally and internationally. In 1996, he was awarded an honorary doctorate of science by the University of Khartoum.

Cyril Maplethorpe, looking back at this period from the 1960s, realised how the ambitions of the 1930s for one register of pharmacists and one qualification were finally being realised. From the situation in the 1940s, when only 10% of pharmacists entered the profession with a degree-standard education, by the end of the 1950s, all pharmacy students had to complete a three-year course at degree standard. From 1958 onwards, all of the "technological universities" apart from Edinburgh provided teaching for the University of London external degree.

At the Charter Inaugural Meeting on 8th October 1952, Professor Berry explained that the new degree which all pharmacy undergraduates had been studying since 1950 would provide pharmacists equipped to work in a new environment, whether as hospital pharmacists within the (new) NHS, in manufacturing, in chemotherapeutic research on new drugs, or in the study of crude drugs and the analytical control of drugs. The degree course was also, importantly, a good grounding to continue into postgraduate research. These aims were bolstered in 1955 when the School put a scheme of vacation work into operation where students gained experience of working in manufacturing laboratories, hospitals or retail establishments for a six-week period. Not only did this provide students with practical experience, it also helped to inform their choices about which sector they would like to work in. In addition, on 20th July 1955, the University's Senate approved the institution of the degree of Master of Pharmacy, which the School hoped would foster research in pharmacy.

> **"The three year's course**
> **Pharmacog still plays its part,**
> **Dispensing's studied from the start.**
> **We know of some old C and Ds**
> **Who thank the Lord on bended knees**
> **They didn't have to work and cram**
> **To pass the present stiff exam …**
>
> **We think this move has done much harm,**
> **Future students will take BPharm**
> **The reason for this awful mess**
> **Seems to be, we must confess,**
> **Because we're dominated from the top**
> **By men whose only take is shop."**
>
> *B.H. Norris, August 1957*

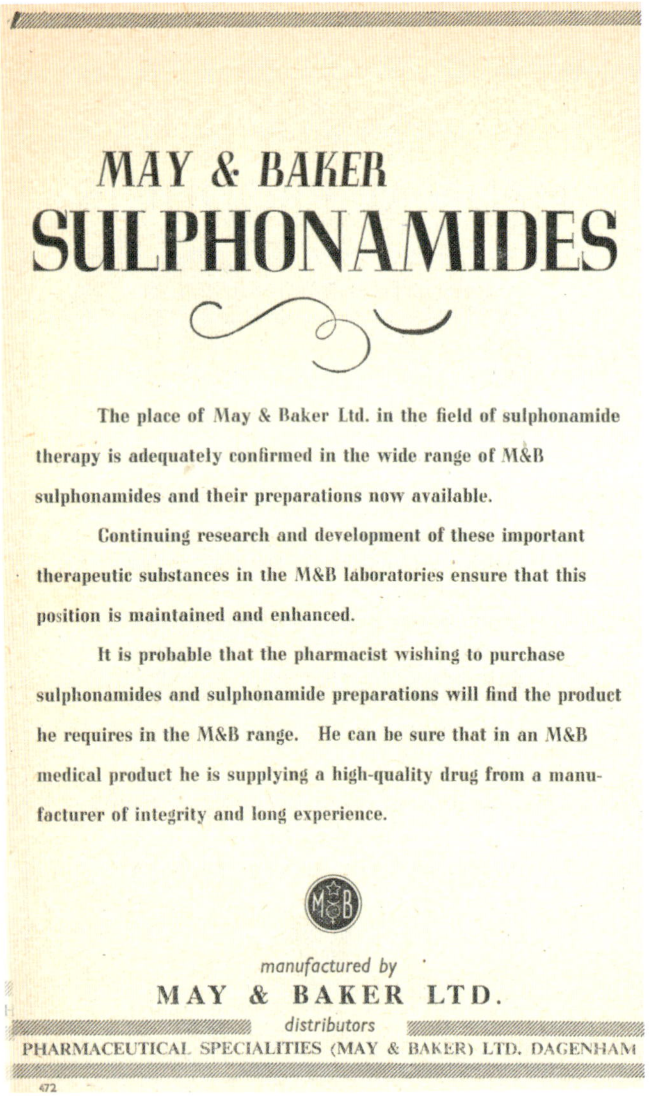

Sulphonamides were no longer at the cutting edge of drug development by the time this advert appeared in the *Square Chronicle* in the late 1940s. They had been the breakthrough products of the 1930s, effective against bacterial infections, and therefore revolutionary in their ability to treat diseases such as pneumonia and meningitis.

UCL School of Pharmacy Library

There had been significant changes in medicines and therapies immediately before, during and after the Second World War, with wartime developments scaled up and developed further for civilian populations. Sulphonamides, penicillin and the use of steroids were just some of the new drug areas, and microbiology was now essential training for a pharmacist because of the new work with parenteral technology, antimicrobial agents and aseptic techniques. Professor Berry also felt that chemical engineering was important in understanding the production of oral dose forms. His interest had been stimulated by meeting Charles Peck, a chemical engineer who was working on tablet machine design, at the British Pharmaceutical Conference. When David Train joined the staff in October 1945, he was persuaded to take a chemical engineering degree at Imperial College. When he returned to the Square in 1949, he was given responsibility for a new area of pharmaceutical engineering which later became a final year option in the honours degree. The University's Faculty of Engineering objected to the use of the word "engineering" in the course title and formally investigated Train and Berry. As a result, the course was to be called "pharmaceutical engineering science". In addition to lectures, the engineering department had a workshop, initially at Bloomsbury Square, and then in the new Brunswick Square building.

In September 1955, *The Pharmaceutical Journal* published an article entitled "School of Pharmacy, University of London. A review of new projects by the dean, Professor H. Berry". Even though the building was far from complete, the article included many photographs of the laboratories, stores and other facilities. Berry explained that the University's Board of Studies in Pharmacy had reviewed postwar practice, and as a result two subjects, pharmacognosy and pharmacology, had "a very drastic overhaul". The situation for pharmacognosy was that "This, our oldest subject, has undergone many changes because so many vegetable drugs have been discarded ... in the opinion of the School, however, it would be wrong to conclude that the subject has no future." Pharmacologists were particularly busy in India, Egypt and Africa, exploring native drugs. In addition, the subject was being reorientated towards plant physiology and its effect on drug production. As such, the new department set-up for pharmacognosy at Brunswick Square included a glasshouse on the roof, to be able to work on plant physiology and biochemistry.

However, the pharmacognosy staff at the Square, notably Wallis, had had to leave much of the subject's history and current research behind. The reason was the reduced importance given to the Society's museum, even while still at Bloomsbury Square. Wallis, in *The Pharmaceutical Journal* of 8th August 1942, had called for the museum to have a new curator so that it "would become a veritable centre of post-graduate instruction and a stimulus of research in all departments of pharmacy." However, the *Chronicle* in April 1948 described the room on the ground floor: "it sets out to be a museum, but ended as a mausoleum." In late 1948, the Society advertised for a full-time curator at a salary of £800 per annum. Professor Jack Rowson was appointed, and Wallis continued as emeritus curator. When the School became part of the University, the museum was drawn in two directions. A curator to promote teaching might sit in the School or in the Society. Rowson, an employee of the Society, continued the research side of the museum's work, alongside talks and exhibitions. He also showed specimens to students from all schools of pharmacy. In fact, in 1954, the *Chemist and Druggist* valued the museum as the only part of the Society promoting scientific research: "Since the Society abdicated responsibility for the training of students by handing over its School to the University of London, the work, incidental to the Museum has been the only scientific work done under its aegis." Professor Rowson left the post in 1957, and Wallis, with the help of a technical assistant, oversaw the collection.

Berry's 1955 article in *The Pharmaceutical Journal* indicated that pharmacology experienced the other significant change in the course. Derek Dunlop, writing in 1948, had said:

> It might be thought that of all scientific subjects pharmacology would be the most important for the pharmacist, to which all their previous scientific study – particularly physiology – would lead. It is, therefore, surprising that pharmacology has practically no place in the syllabus of study or in the examinations for the pharmaceutical chemist. It would seem desirable for this to be remedied in the future.

By 1955, the pharmacy student spent more hours on pharmacology than the medical student. This was particularly important because of the use of animal experiments for new drugs. Berry saw a key role for the pharmacist in keeping up with detailed knowledge of new drugs and acting as an advisor to other medical practitioners. The School was also teaching new techniques in pharmaceutical analysis, using physical instruments. The microanalytical laboratory was able to carry out research work for the School, but also for other University departments.

The new course for pharmaceutics involved pilot-scale production of medicines, before mass manufacture, and made students consider problems of packaging and packaging materials. There was the recognition that fewer medicines were made in individual pharmacies. The Square also developed teaching in pharmaceutical microbiology, particularly important for injections and drugs with aseptic requirements. The pharmaceutical engineering science course was also a unique selling point for the School, promoted as chemical engineering from a pharmacy standpoint.

The students appeared ready to embrace this new world. The *Chronicle* in September 1953 reported that at the International Chemical Exhibition in Paris, a robot chemist was exhibited that prepared medicines. They argued that the School should have one for the pharmaceutical engineers to take to pieces. However, the students were also realistic: "It seems sometimes as though the technological developments must outstrip our ability to keep pace with them in the time at our disposal. It becomes even more than ever important to concentrate on basic principles." Nevertheless, works visits to see current pharmaceutical industry in action continued as a valued part of the programme, either on Wednesday afternoons, the half-day of taught courses, or for a whole day out for visits further afield. In the 1950s, the trips included destinations such as Ransom's at Hitchin and British Drug Houses at Poole.

Of course, the core syllabus across the country was now compulsory and fixed, but this did not exclude various approaches to the component subjects, usually dependent on the interests and qualifications of the staff at each school. At the Square in 1955, BPharm students spent the first two years studying all subjects, then took the Part I exam. In the third year, they could specialise in two subjects out of pharmaceutical chemistry, pharmaceutical engineering science, pharmaceutics, pharmacognosy or pharmacology. The course culminated in the Part II exam. It was also possible to take a Master of Pharmacy for those who wanted to continue above the BPharm level, but not as far as a doctorate.

In his 1955 article, Berry gave some current statistics. The levels of staffing were nine staff for pharmaceutical chemistry (one professor, one senior lecturer, four lecturers, three assistant lecturers), 11 staff for pharmaceutics and pharmaceutical engineering science (one professor, one senior lecturer, five lecturers, four assistant lecturers), four staff for pharmacognosy (one reader, two lecturers, one assistant lecturer) and eight staff for pharmacology (one professor, one reader, three lecturers, three assistant lecturers). As for the allocation of time across the subjects for the students, in the first year, they spent 35% on pharmaceutical chemistry, 35% on pharmaceutics and pharmaceutical engineering science, 15% on pharmacognosy and 15% on pharmacology. In the second year, this changed slightly to 37% on pharmaceutical chemistry and 33% on pharmaceutics and pharmaceutical engineering science. The third year course had the time divided equally between the two subjects chosen.

In 1957, the entrance requirements for the pharmaceutical chemist exam were brought into line with universities. Applicants could either sit the Society's entrance exam, or achieve advanced GCE Chemistry, Physics and Biology, plus English, Mathematics and a language other than English at GCE ordinary level. They did not have to take an approved course. The aim was that this would allow flexibility for all applicants and would encourage students to stay on in the sixth form.

The practical elements of pharmacy training were also altered. Rather than the established two years of preacademic practical training, or one year of postacademic training, from 1958 students only had to do one year's training, which could be carried out either before or after the course, although it was assumed that most would do it afterwards. Articles of pupillage were discontinued and premises for practical training were no longer approved by the Society, although it retained the power to disallow a premises if it proved unsuitable. When the new honours degree was introduced the Society had discontinued its joint inspectorate, run with the University of London, for schools teaching the BPharm.

The pharmaceutical chemist diploma course was extended from two to three years in 1958. These changes had first been proposed by the Council in 1947 to enable more time for a broad range of subjects, and for students to assimilate and understand the subjects they were being taught. It would also allow for the Qualifying exam not to be concentrated into the end of the course. However, the changes were controversial in the profession as some pharmacists thought the longer course would be a deterrent to candidates and create a manpower problem.

With the length of the pharmaceutical chemist course now the same as the degree, students could choose whether to do the diploma or the BPharm. It was considered that most aspiring retail pharmacists would do the diploma, and there was some criticism that the degree level was set too high and would lose potential students to other science subjects. The other criticism was that, having completed the degree, the graduate would remain in research or academia rather than registering as a pharmacist. C.W. Maplethorpe countered these criticisms with a strongly held belief that retail pharmacists should be equipped with an academic qualification. He argued that they needed to be able to understand new drugs and to talk to other medical professionals on the same level. Running a business also required high levels of education as well as practical training. There were a number of letters in *The Pharmaceutical Journal* in this period calling for the course to provide business training, as the multiple pharmacies were already doing for their staff. The Council argued that the three-year course allowed them to include this element.

The role of pharmacognosy in the new syllabus was also problematic, based on differing beliefs about its relevance in the modern pharmacy profession. An initial proposal by the Society's Education Committee in 1955 was that it should only be allocated 100 hours over two years, a dramatic reduction. However, the change to a three-year pharmaceutical chemist course in 1958 meant a new proposal of 180 hours for pharmacognosy in the first two years of the course, and none in the final year. The opposition from many pharmacognosy lecturers led to the final agreement that each school could set its own Part I paper based on material taught in the School. Importantly for the subject's continued vibrancy, the syllabus did not rely on memorising drugs, but included chromatography and chemistry.

"the pharmacist [should be educated to be] ... accepted as the ultimate professional authority on drugs. He becomes the one professional man who has a complete all-round knowledge of the sources, identification, preparation, standardisation, actions and uses of drugs."

C.W. Maplethorpe, 1957

A significant problem for the School was financing the acquisition of equipment to allow the departments to keep up to date in both teaching and research. The Annual Reports show how much they were dependent on external funding. For example, in 1960 the Wellcome Trustees had given a spectrophotofluorimeter to the department of pharmacology, and the British Empire Cancer Campaign had supported research. CIBA, the Distillers Company, Parke Davis, Pfizer, and Smith, Kline and French had all supported research students. Scholarships also encouraged further research. However, the age of endless prizes appeared to be over. The Herbarium competition, established in the early years of the School, was finally ended in 1950.

The research work in the laboratories did continue with many successes in this postwar period. In fact, with the shortage of pharmacologists in teaching schools in London after the war, staff from the Square taught at three medical schools in addition to their research and teaching roles at the School. Some of the key areas of research going on in this period were work by Geoff West on anaphylactic reactions, Mike Rand looking into adrenergic transmission, and George Somers' investigations into the actions and uses of succinylcholine and of glycyrrhetinic acid.

ELEANOR ZAIMIS (1915–1982)

Eleanor Christides was educated in Bucharest and graduated from Athens University in 1938. She then worked there in the pharmacology department. She moved to England after her marriage to John Zaimis in 1943, and worked for a number of research institutions before being appointed reader at the School in 1954. She went on to become head of the pharmacology department at the Royal Free Hospital until 1980. Her specialist research area was neuromuscular blockade. She continued her work on methonium compounds from her previous posts while at the Square, having injected herself with various methonium drugs in the course of her research in the 1940s. She was successful in developing techniques to understand local anaesthetics, and the process of lowering blood pressure. One of her students at the Square commented: "Zaimis's enthusiasm for the elucidation of pharmacological mechanisms was infectious."

THE STUDENT EXPERIENCE

In the *Square Chronicle* of September 1949, the president of the Students' Union, R. Thornton, felt optimistic: "The present lack of facilities will not last for ever. Indeed, the luxury of the new school at Brunswick Square is something that the new students will look forward to, and our search for a hostel and sports ground may yet be successful."

The lack of their own sports ground had become a recurrent theme of student publications. Sharing with other colleges, taking up offers from pharmaceutical manufacturers and trekking long distances to play matches seemed to be the norm. In 1947, the Hockey Club was able to make use of a London County Council pitch in Victoria Park. However, the staff were also well aware that a sports ground specifically for the School would be a valuable development. Professor Berry made his view clear in 1952 that a sports ground was "an essential for any student body if it is to enjoy a proper university atmosphere."

The breakthrough came in May 1954 when the School jointly bought Myddelton House in Enfield as a site for a sports grounds and a botanical garden. The *Chronicle* reported: "The ground is being shared with the Royal Free Hospital Medical School, but when twenty-five acres are available one does not mind doing a bit of sharing." Myddelton House had been in the hands of the same family, the Bowles, since 1724. The last member to own it was the renowned horticulturalist Augustus Bowles. Early in the 1950s, Dr James Fairbairn had been recommended by staff at Chelsea Physic Garden to

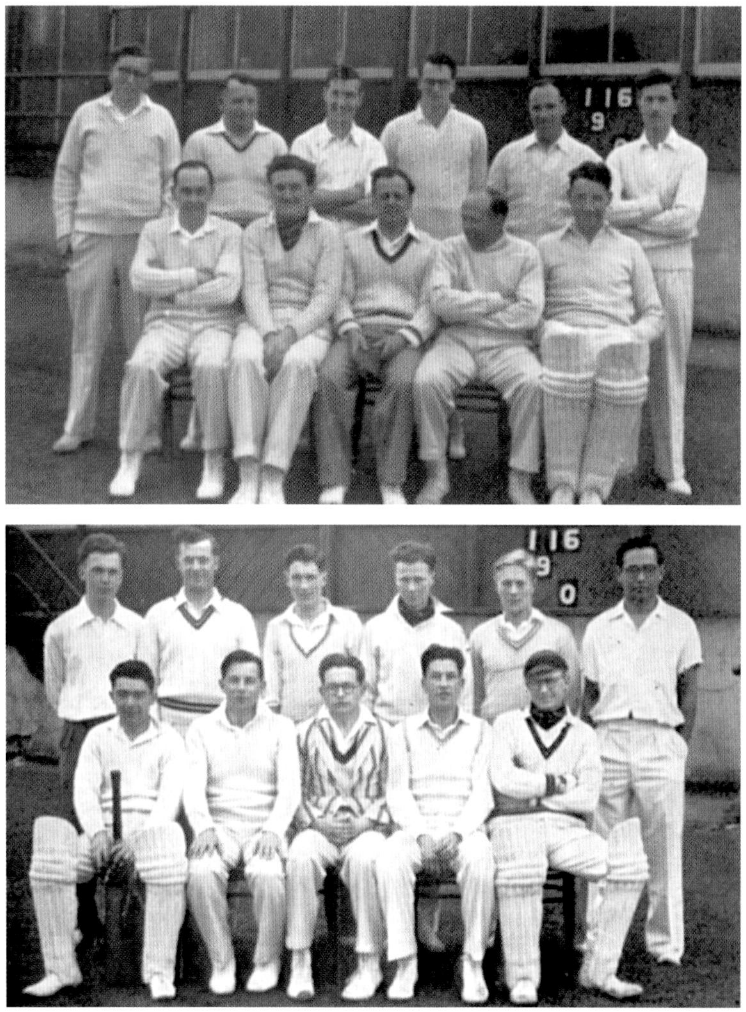

The Association cricket team and their school opponents were pictured in the *Square Chronicle* in September 1954, with an account of the annual match.

UCL School of Pharmacy Library

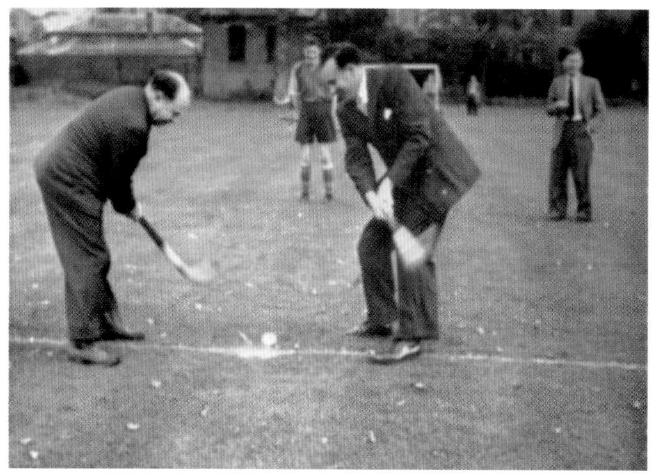

The pitch at Myddelton House was ceremonially opened in 1955 with a bully off between the Dean and the President of the Student's Union.

UCL School of Pharmacy Library

approach Bowles as a potential supplier of rhubarb root for research. Fairbairn obtained his supply but also learnt more about the house and gardens and found that Bowles had no heir to pass Myddelton House to. When Bowles died in May 1954, the School of Pharmacy and the Royal Free Hospital Medical School received a capital grant from the University Court for acquisition, adaption and equipment of the grounds. Berry announced in his 1954 Report that although the grounds were immediately available for use, the "changing accommodation is at present rudimentary." The students were not interested in these facilities, but had other concerns: "Certain vital information is not yet to hand. For example, the distances (in feet) from the ground to the nearest hostelries and the nature of the brews supplied therein."

Having settled in the joint rugby club with the Royal Free (which had been founded in 1953 by Tony Evans, later Professor Evans, the first librarian at Brunswick Square) as a priority, staff and students proceeded to improve the surroundings at Myddelton House. In 1955, six hard tennis courts were installed, and work was undertaken to bring the playing fields' turf up to standard. In 1958, the two student bodies decorated the house, so that it could be used for dances and parties. In 1960, a refectory was set up, as well as an all-weather tennis court that could also be used for netball. Cricket and football were also happily based at the grounds.

Meanwhile, the postwar period saw an explosion in the number of clubs and societies at the Square. In 1947, The Hobby-Horse Club was formed to learn more about others' hobbies and other countries, as there were so many overseas students at the School. Early talks included one on Indian Independence, and another on the Egyptian Pyramids. The Music Club was absorbed by an Arts Club, which widened its remit to include exhibition visits and theatre trips. In 1948, a Chess Club, Camera Club, Bible Study Group, The Socialist Society (affiliated to the Student Labour Federation), and the School of Pharmacy Branch of the London University Conservative Association were all founded. In 1951, a Rag Committee was formed for the School, and in 1952, a new Sailing Club was set up, using the Welsh Harp Reservoir at Hendon to sail its National Firefly boat. In 1954, there was a new Horticultural Society set up, a new Bridge Club, and a Historical and Literary Society, whose first talk was by Agnes Lothian, the Pharmaceutical Society's librarian, on the history of 17 Bloomsbury Square.

The infamous pantomimes really came into the limelight in this period. Productions such as *Walladin* in 1950, *Doris in Mortarland* in 1955, *The Wizard of Pharm* in 1956, *My Pharm Lady* in 1957 and *Peter Pan – the Spore who Wouldn't Grow Up* in 1963 went down into the Square's history and showcased the writing and performing talent of both students and staff.

Unsurprisingly, the social side of the School also became more integrated with that of the University of London. All Student Union members at the School were automatically members of the Square Association, the University of London Union, the British Pharmaceutical Students' Association, the International Pharmaceutical Students' Federation, the National Union of Students and the International Union of Students. In his role as dean, Professor Berry felt that these broad links were valuable: "We are a small and specialised school, and for this reason I think it is of the utmost importance that our students should enter most fully into the wider general life of the University." There was also much fun to be had beyond the walls of the School. In 1949, the Square decorated a lorry with a tableau of pharmacy from 1549 to 1949 as part of the Colleges of the University Carnival, judged in Hyde Park by the Duke and Duchess of Edinburgh (the current Queen and Prince Philip). Although part of the mortar in the nineteenth century section of the float set light to the crêpe paper decorations, the students' efforts were commended. The report in the *Chronicle* confessed: "only the cleaners know how closely the Women's Common Room approached in appearance the studio of an unemployed artist." The Square also participated in other University-wide events, including a fundraising Ball and Rum Fair to raise funds following disastrous hurricanes in Jamaica in 1952.

Perhaps the most enduring relationship formed in this period was the rivalry with Chelsea College. In 1952, the Square held its first official intercollegiate activity with Chelsea for Guy Fawkes' Night. However, setting a precedent for future high jinks, the evening ended with an ex-service member setting off an army smoke bomb in the Chelsea School, causing closure of the entire premises.

In fact, the fun to be had in the wider playing field of the University actually had a negative impact on the School's social life. The *Square Chronicle* of September 1954 reported that there had been a general decline in social activities at the Square because people were taking part in University ones instead. The *Chronicle* itself also suffered in the later 1950s with the establishment of a college newspaper called *Sig*. By December 1960, the editor of the *Chronicle* explained that *Sig* was now a "racy news-sheet" which the current students enjoyed, whilst the *Chronicle* had become "a rather drab perennial".

Meanwhile, the Square Association continued to support the School's links with its past students and staff. Professor Berry was made its patron after his retirement, and Sir Harry Jephcott, Stanley Curtis and Margaret Fleming were made honorary members. The Association's main social event continued to be the annual dinner dance. The old boys' day, which included a hockey match between current students and past students, remained an annual event, and the women students maintained their annual reunion dinner.

A major issue for prospective students at the School was its lack of accommodation. With students no longer serving an apprenticeship with bed and board as part of the deal as their nineteenth century predecessors had done, in the early 1950s they were reliant on lodgings. The prospectus for 1951–2 had details on the back page for lodgings at 32 Philbeach Gardens, Earl's Court, explaining that you had to apply to Miss F. Armsden at that address. The *Chronicle* for that year sheds some light on this arrangement, explaining that this was a hotel run by a former member of the Pharmaceutical Society's staff, who was offering student accommodation for a reasonable charge. Eric Robins, a first year student in 1951, took up residence alongside around 14 other students, mainly first years as well. Robins recalled: "I think we all enjoyed our times at Earl's Court. As we lodged together and ate together we became close as colleagues. This lasted for two academic years and I still remember the names of most of the students who stayed there, some unfortunately no longer with us."

By 1954, students were eligible to apply for the University Halls of Canterbury, College and Nutford for women, and Connaught Hall for men. If unsuccessful, they could approach the University Lodgings Bureau.

Professor Berry was frustrated by the lack of progress in opening a residential hall specifically for the School. However, the University Grants Committee was not forthcoming as they did not want to establish a small hall for a single faculty school. In 1955, Berry wondered if there was the possibility of a joint scheme with another small school. Linnell took up the project in 1956, feeling that pharmacy students having to live separately in lodgings were missing out on "the varied social contacts so important in a university education." However, there was no success in the 1950s. After an "abortive" attempt to obtain a hall of residence in 1957, Linnell appealed in his Dean's Report for a benefactor to finance a shared hall with another school.

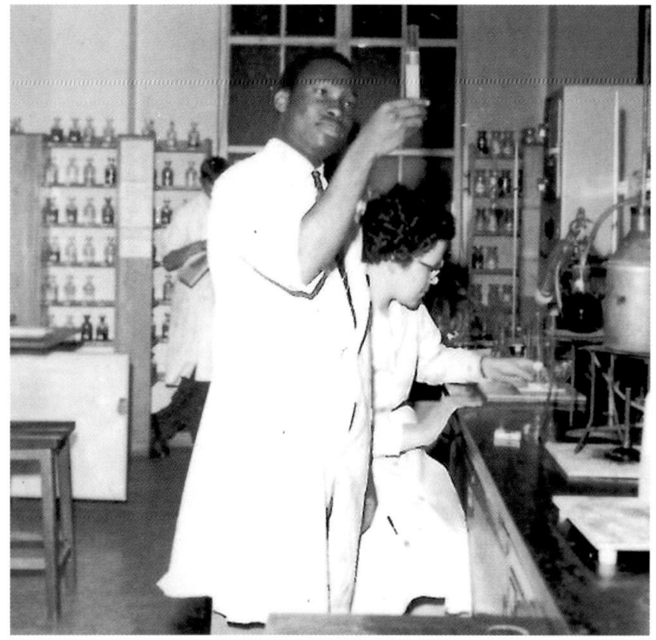

Joshua Oduro-Yeboah from Ghana came to the Square in 1956 and obtained a PhD in 1966. A series of photographs of him working in the pharmaceutics laboratory were taken in 1961.

UCL School of Pharmacy Library

The make-up of the student body was extremely varied, with a growing number of overseas students, particularly coming to the Square to take diplomas or undertake research work. For example, in 1953, Berry reported that, in the last session, there had been five undergraduate and 11 postgraduate students from overseas, from West Africa, the West Indies, South Africa, British Guiana, Egypt, India, Pakistan and Thailand. In addition, a member of teaching staff from the University of Ceylon was enrolled at the School to train as a teacher of pharmacy. Many overseas students received funding for their studies. For example, Joshua Oduro-Yeboah from Mamfe, Ghana, came to the Square in 1956 with a scholarship from the Cocoa Growers' Association. He went on to obtain a PhD in 1966, and settled in Britain, working first in hospital production, and then as a formulation researcher at Beecham's Pharmaceuticals in Worthing.

In contrast to struggles in earlier decades, the School now had to grapple with massively increased applications for its courses. In 1953, there were around 200 applicants for 32 places, and this continued to be the case in 1955. Berry reported "the limitation of our present annual intake to 32 students is becoming a distinct embarrassment when related to a field of over 200 well qualified applicants, who now appear to rate pharmacy very high in their selection of a profession." He put the popularity of the profession down to an increase in demand from the pharmaceutical industry, the need for an expanding supply of pharmacy graduates for the NHS, and the growth of British exports of medicines.

"The limitation of our present annual intake to 32 students is becoming a distinct embarrassment when related to a field of over 200 well qualified applicants, who now appear to rate pharmacy very high in their selection of a profession."

Professor Berry, 1955

By 1959, the student intake had increased to 48 each year because of the completed move into the new building. However, the application numbers had gone up to around 300. The concern for the new dean, Linnell, was that too many of the students, once accepted, failed the first year or were referred because they simply did not work hard enough. In this year, a tutorial system was organised for the first time to try to support the first year students. In 1960, the tutorial system was extended to second year students, and revision classes for first years who had failed were repeated for a second year.

Fees in this decade were £50 per year (or £17 per term), which included tuition, subs for the School and University Student unions and others, and notebooks. The prospectuses made it clear that "Excessive

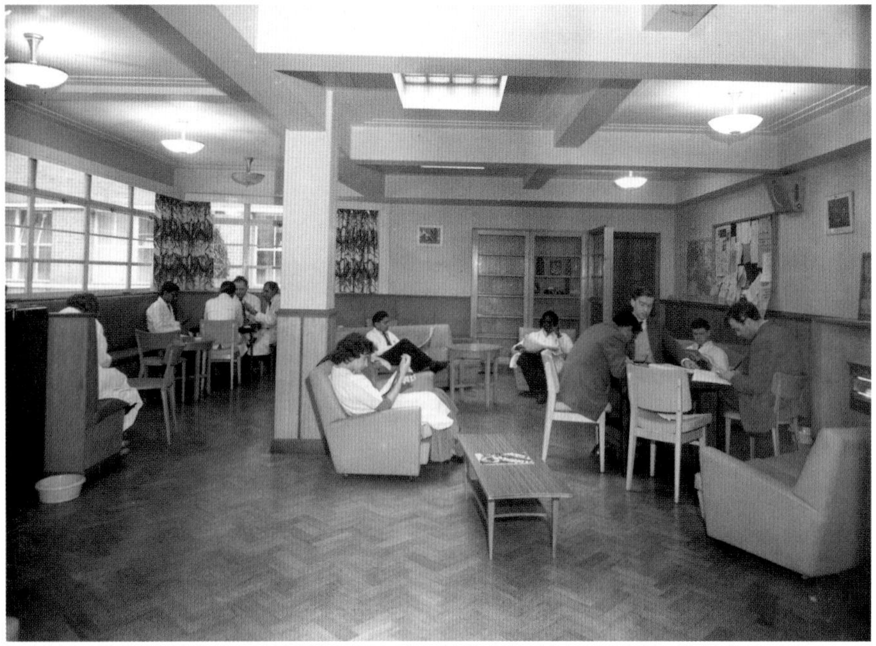

The students' common room in the basement, 1960.

Royal Pharmaceutical Society Museum

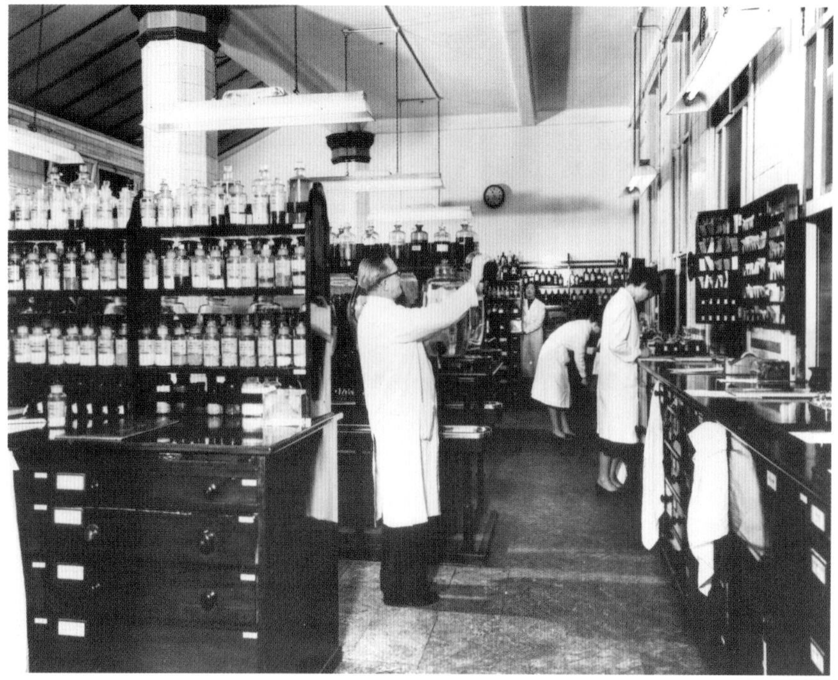

The Pharmaceutical Society commissioned this photograph of "The Pharmacist in hospital: the dispensary" in 1959. It was taken at St Bartholomew's Hospital in London.

Royal Pharmaceutical Society Museum

breakages of apparatus will be chargeable." The Jacob Bell scholarships continued, almost a century after their introduction, as did a number of other awards. They were joined in 1954 by the Greenish Memorial Award, primarily funded by the Pharmaceutical Society in memory of Professor Greenish. The Award provided a free place for a student who had distinguished him or herself in Part I, and was now moving on to Part II.

Pharmacy students in the late 1950s were entering a profession very different from that only a couple of decades earlier. The impact of the NHS on community pharmacy was one of scale rather than a significant change in operation, because of the pharmacist's experience of the National Health Insurance scheme. Nevertheless, the move of the retail pharmacist from the counter into the dispensary was now established. Hospital pharmacists conversely had begun to move from the dispensary to the wards in the light of the Aitken Report of 1958, which had highlighted their responsibility for the safe handling of medicines across the whole hospital. Industrial pharmacists were operating in a rapidly expanding field at an exciting time of drug discoveries, and those in research were at the cutting edge of these developments. The opportunities for pharmacy graduates were widening, and training at the Square meant that its students were able to grasp them.

CHAPTER 6

"WINDS OF CHANGE": 1961–1986

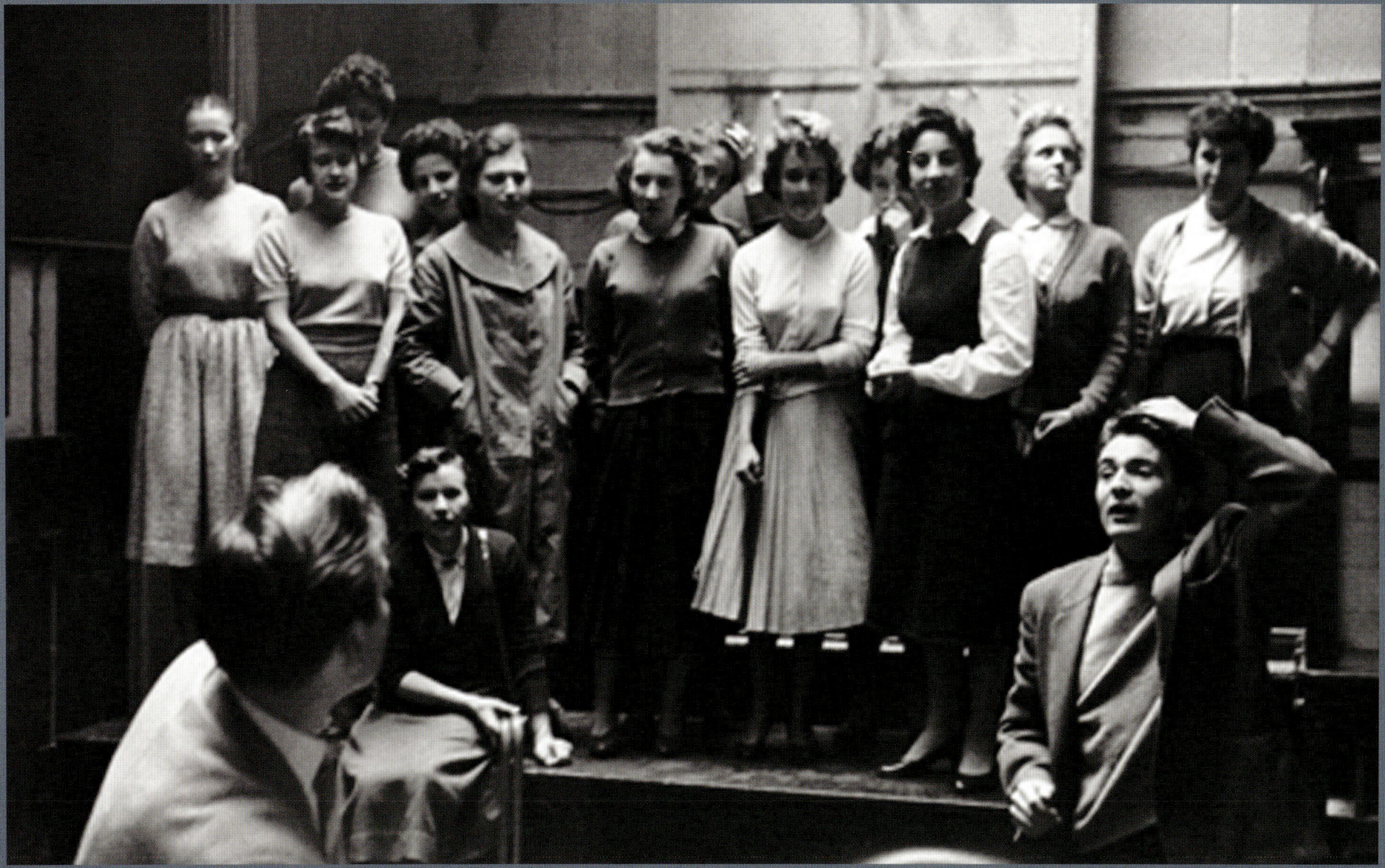

The exact event captured in this photograph has not been recorded. Suggestions include a rehearsal for a female-only performance, a Student's Union initiation, or some kind of strange leg-examination ritual.

Reproduced with permission from Royal Pharmaceutical Society Museum

MILESTONES

Popular Culture

1963 The Beatles hit the big time
1967 The Beatles released "Sgt. Pepper's Lonely Hearts Club Band"
1967 "Summer of Love"
1969 Woodstock Festival
1969 regular colour television broadcasts began on BBC1 and ITV
1969 The Beatles gave their last public performance, on the roof of Apple Records
1971 Michael Jackson launched his solo career
1976 first VHS video recorder launched
1978 first digital camera patented in the USA
1981 IBM PC launched
1982 first album released on CD
1985 Live Aid concerts

London Life

1964 Post Office Tower completed
1965 Barbican complex started
1981 first London Marathon
1981 Brixton riots
1984 Thames Barrier completed
1985 Broadwater Farm riots
1986 M25 motorway around London completed

National News

1965 death of Winston Churchill
1967 British Parliament decriminalised homosexuality
1968 first heart transplant carried out in the UK
1970s energy crisis and shortened working week
1971 decimal currency introduced
1974 first major reorganisation of National Health Service
1979 Margaret Thatcher became Britain's first female prime minister
1981 wedding of Prince Charles and Lady Diana Spencer
1984–1985 miners' strike
1986 "Big Bang" in the Stock Exchange

The Wider World

1960s feminist movement began
1961 Yuri Gagarin became first man in space
1961 Berlin Wall built
1962 Cuban Missile Crisis
1963 assassination of US President Kennedy
1967 Che Guevara executed in Bolivia
1967 Christian Barnard carried out the world's first heart transplant
1967 Arab–Israeli Six-Day War
1968 American troops killed scores of civilians in the My Lai massacre
1968 student unrest across Europe
1968 Martin Luther King killed
1968 Tommie Smith and John Carlos made the black power salute on the Olympic rostrum
1969 start of the Troubles in Ireland
1969 first men landed on the moon
1973 UK joined the European Economic Community
1975 Vietnam War ended
1976 Concorde supersonic Atlantic service launched
1977 Sanger and colleagues published the first sequence of a whole DNA genome
1978 Louise Brown was born, after Steptoe and Edwards developed in vitro fertilisation
1978 World Health Organization Declaration at Alma Alta recognised that health is a wider concept than absence of disease or infirmity
1979 Iranian Revolution
1979 Smallpox eradicated globally
1980–1988 Iran–Iraq War
1981 AIDS recognised as a new disease
1981 first flight of the Space Shuttle
1982 Falklands War

Whilst staff and students settled into the new building, the changes in the wider world gathered pace. It was an exciting time to be a student, with a growing sense of youth culture, particularly in London, and dramatic developments in technology and communication. For pharmacy, new and complex therapies presented interesting challenges for research, teaching and practice. Pharmacists took on a new clinical role, and for hospital practitioners their outlook changed dramatically with a move on to the wards. From the 1960s onwards, the growth of the global pharmaceutical industry was enormous. The parallel growth in medicines and the increased demand within the National Health Service (NHS) put increasing pressure on the expertise required for prescribing. In the 1980s, the massive increases in drug costs had a dramatic impact on pharmacy services, and subsequent cuts, including the "Black List" of products that were no longer to be available on the NHS, were yet another challenge for the profession.

TEACHING

Courses

As pharmacy practice continued to develop, so did the need to keep the School's course up to date and relevant. Linnell, in his Dean's Report in 1961, emphasised the need to increase teaching in biochemistry, but external forces also played a part. In 1962, Linnell surmised that the country's possible entry into the European Common Market maintained the pressure on British pharmacists to qualify at degree level in order to compete successfully with European applicants for jobs. The fact that, in that year, all the universities in the UK combined provided less than half the pharmacists needed to meet the labour requirements of the British profession meant that Linnell foresaw an influx of European colleagues.

The impact of the thalidomide tragedy in 1962 had lasting consequences for the pharmacy profession. As a result of the tragedy, the Committee on Safety of Drugs (CSD) was established from 1st January 1964, working with the pharmaceutical industry to look at toxicity tests, clinical trials, efficacy and adverse reactions during general use. In his Dean's Report in 1964, Professor Hartley recognised that the CSD's actions had had an impact on pharmacy with regard

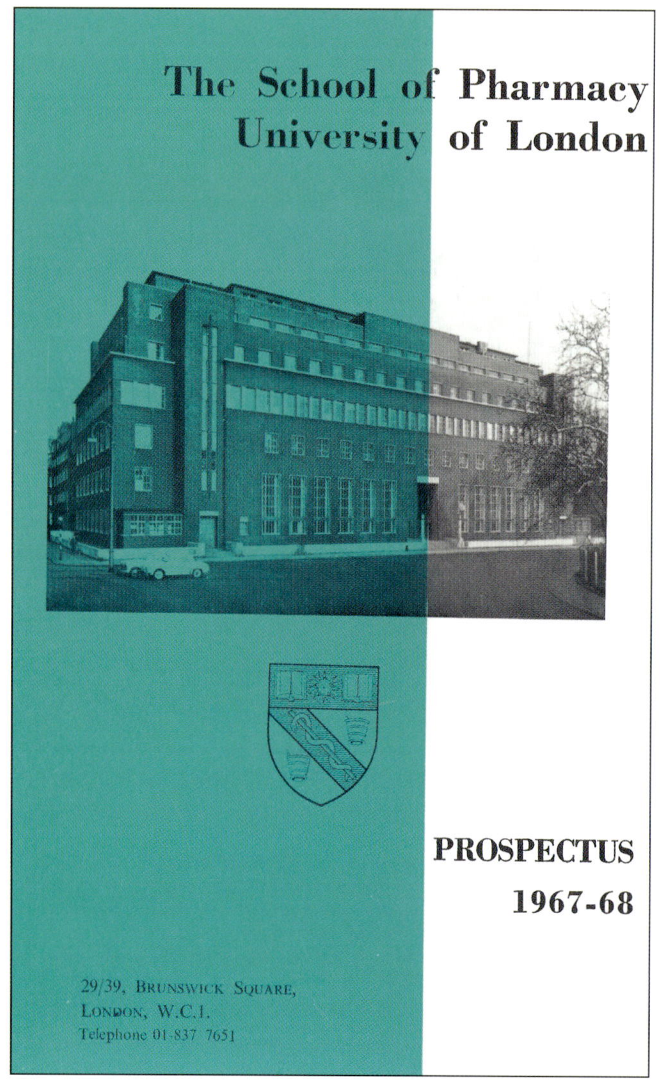

UCL School of Pharmacy Library

to the testing, preparation and handling of drugs. However, he welcomed further work in this area: "The hotch-potch of laws relating to medicines, however, with the consequent detailed and complex regulations made under them necessarily now imposed almost intolerable burdens on memory both for students and practitioner alike and give point to the need for the rationalisations which it is hoped the proposed revision of medicines legislation will provide." The following year, he used his Report to emphasise the need to modify the BPharm course to give recognition to understanding the action and side-effects of drugs, and to reflect the decreasing importance of plant-based medicines. He also called on the Master's course to include more biochemistry, alongside the use of computers, a key skill for pharmacy students to develop. It was not until the 1973–4 session that all second year students had an introduction to computing as part of the course.

Another external influence was the Medicines Act of 1968, which brought together into a single Act everything to do with the control of medicines, for both human and animal use, including their promotion and sales. This Act set up the legislation that, as from 1st September 1971, all medicines already on the UK market had to go through peer review and subsequent approval or be withdrawn. This process was ultimately completed in 1990 with only around 5,000 full licences granted out of the original 39,000 products that existed in 1971. The dean reported in 1972 that a new pharmacology option had been introduced for third year students, which included time at St Bartholomew's Medical School (Barts). His hope was that it would help pharmacy students to cope with changes as a result of the

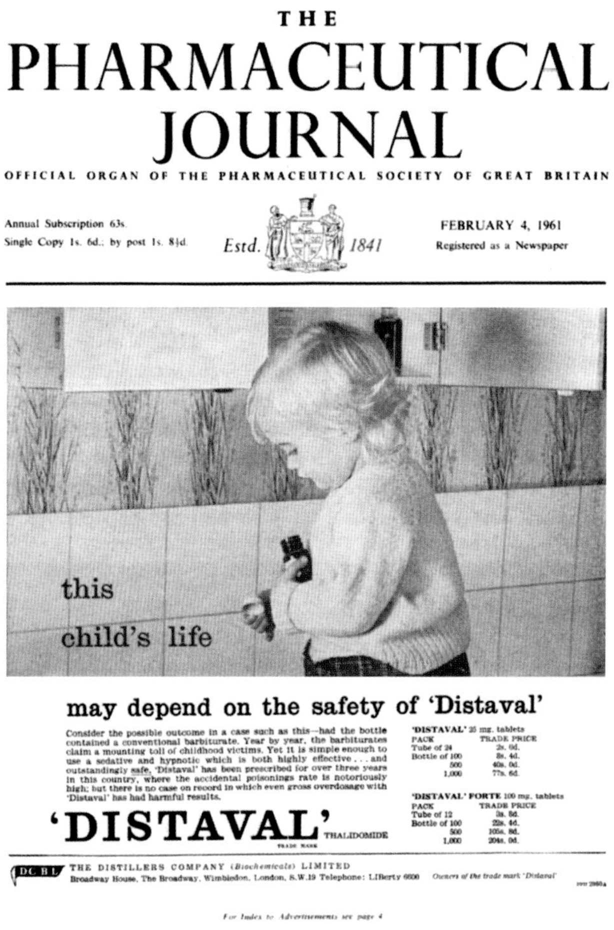

THE
PHARMACEUTICAL
JOURNAL

OFFICIAL ORGAN OF THE PHARMACEUTICAL SOCIETY OF GREAT BRITAIN

Annual Subscription 63s.
Single Copy 1s. 6d.; by post 1s. 8½d.

Estd. 1841

FEBRUARY 4, 1961
Registered as a Newspaper

this
child's life

may depend on the safety of 'Distaval'

Consider the possible outcome in a case such as this—had the bottle contained a conventional barbiturate. Year by year, the barbiturates claim a mounting toll of childhood victims. Yet it is simple enough to use a sedative and hypnotic which is both highly effective . . . and outstandingly safe. 'Distaval' has been prescribed for over three years in this country, where the accidental poisonings rate is notoriously high; but there is no case on record in which even gross overdosage with 'Distaval' has had harmful results.

'DISTAVAL' 25 mg. tablets

PACK	TRADE PRICE
Tube of 24	2s. 6d.
Bottle of 100	8s. 4d.
500	40s. 0d.
1,000	77s. 6d.

'DISTAVAL' FORTE 100 mg. tablets

PACK	TRADE PRICE
Tube of 12	3s. 8d.
Bottle of 100	22s. 4d.
500	105s. 8d.
1,000	204s. 0d.

'DISTAVAL' THALIDOMIDE
TRADE MARK

DCBL THE DISTILLERS COMPANY (Biochemicals) LIMITED
Broadway House, The Broadway, Wimbledon, London, S.W.19 Telephone: LIBerty 6600 Owners of the trade mark 'Distaval'

For Index to Advertisements see page 4

On February 4th 1961, the advertisement on the front cover of *The Pharmaceutical Journal* was for Distaval, or thalidomide.

The Pharmaceutical Journal

> **"Without this fundamental knowledge the pharmacist cannot play his part in the National Health Service and neither can he act as an adviser on drugs to the medical profession, or as one who can protect the public from the dangers inherent in many of the new chemical compounds."**
>
> *C.W. Maplethorpe, 1966*

Drug Developments

1962	Valium (diazepam), for depression
1962	Anovlar (norethisterone/ethinylestradiol), the first oral contraceptive
1963	Penbritin (ampicillin), a major antibiotic
1965	Inderal (propranolol), a beta-blocker
1966	Zyloric (allopurinol), for gout and arthritis
1967	Propaderm (beclometasone dipropionate), for skin, then Becotide, inhaled for asthma
1969	Brufen (ibuprofen), for arthritis and inflammation
1969	Ventolin (salbutamol), for asthma
1970	levodopa, for Parkinson's disease
1971	method of action of aspirin discovered by John Vane
1973	Nolvadex (tamoxifen), for breast cancer
1975	monoclonal antibodies discovered by Köhler and Milstein
1975	Clozaril (clozapine), for schizophrenia, entered clinical trials
1976	Tenormin (atenolol), a beta-blocker
1976	Sandimmune (ciclosporin), an immunosuppressant, for transplantation
1976	Tagamet (cimetidine), for peptic ulcers
1981	Capoten (captopril), angiotensin-converting enzyme inhibitor for hypertension
1981	Zantac (ranitidine), for gastric and duodenal ulceration
1982	Humulin (human insulin), first pharmaceutical product of recombinant DNA
1982	Zovirax (aciclovir), an antiviral against herpes simplex
1983	Imigran (sumatriptan), for migraine
1984	Augmentin (co-amoxiclav), a mixture of amoxicillin and clavulanic acid used for resistant micro-organisms
1985	Protropin (human growth hormone), for dwarfism
1986	Orthoclone (muromonab-CD3), first licensed human monoclonal antibody, for transplantation

Pharmacy Milestones

1961	thalidomide disaster
1963	Committee on Safety of Drugs set up, to start work in 1964
1964	introduction of the adverse drug reaction "yellow card" scheme in response to the thalidomide tragedy
1968	Medicines Act established three categories of medicines: general sale (available from any shop), pharmacy (to be sold only with a pharmacist in attendance) and prescription only
1968	Trades Description Act restricted extravagant advertising
1969	metrication introduced into pharmacy
1971	Misuse of Drugs Act
1971	all medicines already on the UK market had to go through peer review and subsequent approval or be withdrawn; this process was completed in 1990 with only around 5,000 full licences granted out of the original 39,000 products that existed in 1971
1971	all new medicines subject to premarketing assessment for safety, quality and efficacy
1972	Poisons Act
1976	Pharmaceutical Society moved out of Bloomsbury Square to its current location at 1 Lambeth High Street
1977	Lambeth High Street headquarters of the Pharmaceutical Society of Great Britain (PSGB) officially opened by the Queen Mother
1983	"Ask Your Pharmacist" campaign started by the Royal Pharmaceutical Society of Great Britain, the National Pharmaceutical Association and the Family Planning Association
1984	green cross adopted as the official symbol for pharmacy by the PSGB
1984	NHS Black List proposed; introduced in 1985

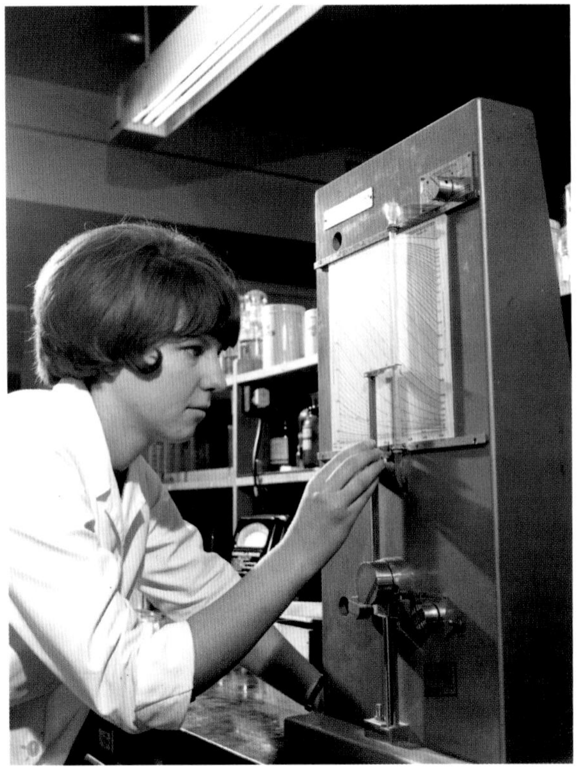

UCL School of Pharmacy Library

PATRICK PAUL ANTHONY HUMPHREY (1946–)

Patrick Humphrey graduated from the Square in 1968, and obtained a PhD in Pharmacology at St Mary's Hospital Medical School. He joined Allen & Hanburys to start a project on migraine initiated by Sir David Jack, and was part of the team which developed sumatriptan, the first of a new generation of selective serotonin receptor agonists. It took 15 years of research to find a drug that constricted only cerebral blood vessels. He went on to become director of the Glaxo Division of Pharmacology, and during his time in the post, oversaw the development of naratriptan (for migraine), alosetron (used to treat irritable bowel syndrome), ondansetron (to treat nausea) and salmeterol (for asthma).

In 1999, Humphrey was awarded the OBE for "services to migraine research". He went on to work as head of research at Theravance in San Francisco from 2001 to 2008. In 2008, he was awarded the Society's Harrison memorial medal. He has published more than 300 scientific papers and book chapters. He is currently a non-executive director on the board of Verona Pharma plc.

Act, but also that teaching alongside medical students should help the relationship between doctors and pharmacists in the future.

However, the School also recognised the need for students to use their time at university to broaden their outlook beyond the medical world. Starting in 1962, the staff organised a programme of liberal studies by outside lecturers, "as part of our effort to diminish the educational risks of isolation for our undergraduates." The timetable for all three years included sessions such as appreciation of art, architecture and sculpture, appreciation of music, archaeology, politics, and religions of the world. The *Square Chronicle* recognised that the prompt for this broader curriculum had come from newer universities, particularly Keele.

In 1976, the dean, Professor Swarbrick, and senior staff went on a faculty retreat to consider the School's future, particularly the curriculum. The following year, a new curriculum was approved by the School and University, which included the introduction of a common practice-based core which formed 50% of the final year. For the other half of the course, students could choose from seven specialist subjects. They also introduced two new interdepartmental subject areas. In the first year, students were taught pharmaceutical biology and chemistry, and in the second year they covered pharmaceutical microbiology and chemotherapy. The School also hoped to obtain approval for Master's of Science courses in Clinical Pharmacy, Toxicology, and Industrial Pharmaceutical Quality Control.

In the late 1970s, the *Chronicle* took a retrospective look at the courses over the past decade. For pharmacology, one of the major issues was that many students arrived without O or A levels in Biology, but the ability to take a crash course at the Royal Free Hospital Medical School next door enabled them to catch up. Another practical issue was overcrowding, such that it was impossible to examine the students practically, and individual practical work was only possible in the third year. In terms of the subject itself, the biggest change in the decade had been the greater emphasis on central nervous system pharmacology, membranes, receptors and pharmacokinetics. For pharmaceutical chemistry, the greatest contrast with the late 1960s was in instrumental methods of analysis. First year students were now introduced to infrared spectroscopy and the third year course included experiments to illustrate the theory of fast reaction kinetics, protein binding and light scattering.

The pharmaceutics course had seen some reorganisation over the decade: the number of dispensing lectures in the first year had been reduced and a course on tablet and powder technology started at the end of the first year. Second year students started a course on drug release which carried on into the third year. Exams had been replaced by continuous assessment and a series of tests across the course for practical work. The second year course included practicals on emulsions, tablets and radioisotopes. All third year students chose a specialist course rather than a general third year pharmaceutics course. The options were formulation and stability, powder technology and rheology, or microbiology, particularly bacterial resistance. In pharmacognosy over the past 10 years, the course had moved away from the plant itself to the chemical constituents responsible for its medicinal action. Chromatographic assays, chemical tests and quantitative analysis of extracts had taken over from microscopical and macroscopical examination of specimens. The staff had introduced project work, and looked to connect the course as much as possible with the pharmacy profession. The third year option for pharmacognosy included isolating drugs from plants, using mass spectrometry and nuclear magnetic resonance spectroscopy. Other topics in the course were more vocational, such as crop protective agents, drug discovery and toxic natural substances. However, the third year option also included routes of biosynthesis, metabolism of secondary plant metabolites and chemotaxonomy.

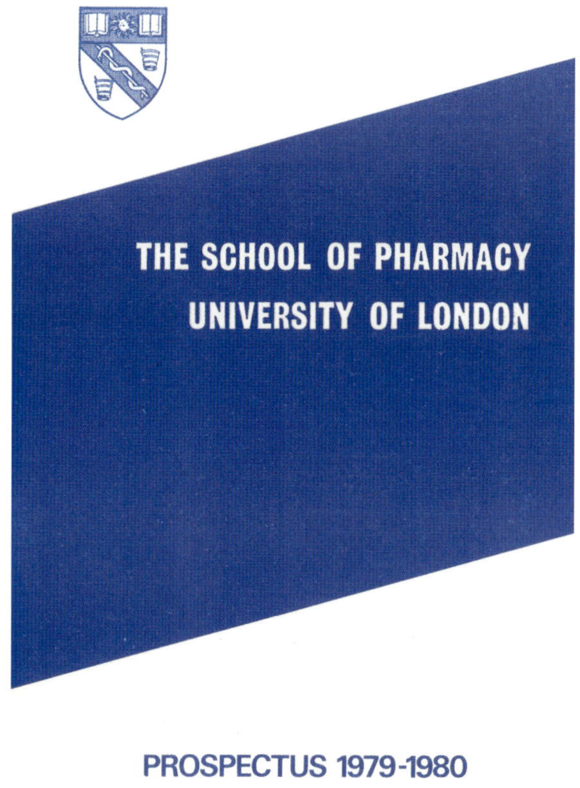

UCL School of Pharmacy Library

The University accepted the new MSc in Clinical Pharmacy, with the first intake of students in October 1980. This was a pioneering development for pharmacy teaching. It had emerged from a steering group, set up in the North Thames regions in 1977, to discuss a strategy for the development of hospital pharmacy, particularly in the area of drug usage. The group recognised that pharmacists would only be appreciated for their contribution if they had increased clinical knowledge. The group approached the Square with a proposal for a Diploma in Clinical Pharmacy, knowing that staff at the School were also keen to establish a course in this area. The School suggested that the qualification should be at Master's level. All of the students had to be existing qualified pharmacists, and the course was set within a clinical practice context with instruction at Northwick Park Hospital in Middlesex. A syllabus was established to meet the needs of an agreed job description for a clinical pharmacist of the future. The School appointed a practitioner supervisor for the course, shared with the North-West Thames Regional Health Authority. Teaching staff on the course also worked at the Medical Research Council (MRC) clinical research centre. The first intake of students for the 12-month course was restricted to practising hospital pharmacists working in the North-West and North-East Thames Regions. In 1985, Dr Soraya Dhillon was appointed as honorary lecturer at the School, alongside her post as staff pharmacist in the Clinical Pharmacy Unit at Northwick Park Hospital, cementing the relationship between the two organisations.

The School also saw the benefits of teacher practitioners in other areas. In 1980, they appointed three members of staff who also continued to hold positions within pharmaceutical practice, plus a number of hospital pharmacists who worked as demonstrators for practical work in pharmaceutics. In 1981, Professor Fish reported that they had introduced "patient orientated pharmacy, especially as it relates to community pharmacy practice" into the core course of the final year of the BPharm. This included making video-recordings as teaching aids to illustrate interviewing techniques for dealing with patients' enquiries.

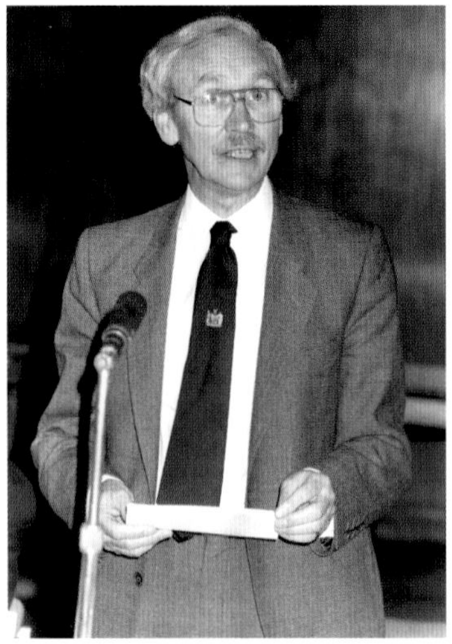

FRANK FISH (1924–2011)

UCL School of Pharmacy Library

FRANK FISH (1924–2011)

Frank Fish was born in County Durham and apprenticed to a local pharmacist before studying pharmacy at Sunderland Technical College. He was awarded his London BPharm in 1946. He took the post of assistant lecturer in pharmacognosy at the pharmacy department in Glasgow, where he gained his PhD on digitalis in 1955. He stayed at the School of Pharmaceutical Sciences at Strathclyde, becoming dean in 1977. During his time there, he set up an MSc course in Forensic Science, the only postgraduate course on the subject in the UK.

In 1978, he moved to London to take up the post of dean of the School of Pharmacy. In his 10 years as dean, he oversaw the introduction of the degree course in Toxicology and Pharmacology, and the establishment of the Master's in Clinical Pharmacy. He also steered the School through a period of extreme cuts, and threats such as a move to the medical school at St George's Hospital in Tooting. In response to the possibility of more drastic cuts, he wrote to the UGC in May 1985: "We must continue in the knowledge that if and when the clouds clear the view will still be best from the top!"

He also served on the Committee on Safety of Medicines, the *British Pharmacopoeia* Commission, the DHSS Standing Advisory Committee, the University of London Senate and the Nuffield Committee of Inquiry into Pharmacy. He was awarded the Harrison memorial medal in 1982 and the Society's Charter gold medal in 1987, and was made an OBE in 1988.

The need to focus on clinical pharmacy and pharmacy practice was more than a fashionable trend. The founders of the Pharmaceutical Society spent significant amounts of time and effort distancing the profession from what we now know as clinical pharmacy, owing to the territorial disputes between themselves and the apothecaries. However, by the twentieth century, the potential for the pharmacist's role within the medical landscape to become more integrated was identified by a number of key players, notably Cyril Maplethorpe, chair of the Pharmaceutical Society's Education Committee, and Society president from 1963 to 1965. In an article in *The Pharmaceutical Journal* in 1957, he had assessed that pharmacists had a much greater role to play in the healthcare team, as advisers to other professionals as well as the public on drugs and medicines. This role had been particularly highlighted with the therapeutic revolution, the introduction of the NHS, and the thalidomide tragedy and its consequences. A shift of hospital pharmacists from the dispensary to the wards was key to this development. Pharmacists such as Chris Barrett were prime movers in this area, from the mid-1960s onwards. However, it took until 1977 for the first pharmacy practice research session to be introduced into the British Pharmaceutical Conference. This first session included papers on reporting adverse drug reactions, child-resistant closures, and the role of the pharmacist in health education and community health.

The key milestone, however, was the Nuffield Report, published in March 1986. In 1983, the Nuffield Foundation set up a committee "to consider the present and future structure of the practice of pharmacy in its several branches and its potential contribution to healthcare and to review the education and training of pharmacists accordingly." The Report's 96 recommendations covered a wide range of topics, including an extended role for the community pharmacist. However, in terms of undergraduate education, the committee concluded that the traditional set-up of pharmacy departments into four areas, each with its own allocated staff, space and funding, was restricting development. They proposed that subjects should be grouped, and that teaching should also concentrate on other key skills such as communication. As a result of the Report, 16 pharmacy practice chairs were established in the following 10 years, and the BPharm course was altered radically. At the Square, Professor Fish reported that the School would look at what they taught but also how they taught it. However, staff had already introduced new teaching methods such as video, tape-slide and film presentations, plus computer-assisted learning. Fish assured the audience for his Dean's Report in 1986 that in practicals, "recipe-following was abandoned in favour of problem-solving."

Of course, with the already established MSc in Clinical Pharmacy, the School had travelled some way in the direction that the Nuffield Report proposed. Its recommendation that schools of pharmacy should establish academic units in hospitals to act as a base for teaching and research, and to promote contact with other healthcare professionals, had been pre-empted by the School with its established links with the Clinical Pharmacy Unit at Northwick Park Hospital from 1980 and other links with many hospitals in the London region. For example, from as early as 1971, an option had been available for third year students in applied pharmacology, which had joint teaching at the School and in the clinical pharmacology department at St Bartholomew's Hospital. The School had also broken down some departmental barriers by teaching biochemistry, microbiology, immunology and chemotherapy as integrated non-departmental courses from the 1970s, alongside the interdisciplinary nature of the final year core course. The old dispensing course had become an integrated three-year education in modern pharmacy practice. The difficulty faced by the School, and many others in the period, was not any reluctance to embrace change, but the time to include all of the potential courses. What was needed was a four-year course, but this was more than a decade away.

The other major development for the Square's teaching was their introduction of a BSc in Toxicology and Pharmacology in 1981, the only course of its kind in Britain. As a four-year "thick sandwich" course, students could spend their third year working outside the School in placements throughout the UK and also abroad. The areas of the building previously part of university examinations laboratories were converted for teaching the course, and specialist staff were appointed. The opportunity to undertake toxicology research at the School was also particularly exciting. The aim was that the taught course would enable students to undertake careers in a broad range of chemically based industries, plus in environmental, regulatory and law enforcement authorities. However, in the late 1990s, the School decided that its teaching should be focused solely on the undergraduate Pharmacy degree, and the BSc in Toxicology and Pharmacology was abandoned.

Staffing

These exciting developments in the curriculum were achieved against a very difficult financial backdrop. In the first year, the move to the new building had enabled an increase in the student numbers from 116 to 204, but academic staffing had only increased by one post. Professor Hartley reported in the mid-1960s that the

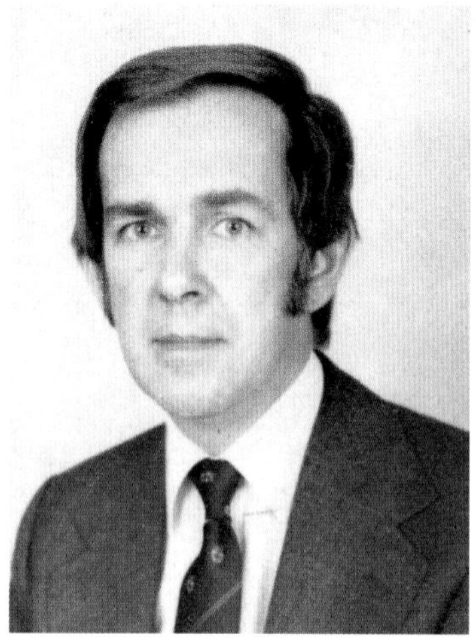

JAMES SWARBRICK (1934–)

UCL School of Pharmacy Library

JAMES SWARBRICK (1934–)

James Swarbrick gained his BPharm at Chelsea College in 1960 and stayed there as a lecturer until moving to the USA in 1964 to take up posts at Purdue University and then the University of Connecticut. He was the director of product development for Sterling-Winthrop from 1972 to 1975 before moving to become the first holder of a new chair in pharmaceutics at the University of Sydney from 1975 to 1976. In 1976, he returned to England when he was appointed as dean of the School. However, he returned to the United States in 1978, first as professor of pharmacy at the University of Southern California, and then the University of North Carolina, the latter post until 1993. Since then, and during his earlier career, he has worked as a consultant and visiting scientist for a number of pharmaceutical companies and government departments, primarily in the United States.

He is the author of around 70 scientific articles, as well as *Physical Pharmacy* (2nd and 3rd editions) and *Drug Delivery and Targeting* (2001), and the editor of *Biopharmaceutics, Dosage Form Design and Bioavailability* and *Drugs and the Pharmaceutical Sciences*.

School was facing problems recruiting technicians, and also that there was a need for more secretarial staff to support research so that research assistants were not spending time doing administrative work. However, by the time that Hartley retired in September 1976, to be replaced by Dr James Swarbrick, the situation was much more critical. Swarbrick reported in 1977 that there was a 10% drop in real terms of funds available to the School. As a result, he had frozen 17 posts out of total staff of 195, including four academic posts. All non-salary budget headings had been reduced by 10%, apart from the library which had retained its purchasing power in the current budget. However, a year later, five academic and 22 non-academic posts were frozen owing to the financial situation.

Unsurprisingly, the School was keen to take the opportunities offered by the "New Blood" lecturers scheme, first introduced in 1983. In spring 1984, they were successful in applying for a new lecturer in chemistry and biochemistry of peptides, and Dr Paolo Mascagni was appointed to support the existing plans to develop biochemistry as a significant component in the pharmaceutical chemistry course. The School had already successfully appointed Dr Trevor Smart as a new lecturer with special interests in neuropharmacology. In the following year, they were successful in gaining funding for a new lecturer in neurotoxicology, Dr Elizabeth Moss.

Equipment

The precarious funding environment put much pressure on the School to find external funding for the expensive equipment that was needed to keep up to date with new technologies and new subject areas. The departments continued to report their successes in this arena through the Annual Report. In 1962, the Wellcome Trust provided two large research grants of £4,850 to pharmaceutics for a Weissenberg rheogoniometer, and more than £10,000 to pharmaceutical chemistry for a nuclear magnetic resonance

(NMR) machine, which they shared with Birkbeck College and Chelsea pharmacy department.

Hartley made it clear in his Report of 1964 that in order to bring the new one-year MPharm course into effect, new laboratory facilities were needed which would depend on more benefactions to afford the equipment needed for research. The 1967–8 session seems to have been a particularly successful year. The School installed a new animal house on the roof, and established a cat breeding unit at Myddelton House jointly with the Royal Free Medical School. They received grants of £30,000 from the MRC and University Grants Committee (UGC), bought a MS902 mass spectrometer with a grant from the Science Research Council (SRC) for £36,425, a vapour pressure osmometer for physicochemical investigations with a special grant of £1,000 from the University Court, and an Olivetti Programma 101 electronic calculating machine to relieve pressure on the University's central computers, with funding of £1,680 from Smith Kline and French. In addition, they received a grant of £7,250 from the SRC for a Varian A-60-A NMR spectrometer for use in pharmaceutical chemistry to investigate NMR spectra in organic compounds.

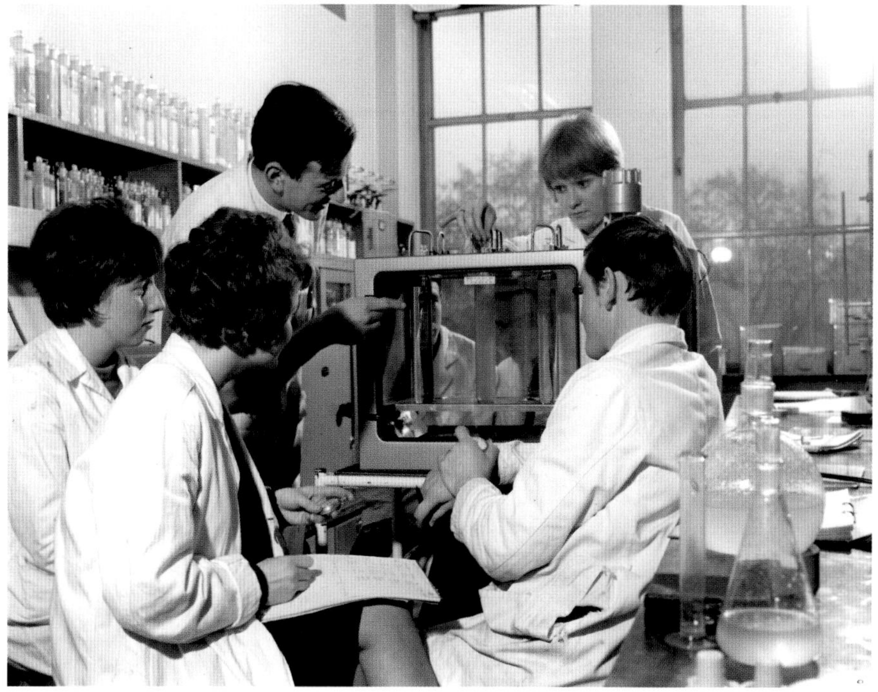

UCL School of Pharmacy Library

The School also received funding from the University for new equipment, and support for technological developments. In the 1969–70 session, with help from the University, staff started using some audiovisual resources in teaching, especially for biology experiments, but they reported that they needed higher quality recording equipment to be more successful with this. Staff also started working with the controller of the University's central CDC 6600 computer, and introduced a short programming course for third years. The School was also working towards computerising their accounts procedures in the early 1970s.

The equipment that the School gained could also be shared across the University. In 1984, Professor Fish reported that a Varian X-L 300 superconducting high-resolution NMR spectrometer had been bought with a grant to the head of pharmaceutical chemistry from the Science and Engineering Research Council. In explaining that this new spectrometer would be housed next to the existing mass spectrometry laboratory, Fish also reported that the School provided the University of London Intercollegiate Research Service with mass spectrometry services for chemistry and related sciences. This arrangement had been in place since the early 1970s, and the School received work in circular dichroism X-ray crystallography and electron spin resonance from other schools in return. In 1985, the University provided funding for a VG ZAB-SE high-field mass spectrometer, to sit alongside a new 12–250 quadropole instrument for mass spectrometry linked with chromatography.

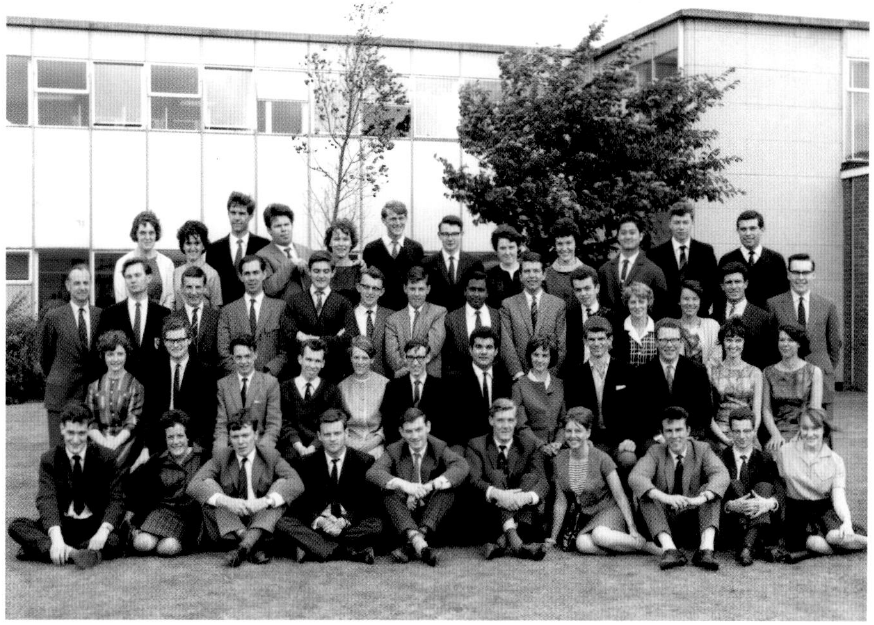

Student visits to manufacturing sites continued to be a feature. These first year students visited Allen and Hanburys plant at Ware, Hertfordshire in 1962.

UCL School of Pharmacy Library

Facilities

The School's library continued to provide support for students and staff through this period, in spite of suffering from the same restrictions on space and funding as the rest of the organisation. In 1961, Linnell reported that the appointment of an assistant to the librarian meant that the library could stay open until 9pm on every working day, and the demands on the facility are shown by the report in 1964 that it was hoped to extend the library by four desks. By 1967, the situation was difficult: "With the increase in the number of students the lack of reading space, adequate shelf space for books and journals and room for display of current periodicals have become serious problems. The new study room is in constant demand by post-graduates, and there is a waiting list for the reserved desks." A library extension was completed in 1971, providing 10 extra seats for readers and shelf space for an additional 1,200 books.

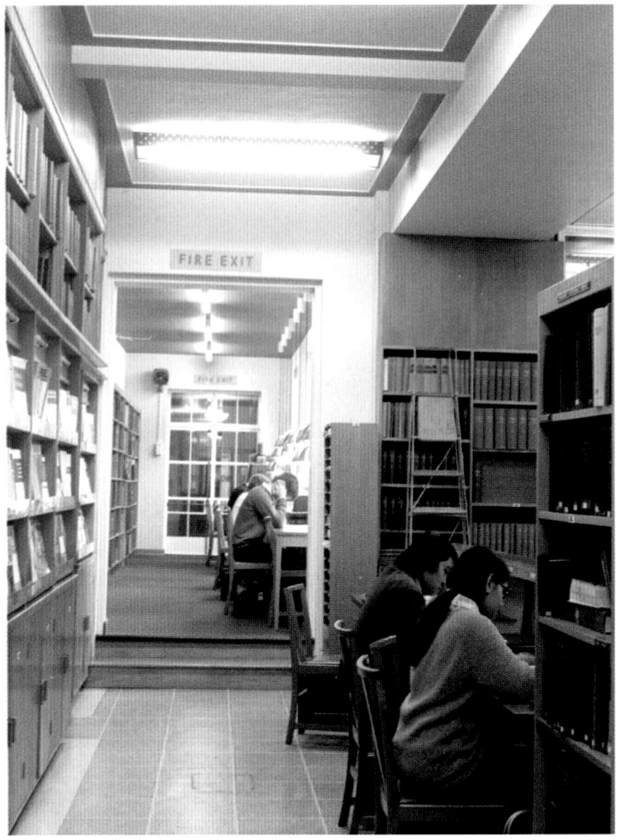

The new-look Library in the early 1970s.

UCL School of Pharmacy Library

The situation for the museum in the new building was very much tied to the attitudes towards pharmacognosy. Although specimens had been moved to Brunswick Square before the move to the new building had taken place, the original materia medica collections had fallen out of favour. Although their research potential was still recognised, changes in pharmacy and pharmacy education meant that the museum's original purpose, its "practical utility" for students, was in an irreversible decline. The herbarium and materia medica were transferred to the University of Bradford in 1965, and then to the Royal Botanic Gardens, Kew, in 1982. The "Pharmaceutical Society" collection now forms part of the Centre for Economic Botany at Kew and is used for displays and research.

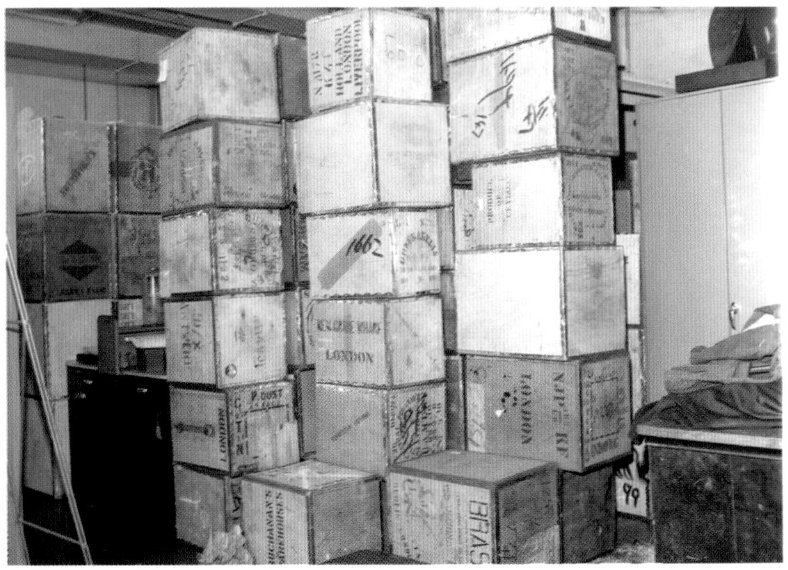

In 1965, the Museum collection was boxed up and moved to the University of Bradford.

Royal Pharmaceutical Society Museum

Meanwhile, microbiology was a new area that the School was very keen to develop. In the 1980–1 session, the School received a grant from the University to upgrade its facilities for the teaching of pharmaceutical microbiology. In March 1986, the School opened a sterile products unit, with funding from the University and from Glaxo Holdings Ltd. The suite of rooms allowed students to work in groups to produce batches of sterilised solutions and aseptically prepared products, to check and validate data and conditions relating to the products, and to monitor particulate and microbial contamination levels. Dr David Jack, a director of Glaxo, officially opened the suite, which had been equipped to comply with the requirements of the Department of Health's *Guide to Good Manufacturing Practice*.

Research

The research carried out at the School was obviously linked to the same funding pressures and the development of new facilities. Staff looked widely for external funding, for example from the Tobacco Research Council, and the Egg Marketing Board for pharmacology research in 1964. All departments developed partnerships with external organisations including hospitals, other university departments, and research departments in industry, both at home and abroad. The research side of the School's activity continued to be very

ROY BRITTAIN (1930–)

Having studied at the Square, and registered as a pharmacist in 1961, Roy Brittain was part of the team put together by Sir David Jack to develop a range of drugs at Glaxo, where he took the post of head of pharmacology. In 1966, they achieved a major breakthrough with the development of the bronchodilator salbutamol, a new treatment for asthma. It was launched as Ventolin in 1969 and is still incredibly successful. Brittain and Jack went on to discover salmeterol, which extended the duration of the drug's action for asthma sufferers.

In competition with James (later Sir James) Black, who was working for Smith Kline and French, Jack wanted his team to discover a treatment for duodenal and gastric ulcers. Black had published a paper on histamine H_2 antagonists, and Jack brought together a group to investigate them for Glaxo. In 1976, Black produced cimetidine (launched as Tagamet), but Jack's team developed a more effective drug, ranitidine hydrochloride, launched as Zantac in 1981, which inhibits stomach acid production. It became the first drug to achieve sales of more than $1 billion a year.

Brittain became Glaxo's research director at the Allen & Hanburys plant at Ware in 1983, and remained with the company until 1992.

successful in spite of the pressures. In the 1967–8 session, Professor Hartley reported that 18 PhDs had been awarded, the most so far in one year.

The pharmacological laboratory celebrated its 50th anniversary in 1976 with an event and reunion, and a special supplement in the *Journal of Pharmacy and Pharmacology*. The same year saw the installation of an electron microscope with a grant from the MRC for £40,000. It was planned to be used for studies of the liberation of nerve transmitters, factors affecting the transfer of drug resistance in micro-organisms, and intercellular aspects of the biogenesis of plant constituents.

On 30th July 1983, an article on the School written by Frank Fish was included in a special supplement of *The Pharmaceutical Journal* for the London British Pharmaceutical Conference. It provides a valuable snapshot of the research work currently undertaken at the Square. Fish particularly highlighted the impressive contributions to pharmacology that the School had made since its move to the new building, but also paid tribute to the leading work that had been carried out and was still ongoing by Wallis, Berry and Linnell, and then Fairbairn in pharmacognosy, by Shotton in pharmaceutics, and by Whalley and Saunders in pharmaceutical chemistry. Fish identified the key current research areas as neuroscience and chemical transmitter systems, toxicology with toxicity testing and selectively toxic anticancer drugs, chemistry and biochemistry of peptides and proteins of endocrinological and pharmacological importance, and structure and function of membrane ionophores.

However, the financial situation continued to overshadow developments. In his Dean's Report for the 1985–6 session, Professor Fish explained that the result of the UGC's deliberations over funding for the late 1980s, the outcome of the first research assessment exercise in 1986, was that School's research was judged as "outstanding". Ironically, a new formula for funding meant that there was less government money available.

The building

Although it was obviously both exciting and refreshing for staff and students to settle into the new Brunswick Square building, the issue of space and facilities was not one that disappeared. A key feature of the new building was that outside organisations could continue to book the School's facilities for weekly meetings and special events. Pharmaceutical gatherings were also keen to view the new School and to use its modern facilities. For example, in 1969, delegates at the inaugural Commonwealth Pharmaceutical Conference spent some time at the Square. The School hosted the scientific sessions of the British Pharmaceutical Conference in London in September 1973. In the 1977–8 session, the School hosted the inaugural meeting of the Committee of Heads of Schools of Pharmacy.

"The investment of money, time and effort represented in this building can only be justified by constant activity at maximum pressure."

Professor Linnell, 1962

But for everyday use, the building was too small. Professor Linnell reported in 1962 that "The investment of money, time and effort represented in this building can only be justified by constant activity at maximum pressure." He was still hopeful that it might be possible to expand into the building vacated by the Royal Free Hospital Medical School next door. By 1966, the School was moving forward with plans for a third and fourth floor extension of the Hunter Street wing which would provide 2,400 square feet of additional laboratory space. However, even this was not really sufficient, and Linnell reported that the School really needed an additional 20,000 square feet to accommodate postgraduate work too.

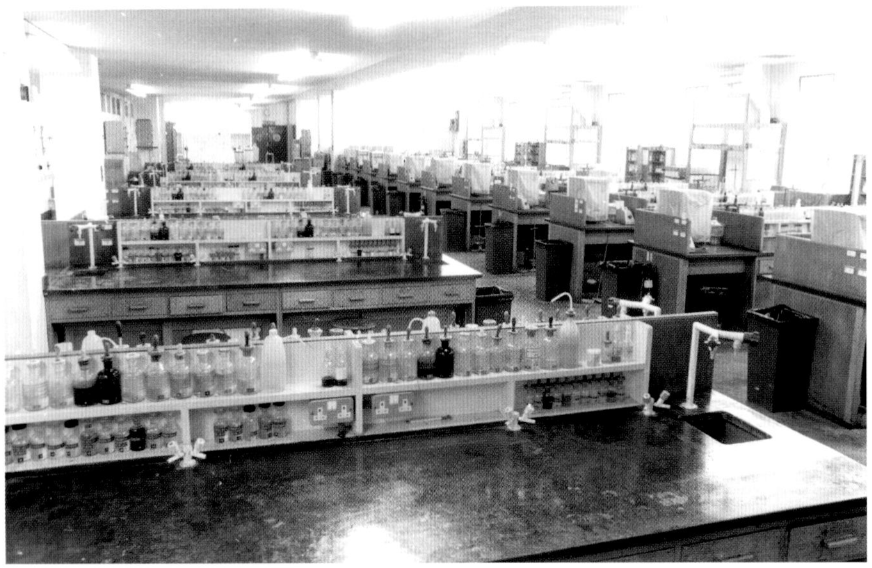

The chemistry labs on the second floor, overlooking Brunswick Square, had been part of the University Exam Department until the early 1980s.

UCL School of Pharmacy Library

There was a glimmer of hope from the Thomas Coram Foundation, next door to the School, which offered 2,500 square feet on a long lease of 15 years. This building, previously a swimming pool, was converted into a lecture block during 1967–8. As a result, about 2,000 square feet of lecture rooms in the main building were freed up and the plan was to convert them into laboratories. The School used this building until 1984, when a new large lecture theatre within the main building was completed on the second floor of the north-west corner. Professor Hartley reported in 1969 that the alterations in the Coram building had been completed to create two new lecture theatres and two seminar rooms. Back in the main building, the space freed up had been converted into two laboratories, one for physical measurements which was installed in the summer of 1971 with funding from the SRC, the MRC and industrial organisations, and one for biochemical pharmacology. These could be used both for the third year course and postgraduate research. Meanwhile, the plans for the third and fourth floor extensions to the Hunter Street wing had come to nothing as the scheme was just too expensive. However, in the 1973–4 session, the School received funding of nearly £25,000 from the UGC to reorganise and update the sixth floor for the pharmacology department.

Further laboratory space was made available when the examination laboratories within the Brunswick Square building were handed over from the University to the School from 1st August 1976. Initially, the School managed the remaining University use of the laboratories, but by 1982, this activity had declined so that the School could take over full use of them for teaching. The work was finished in the summer of 1983 with the addition to the School of a joint teaching laboratory for pharmaceutical chemistry and pharmacognosy, and then separate laboratories for third year teaching and research in pharmacognosy.

Technological developments also prompted the need for more space. In 1975, the School rented accommodation from the local United Reformed Church to enable them to fit out a 200-user terminal computer room linked to the main University computer centre in Guilford Street, which they boasted was connected by a special Post Office cable. Even before this room was available, the School proudly showed off its computer facilities to the 500 delegates at an open day on 5th March 1975. In 1986, a new computer unit was created, with a PDP-11/44 computer linked to several centres, including a staff and postgraduate computer room, and an undergraduate computer room for teaching.

Another modern development reared its head in the 1976–7 session with the formation of the School's first Safety Committee. Dr Frye acted as the inaugural School Safety Officer. The School's activities had come on a long way from the previous safety measure reported whilst still at Bloomsbury Square when, in 1924, red fire buckets with framed instructions were installed around the stairs and corridors of number 17.

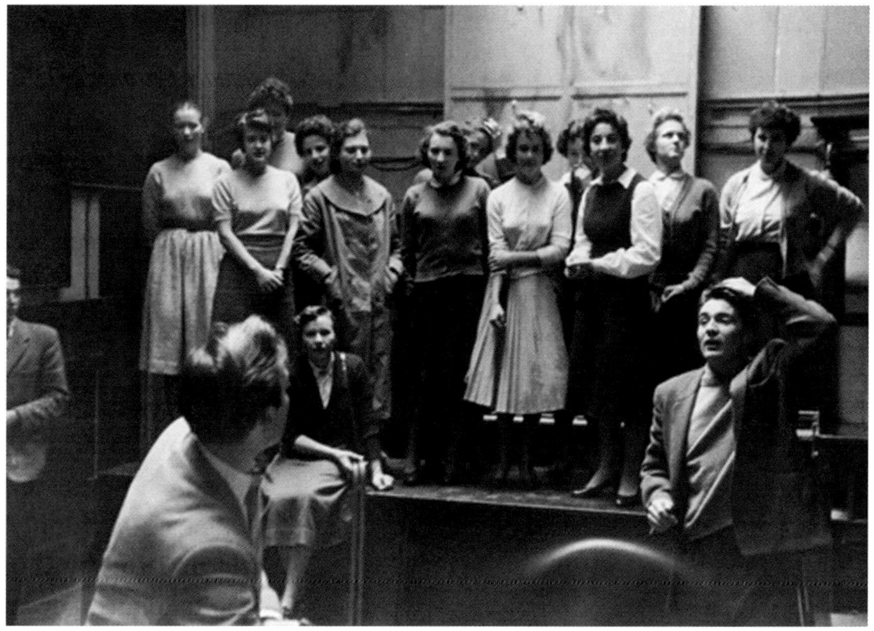

The exact event captured in this photograph has not been recorded. Suggestions include a rehearsal for a female-only performance, a Student's Union initiation, or some kind of strange leg-examination ritual.

Royal Pharmaceutical Society Museum

THE STUDENT EXPERIENCE

Student numbers

At the beginning of the 1960s, in the new building, the student intake could increase, and the total student numbers went up from 116 to 204. However, the School was only able to accept one in ten applicants to their courses. By 1963, around 600 applications were received for the 48 available places in the first year of the BPharm. In 1961, Linnell expressed the desire to double the number of both undergraduates and postgraduates at the Square. After the Robbins' Report on Higher Education in 1963 (see *Examinations*, below), the School was invited by the UGC to formally propose the doubling of the undergraduate intake. From October 1964, having received the necessary funding to adapt rooms and laboratories, purchase additional equipment, and fund the required academic and technical staff, the first year intake was increased to 72 students. The total student population by the time this filtered through to all three years in the 1966–7 session was 217 students, and the School hoped to increase the annual intake of postgraduate students within the next five years to 84, again following the Robbins' Report recommendations. In the 1969–70 year, Professor Hartley was able to report a School record for the number of students graduating in a session, of 75 students. The annual intake went up to 84 students in the 1971–2 session, and for the 1972–3 session, the intake for the BPharm was increased to 100, with 1,100 applications received for those places in that year.

> **"The BPharm course has been accused of churning out nothing more than efficient dispensers … The truth of it is, that in this Television Age, students want not only their Pharmaceutical education fed to them on a plate but all their other activities including culture, as well … The thought that it is their duty to help educate themselves does not appear to have occurred."**
>
> *Square Chronicle, 1961*

Professor Fish reported in 1981 that a "UGC bombshell" had been dropped in July with pharmacy a target for "particularly savage cuts". The UGC had advised universities to reduce home student numbers by 25% for subjects related to medicine in order to preserve excellence. The University of London included pharmacy in this proposal, which meant that the Square suffered harsher cuts than other schools of pharmacy. Fish reported that the allocation of places to the new BSc in Toxicology and Pharmacology would slightly offset the loss of numbers in the BPharm, but he clearly could not see how these measures would maintain the high standards at the School. The following year he could report that the threatened 25% cut in student numbers was subsequently reduced to around 5% for the BPharm.

The School also experienced an increasing trend in the number of overseas students in this period. However, at the beginning of the 1960s, the numbers dropped, perhaps because more pharmacy courses were opening in other countries, often staffed by Square alumni. In 1961, there were 49 students from other countries, of which 28 were research students. This dropped to 32 students in the following year. Nevertheless, Dr L.K. Sharp was appointed to a new post to act as an advisor to overseas students. The mid-1970s saw discussions about workforce issues in pharmacy, partly because of the entry of so many women into the profession with more part-time working and a pattern of career breaks. By the 1979–80 session, Fish reported that there were more women than men students admitted into the first year (63 women to 41 men), presumably mentioned because this was the first time that this had been the case.

An interesting snapshot of the destination of Square students was provided by an enquiry carried out by the librarian, Dr A.J. Evans, in 1963. Of 385 students graduating from School in 1949–1962, 293 replied (76%). Of these, 15% had begun postgraduate work for higher degrees, 23% went into industry, 9% began teaching, 32% went into the hospital sector and 18% went into retail pharmacy. The positions held in 1963 by those graduating in 1949–1959 comprised 25% in industry, 20% in teaching, 9% in hospital pharmacy and 23% in the retail sector. Of the 23% not employed in pharmacy, the majority were married women.

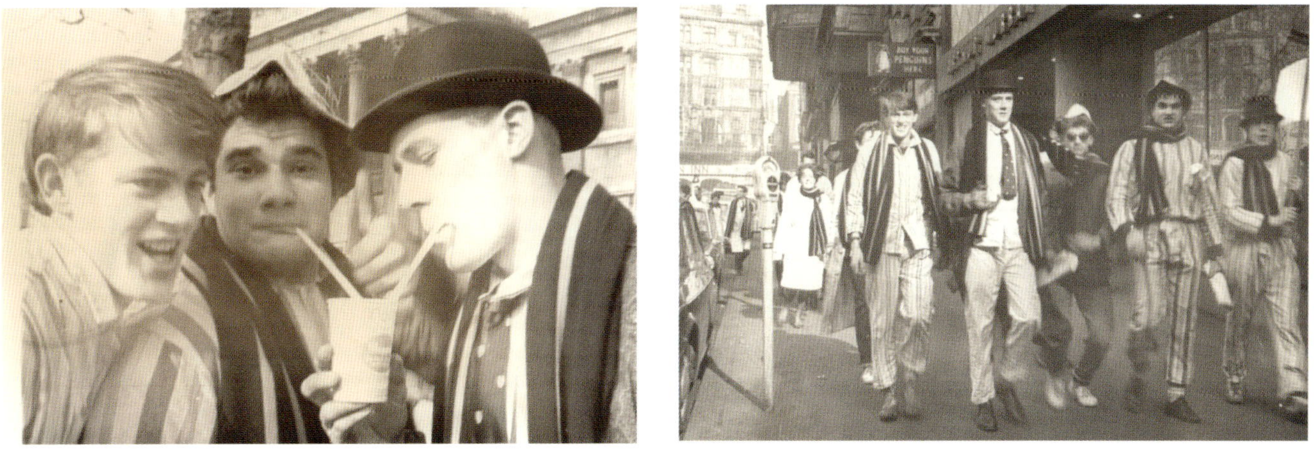

The Students' Union presidential hustings for 1963 seem to have been particularly lively. Derek Bush and Howard Rice are amongst those pictured in their pyjamas.

UCL School of Pharmacy Library

Pastoral care

Although the demand was high for places at the Square, the performance of the successful applicants caused the staff concern. In 1962, Professor Linnell reported that the 16% failure at the Part I examination seemed to be due to a lack of self-discipline. This was still an issue a decade later, and in the 1976–7 session, the staff reintroduced a personal interview system for applicants, including an interview by the dean, and a tour of the building by a current student. Concern was raised about the calibre of applicants, and so the School set up a scheme for representatives to visit schools in London to encourage good science students to go into pharmacy, and to study at the Square. The School had been holding an open afternoon for fifth and sixth formers since the 1960s, and distributing prospectuses to schools across the country.

However, whatever the concerns of the staff, the students at the Square did not choose to take part in the waves of protest and riots against universities happening across Europe in 1968. In his report for the year, Professor Hartley felt that this was worthy of mention:

> Perhaps the most important [achievement] is the retention of happy relations with our students. In a world where there is much student unrest it is an interesting fact that rarely have students and institutions in the physical and applied sciences become involved. This is, I am sure, not because science and technology students are any the less interested than their colleagues in the arts and social sciences in creating better societies. They are just as much interested in eliminating defects in curricula, in teaching methods, in examination procedures and in the ways in which authority is exercised by others. They have however less time to devote to discussion of such matters and I think they use existing channels of communication better.

> **“Perhaps the most important [achievement] is the retention of happy relations with our students. In a world where there is much student unrest it is an interesting fact that rarely have students and institutions in the physical and applied sciences become involved. This is, I am sure, not because science and technology students are any the less interested than their colleagues in the arts and social sciences in creating better societies … They have however less time to devote to discussion of such matters and I think they use existing channels of communication better.”**
>
> *Professor Hartley, 1969*

> **“a firm rock of scientific knowledge and ethical principles in today’s rough sea of pharmaceutical dangers and difficulties.”**
>
> *Lord Porritt, 1983*

An article in the *Square Chronicle* in 1969 defended the students’ right to protest as democracy in action, but did not defend the violence. It agreed with Professor Hartley’s conclusion that students at the Square were unlikely to revolt because they were more conservative than other “militant colleges”, and also as a small college communication between students and staff was easier. The formation of a consultative committee between the Academic Board and students made any protest even more unlikely. In 1977, the students were given a formal voice within the School when, for the first time, students sat as voting members of the School’s Academic Board. The closest that the student body seemed to get to protest was in 1962 when they threatened a boycott of the refectory due to rising prices. However, once the financial situation had been explained, the protesters backed down.

The School also continued to take opportunities to improve students’ experiences and particularly to make links to enhance their subsequent careers. For example, in 1984, the North Metropolitan Branch of the Pharmaceutical Society launched an “Adopt-a-Student” scheme to provide a forum for first years at the Square to meet practising pharmacists and to make visits. In the same year, the Foundation Day ceremony speaker was Lord Porritt, former surgeon to the Royal Family. His message to the student body was to appreciate their time at the School, calling it “a firm rock of scientific knowledge and ethical principles in today’s rough sea of pharmaceutical dangers and difficulties.”

Halls of residence

The enduring lack of a hall of residence for the School was not resolved in this period, although the opening of the University’s International Hall in Brunswick Square in 1962 slightly improved residential issues for overseas students. Professor Hartley identified for the 1965–6 session that only 25% of students could obtain accommodation in halls of residence, so that many who did not live in London were travelling up to two hours each day to get into their classes. Plans for a joint residential hall with the Royal Veterinary College did not materialise. The situation had improved slightly by the late 1970s, although Professor Swarbrick, in his Dean’s Report for 1977–8, thought that some good School students were put off applying because of negative feelings about being in London, particularly issues around accommodation and the high cost of living. However, by this point generally all the students that applied for places in halls got them, and the School had also leased space from the neighbouring Coram Foundation to provide six self-catering units for students.

Sport and clubs

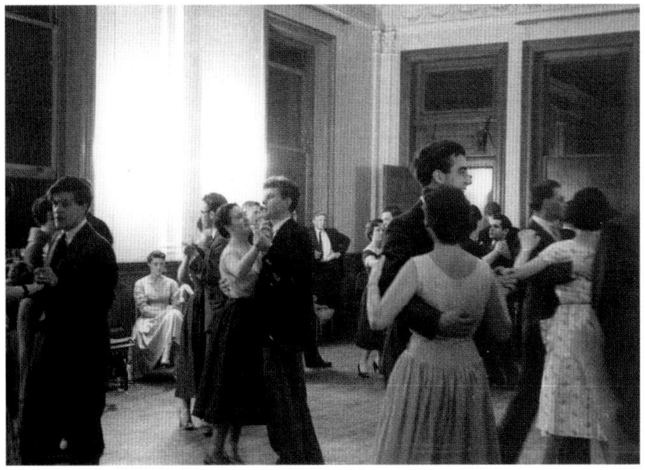

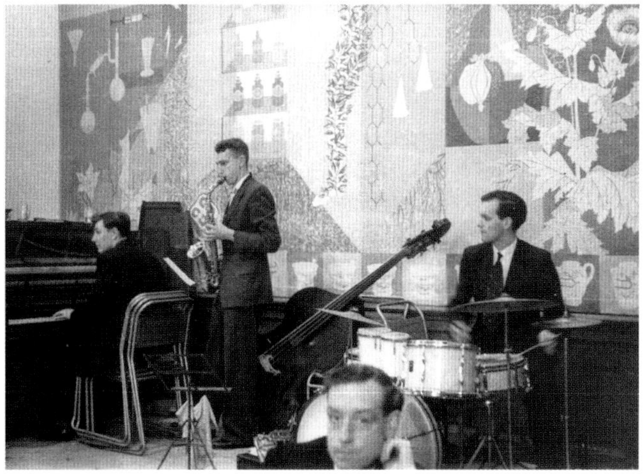

Dancing to the band at an event held at 17 Bloomsbury Square in the early 1960s.

Royal Pharmaceutical Society Museum

The "Swinging Sixties" meant fortnightly dances at the Square for most of the decade. Otherwise, the usual range of clubs and teams continued. A new Jewish Society, incorporating students from the Royal Free Medical School, was formed in 1961. Other new clubs in this period included an Overseas Club established in 1962, which organised film shows and visits to restaurants providing foreign food, and a Postgraduate Society, set up in the mid-1980s. In 1964, Margaret Jones became the first woman president of the Students' Union, although of course the Square Association had had female presidents in much earlier decades.

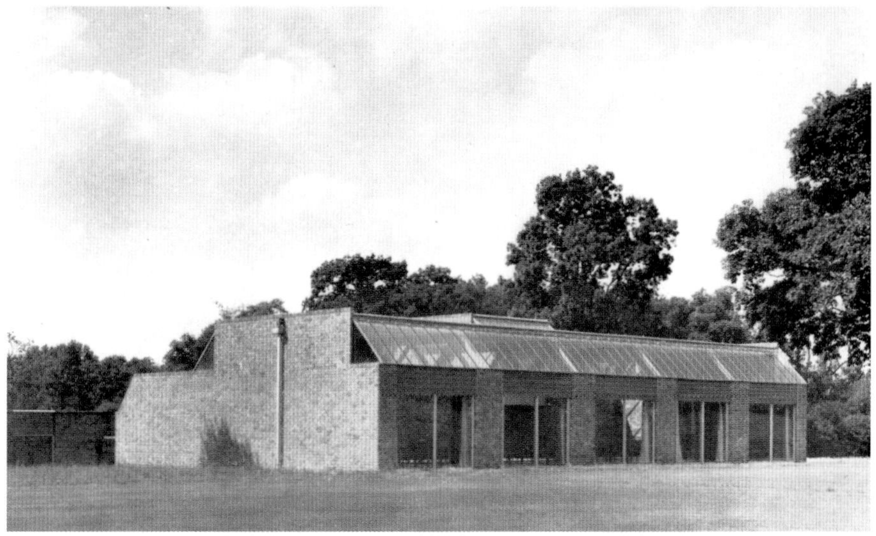

A new pavilion at Myddelton House was completed in June 1969.

UCL School of Pharmacy Library

The Association struggled in this decade, although annual garden parties continued to be held at Myddelton House. In 1961, the event also included a cricket match and "American" tennis tournament. However, by 1969, the *Chronicle* stated that both the Association and its publication were suffering from a lack of support. Nevertheless, both continued, albeit with some erratic intervals between editions of the *Chronicle*. In 1970, the editor remarked on Association events: "The style of dress and hair may vary with the years and the music seems to get louder annually, but the spirit seems remarkably constant." In 1977, Mr H. Loton, beadle at the Square for nine years, had his contribution to School life recognised by being made an honorary member of the Square Association on his retirement.

At the end of 1966, the School sold Myddelton House and the ornamental gardens to Lee Valley Regional Park Authority and used the proceeds of the sale plus a grant from the University Court to build a new pavilion. The pavilion came into use in June 1969, and was inaugurated by a hockey bully-off by Professor

Hartley and the president of the Students' Union. Meanwhile, the Square's football team had been forced to merge with the Royal Free as neither institution had enough players to field a team each. In 1970, the *Chronicle*'s "Sports Round Up" announced a new Judo Club, but that it was not very well supported. Cricket was described as "almost extinct" and rambling had not taken place for about three years. Another new club, "ten-pin bowling had a meteoric rise followed by an equally rapid decline and eventual extinction."

What were the students getting up to? There was a new union mascot, Oni, "a dirty brown stuffed alligator badly in need of a set of NHS teeth. A visit to the taxidermist will soon be called for as Oni's gut is protruding through his stitched abdomen ... Oni's sex is doubtful." And in 1971, the Students' Union opened a bar next to the junior common room. The *Chronicle* suggested that it helped socialising between undergraduate and postgraduate students, and presumably provided an alternative activity to sport in this period.

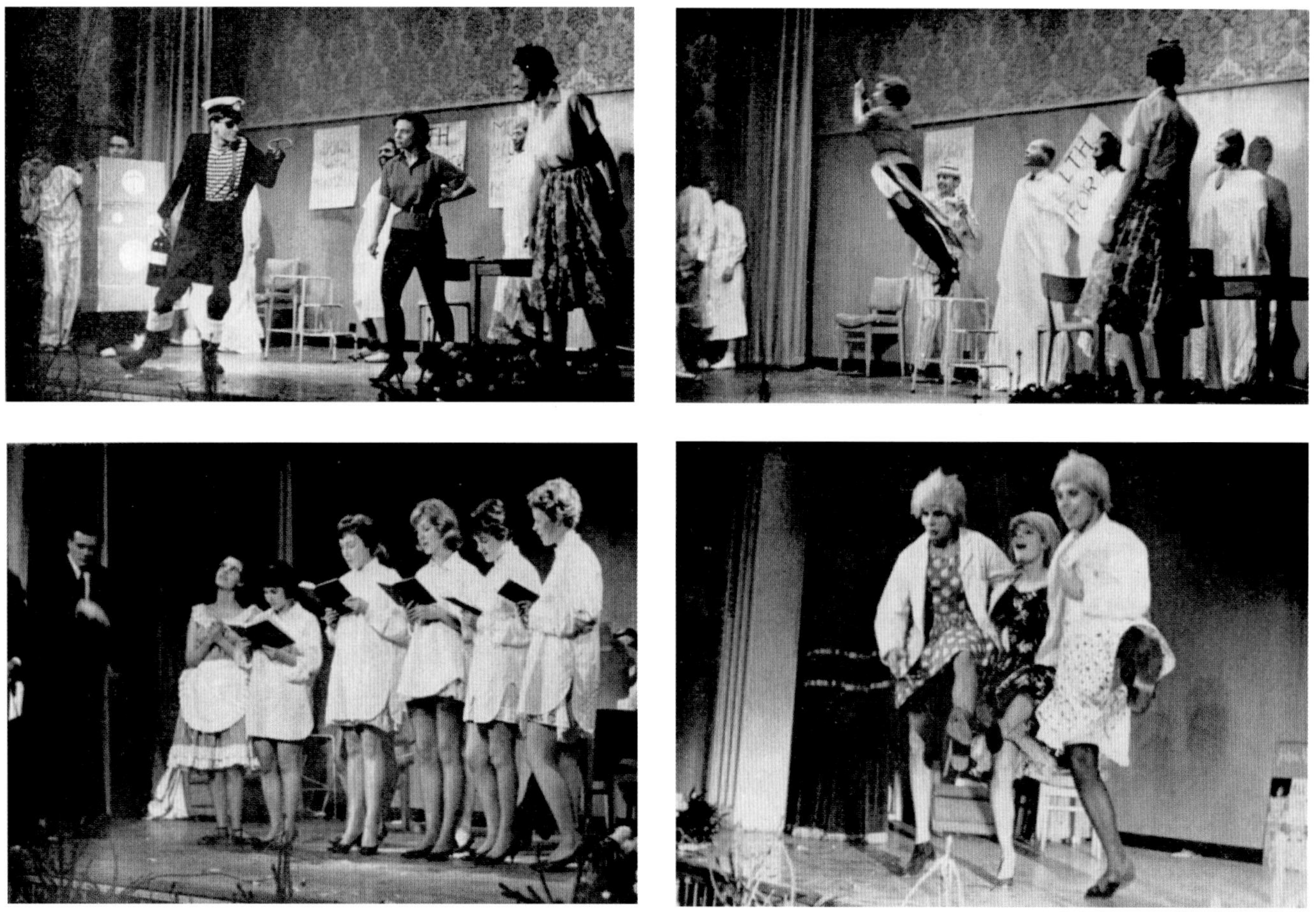

In 1962, the pantomime was *Peter Pan (the spore who would not grow up)*, set in Neversteriland. Captain Cook [sic] was played by Peter Holloway with an evil henchman, Mr Steam the autoclave, played by Colin Lewis. Peter Pan, played by Dr Rosemary Cass, even flew across the stage.

UCL School of Pharmacy Library

EXAMINATIONS

In 1961, the Government commissioned a review of higher education by a committee chaired by Lord Robbins. The Robbins' Report, published in 1963, led to the creation of new technological universities. A number of these had pharmacy departments, and were now able to develop their own degrees to be approved by the Pharmaceutical Society, rather than teaching for the University of London external degree. Chelsea College, as part of the University, was the only exception. Those departments that remained within technical colleges still did the external degree (in 1965, these were Aberdeen, Brighton, Leicester, Liverpool, Portsmouth and Sunderland). However, this meant that from 1967 everyone wanting to practise pharmacy could be required to have a degree because the university standard course was available across the country. The Pharmaceutical Society relinquished its role as examining body, but retained powers to approve the structure and content of degree courses. From 1967, in order to register as a pharmacist with the Society, each person had to hold a pharmacy degree from a course approved by the Society, and to complete a satisfactory period of preregistration experience. The new university status for all schools increased the amount of research being done, but it also introduced issues for pharmacy staff attempting to balance research and teaching for the first time, something that the staff at the Square had been grappling with for decades.

A new undergraduate syllabus was taught for the first time at the School in the 1966–7 session. It led to the First University Examination, which replaced the School's own exam at the end of the first year. This was also the first year of the Pharmaceutical Engineering Science Master's degree by examination. However, the course only ran for three years because the School was unable to obtain funding support for students who could not pay their own fees. Staff hoped to start a Master's course in the Physical Aspects of Pharmaceutics in the following session, although this did not materialise.

Writing in 1966, Cyril Maplethorpe reviewed the importance of a high standard of pharmacy education during this significant period of change, both within the profession and in its relationship with the outside world: "Without this fundamental knowledge the pharmacist cannot play his part in the National Health Service and neither can he act as an adviser on drugs to the medical profession, or as one who can protect the public from the dangers inherent in many of the new chemical compounds."

THE UNIVERSITY

The School's position within the University brought it advantages and disadvantages. Professor Hartley, in his Dean's Report in 1964, concluded that its "status and prestige throughout the world have undoubtedly been steadily enhanced in the post-war years almost wholly through its admission as a constituent School of the University."

The School was definitely able to take advantage of joint working with other institutions in the University. For example, the Dean's Report for 1969 reported on work on the metabolism of drugs with Barts, on the role of prostaglandins in

> **"[The School's] status and prestige throughout the world have undoubtedly been steadily enhanced in the post-war years almost wholly through its admission as a constituent School of the University."**
>
> *Professor Hartley, 1964*

controlling gastrointestinal function with Queen Charlotte's Hospital, Hammersmith Hospital and Central Middlesex Hospital, and on phospholipid research and ultracentrifugal studies with the Royal Free Hospital Medical School and King's College. Teaching facilities for biology had been made available to students by the neighbouring Royal Free Hospital Medical School. Professor Hartley concluded, "This is a modest but nevertheless real example of the kind of rational use of resources which must increasingly occur in this University if we are all to benefit from its magnificent aggregation of special facilities and expertise."

However, there were discussions in the following decades about whether the School should retain its independence within the University. In 1974, it was agreed that the School should retain its autonomy even though it was a small organisation. In the early 1980s, a Joint Planning Committee's Working Party on Pharmacy at the University investigated the possibility of amalgamating the Square and Chelsea to form one pharmacy department within the University. However, this proposal was rejected. The School's relationship with the University was undoubtedly strengthened by the interrelationships it fostered, including the staff. In the 1974–5 session, Hartley was re-elected as deputy vice-chancellor of the University and acted as vice-chancellor when Sir Cyril Philips was ill for two months.

In 1985, HRH Princess Anne attended the School's Foundation Day on 6th March. As chancellor of the University, she was given a tour of the building with displays and demonstrations of current work. She was particularly impressed with research work on tropical diseases, as president of the Save the Children fund. She gave an address, and said of the School:

> We are aware of the sense of pride which rightly exists here among staff and students; and we recognise the influence which The School of Pharmacy continues to exert, not only inside the profession which founded it and the university which adopted it but also outside, in the wider national and international circles where its activities impinge and influence is felt. Long may it be so.

Nevertheless, in an environment of funding cuts and proposals for amalgamations and relocations, including a proposal to move the School to St George's Hospital, Tooting, Professor Fish, dean in 1981–2, made a heartfelt plea in his Annual Report: "Hopefully, by the time this is read the mists of uncertainty ... will have been swept away and the winds of change blowing through the University will not have moved us from the well-earned and strongly-established position which we presently occupy. All we ask is to be allowed to settle to the twin job of teaching and research – a job which this School does so well."

"Hopefully, by the time this is read the mists of uncertainty to which I alluded at the start will have been swept away and the winds of change blowing through the University will not have moved us from the well-earned and strongly-established position which we presently occupy. All we ask is to be allowed to settle to the twin job of teaching and research – a job which this School does so well."

Professor Fish, 1982

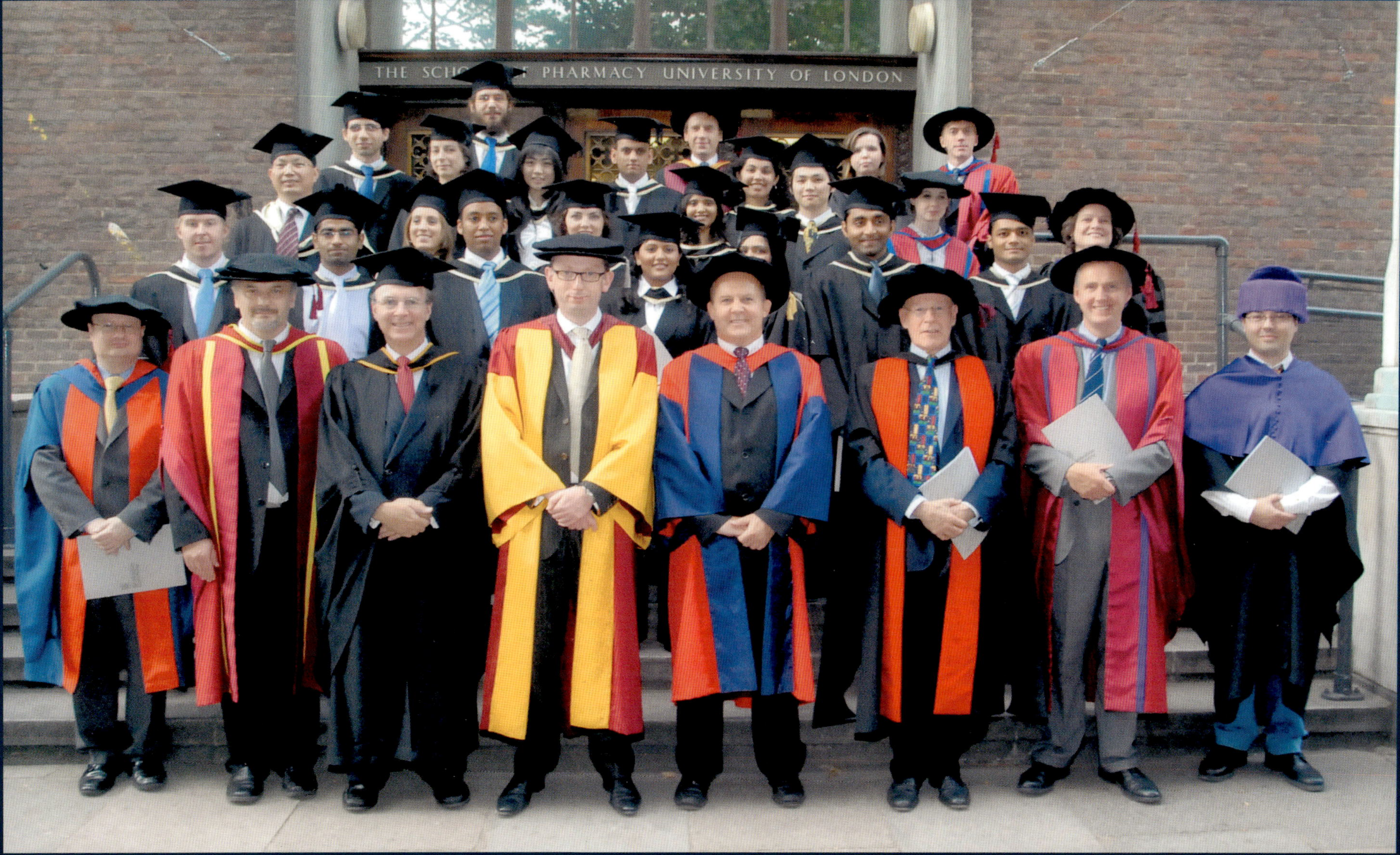

Staff and students at the graduation for MSc in Drug Discovery, 2007.
© UCL School of Pharmacy Library

MILESTONES

Popular Culture

1989	MP3 player patented by its German inventors
1992	one million computers connected to the internet
1996	Hotmail email service launched
1997	Channel 5 launched in the UK
2000	*Big Brother* first screened on British television
2000	Google became the world's largest internet search engine
2004	Facebook launched
2010	Apple's iPad tablet launched

London Life

1987	Docklands Light Railway opened
1988	construction of Canary Wharf begins
1990	Poll Tax riots
1991	Charing Cross Station completed
1994	Eurostar service launched
2000	Tate Modern opened
2000	London Eye opened
2000	Ken Livingstone appointed as London's first elected mayor
2003	congestion charging introduced for central London during peak hours
2005	London bombings
2011	wedding of Prince William and Catherine Middleton
2012	Queen Elizabeth II celebrated her Diamond Jubilee
2012	London hosted the Olympics and Paralympics

National News

1988	a Pan-Am jumbo jet crashed on to the town of Lockerbie in Scotland
1994	first National Lottery draw
1997	death of Princess Diana
1997	Tony Blair became prime minister after a landslide victory for the Labour Party
1998	Good Friday Agreement signed in Belfast
2010	David Cameron became Conservative prime minister in a coalition government with the Liberal Democrats

The Wider World

1987	Black Monday stock market crash
1990	Hubble Space Telescope launched
1997	Kyoto Agreement, to reduce emissions of greenhouse gases
2000	International Space Station hosted its first resident crew
2001	start of Afghanistan war
2001	9/11 attack on World Trade Center and Pentagon
2002	Euro currency introduced
2003–2012	Iraq War
2003	13-year Human Genome Project completed
2007	Eurostar high speed service started
2008	Banking crisis and subsequent recession

Drug Developments

1987	AZT (zidovudine), drug treatment for AIDS
1989	Zocor (simvastatin), for lowering blood lipids
1989	Prozac (fluoxetine), for depression
1990	first gene therapy experiment in a person with adenosine deaminase deficiency

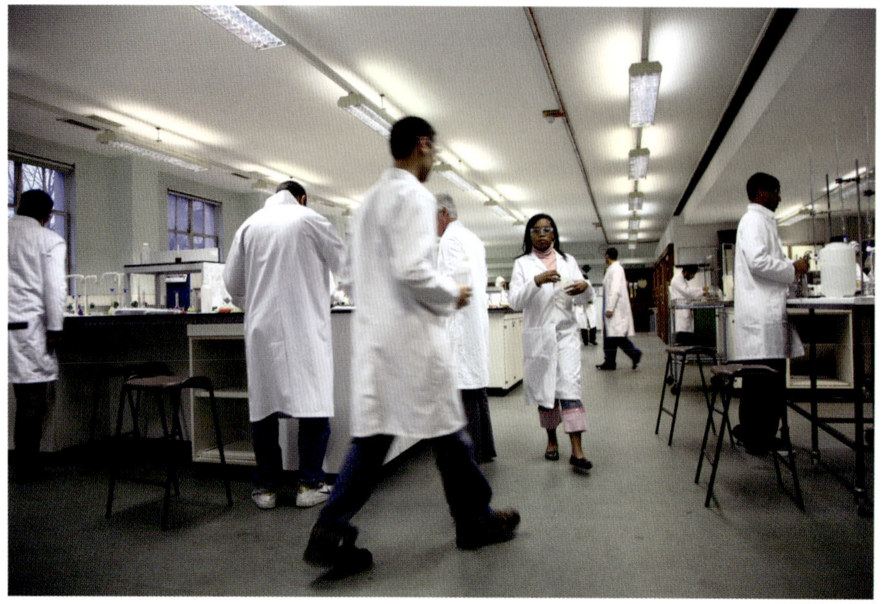

In recent years, the pace of drug development and the increasing complexity of pharmaceutical science have proved both a challenging and exciting backdrop for pharmacy students and practitioners.

Questions about the pharmacy profession itself have also been a key feature of the last decade in particular, not least with the demerger of the Royal Pharmaceutical Society. In 2008, the Health and Social Care Act enabled the General Pharmaceutical Council to be established as a regulatory body for the profession, separate from the Royal Pharmaceutical Society, an event that took place in September 2010. The Society faced a difficult period as it re-established itself as a purely voluntary membership body. Discussions around the status of pharmacists as health professionals, their relationship with a national organisation, and their reputation with both the Government and the public produced remarkably clear echoes of the Society's early days in the mid-nineteenth century.

In addition, the Pharmacy White Paper, *Pharmacy in England – Building on Strength, Delivering the Future*, published in 2008, advocated a more effective role for pharmacists embedded in an integrated healthcare team. Building on the enhanced role for pharmacists laid out in the National Health Service (NHS) contract in 2005, the White Paper in 2008 proposed that they are perfectly placed to meet the public health challenges envisaged for future decades: obesity, alcohol use, sexual health and smoking-related conditions, alongside a significant growth in the number of patients suffering from long-term conditions such as diabetes and asthma. The accessibility of the community pharmacist, it argued, should enable better medicines adherence and allow targeted interventions to improve public health. The subsequent establishment of Medical Education England (MEE) and the Modernising Pharmacy Careers Programme explored how the White Paper's aims could be achieved through pharmacy education, particularly by providing a meaningful clinical context to the science of medicines. The White Paper was led by an alumnus of the School, Dr Keith Ridge, with the subsequent educational element championed by the School's dean, Professor Anthony Smith. In addition, many of the proposals put forward by the Paper were strongly supported by work carried out by staff at the Square over the previous decade.

A CHANGING UNIVERSITY SECTOR

The 1990s and early 2000s were a transformational period for higher education generally in the UK. The School's experience reflected the wider picture including the occasional rollercoaster moment of sudden

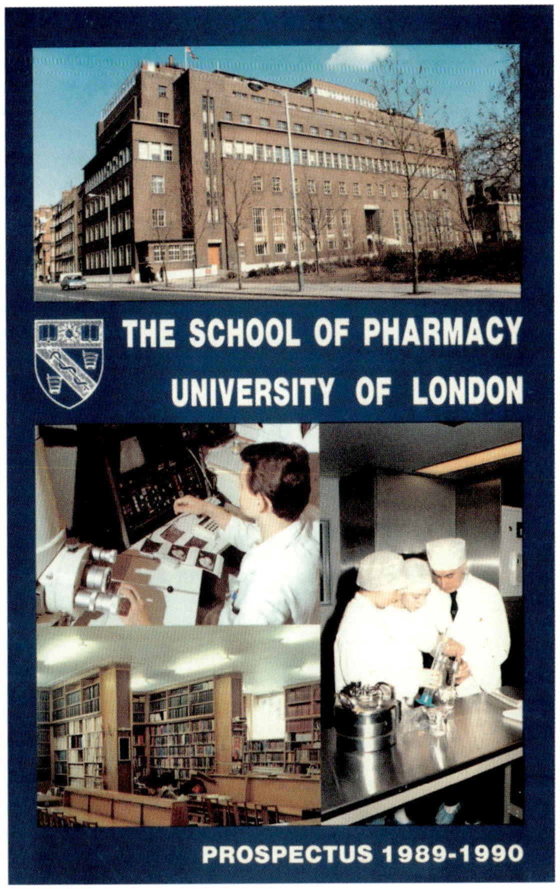

UCL School of Pharmacy Library

changes in national funding policies. After the cuts of the early Thatcher years (around 11% was removed from the national higher education budget in 1982–1984), higher education had recovered. It continued to grow through the 1980s and 1990s, albeit more slowly and (until 1992) across the binary line of universities on the one hand and teaching-led polytechnics on the other. In 1992, this binary line was abolished when polytechnics gained university status, and a long period of transition started, intended in principle to level the funding playing field between the university and polytechnic sectors.

In practice, when it came to teaching, the overlap between the sectors had been extensive, but "blue skies" research and training for most professional careers, including medicine, had remained almost exclusively in the universities. Pharmacy was an exception, with several departments established in the polytechnics. The polytechnics' core mission to provide high-quality teaching had an immediate impact on the older university sector, however, which now had to face external quality assurance systems similar to those which had always regulated the polytechnic sector. From 1993 the Higher Education Quality Council (HEQC) (later replaced by the Quality Assurance Agency, QAA) started to review single academic subjects and whole institutions, and began to provide a national-level comparative and public insight into teaching provision across the sector. It took until 1997 and the Dearing Report into Higher Education (the first major review since the 1960s) for a national qualifications framework to be introduced, with the creation of the QAA.

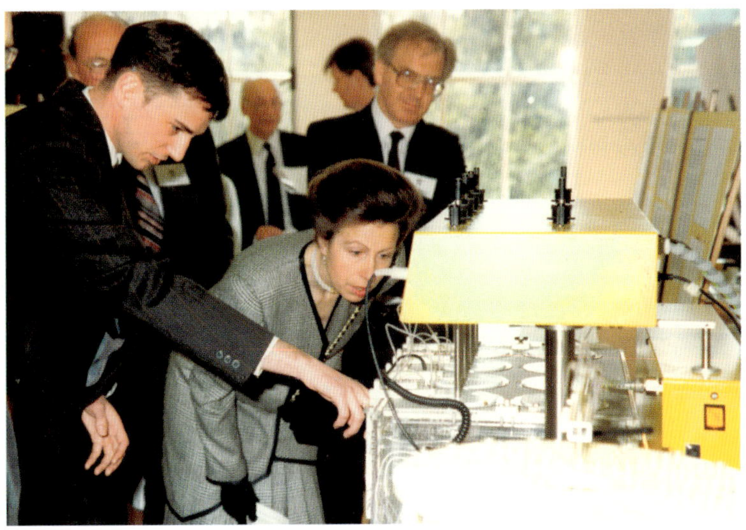

HRH Princess Anne visited the School as Vice Chancellor of the University in 1992, as part of the celebration of its 150th anniversary.

UCL School of Pharmacy Library

The School successfully passed through its first institutional review in 1994, albeit with the following wry comment in the formal report of the event by the HEQC:

the School of Pharmacy was established 150 years ago by the then newly formed

- 1990 cyclo-oxygenase-2 (COX-2) discovered by scientists, revealing a major new focus for anti-inflammatory drugs
- 1992 Taxol (paclitaxel), for breast and ovarian cancer, and for lung cancer
- 1992 Didronel (etidronate), first bisphosphonate in the UK for osteoporosis
- 1993 Glucobay (acarbose), alpha-glucosidase inhibitor for type 2 diabetes
- 1994 Zantac (ranitidine), for acid indigestion
- 1995 Betaferon (interferon beta-1b), treatment for multiple sclerosis
- 1996 Invirase (saquinavir), first protease inhibitor for AIDS in the UK
- 1996 Cozaar (losartan), angiotensin 2 receptor antagonist for high blood pressure
- 1997 Malarone (atovaquone/proguanil), new treatment for malaria
- 1998 Viagra (sildenafil), for erectile dysfunction
- 1998 Singulair (montelukast), a new class of oral medication for asthma
- 1999 Relenza (zanamivir), neuraminidase inhibitor for influenza
- 2000 Herceptin (trastuzumab), for breast cancer
- 2001 Zyvox (linezolid), first entirely new class of antibacterial in 30 years
- 2001 Cancidas (caspofungin), a new class of antifungal agents
- 2002 Varilrix (Varicella zoster vaccine), vaccine against chickenpox
- 2002 Lantus (insulin glargine), long-acting insulin analogue for diabetes
- 2003 Fuzeon (enfuvirtide), fusion inhibitor for antiretroviral-resistant HIV infections
- 2003 Ezetrol (ezetimibe), a new type of cholesterol-lowering agent
- 2004 Cymbalta (duloxetine), medical treatment for stress incontinence in women
- 2004 Velcade (bortezomib), for multiple myeloma
- 2005 Tarceva (erlotinib), oral treatment for advanced or metastatic lung cancer
- 2005 Exelon (rivastigmine), treatment for dementia in Parkinson's disease
- 2005 Erbitux (cetuximab) and Avastin (bevacizumab), monoclonal antibodies for colorectal cancer
- 2006 Tygacil (tigecycline), a new type of antibacterial for skin and abdominal infections
- 2006 Remicade (infliximab), biological agent for severe ulcerative colitis
- 2006 Exubera (inhaled insulin), inhaled insulin for diabetes
- 2006 Rotarix (rotavirus vaccine), vaccine for infants against gastroenteritis caused by rotavirus

Pharmacy Milestones

- 1988 the Pharmaceutical Society becomes the Royal Pharmaceutical Society
- 1989 Medicines Division of the Department of Health and Social Security becomes the Medicines Control Agency
- 1995 European Medicines Agency (EMEA) set up to co-ordinate and provide regulatory support to EU member states and the European medicines advisory committees for both human and veterinary medicines
- 1999 National Institute for Clinical Excellence (NICE) (later National Institute for Health and Clinical Excellence) set up
- 2001 resale price maintenance for medicines abolished
- 2002 Primary care trusts (PCTs) set up their first pharmacy contracts
- 2003 Medicines Control Agency becomes Medicines and Healthcare products Regulatory Agency (MHRA)

2004 Supplemental Charter granted for the Royal Pharmaceutical Society of Great Britain (RPSGB)
2004 membership of RPSGB reduced from five categories to two: practising and non-practising
2004 first pharmacist prescriber registered with the RPSGB
2005 RPSGB operated a voluntary register for pharmacy technicians from 1st January
2006 reciprocal registration of pharmacists from Northern Ireland, Australia, New Zealand and South Africa ended
2007 RPSGB launched online pharmacy registration, and an accompanying logo
2008 Health and Social Care Act amended the Health Act of 1999, and enabled the General Pharmaceutical Council to be established as a regulatory body for the profession, separate from the Royal Pharmaceutical Society
2010 RPSGB demerged to form the General Pharmaceutical Council and the membership body, the Royal Pharmaceutical Society (RPS)

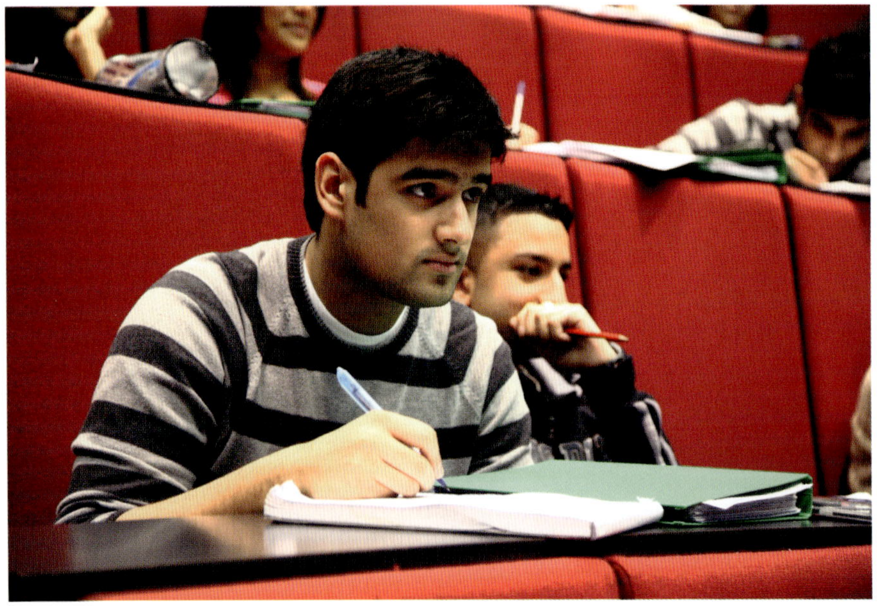

Pharmaceutical Society "for the purpose of advancing Chemistry and Pharmacy and promoting a uniform system of education of those who shall practise the same", the Corporate Plan of the School (June 1992) states that "there has been little reason over the years to deviate from this brief."

For an institution used to facing reaccreditation of its degree on a regular basis, the HEQC and its successor body QAA perhaps posed less of a shock to the School than for many others, but the emergence of national quality assurance agencies was the start of a powerful movement to make universities' teaching provision open to scrutiny.

At much the same time, through the 1990s, the financial governance of universities – along with that of many other publicly funded organisations – started to be closely audited. National bodies were developed with authority to set anything from benign threshold standards through to very demanding accountability regimes. After 1992, all of English higher education was funded from a common pot, managed though a single funding body (the Higher Education Funding Council for England, HEFCE), and the Government not unreasonably wanted to know how these highly autonomous institutions were spending the public investment.

In essence, each university's income derived from the number of UK and European Union (EU) undergraduate students it had contracted to teach, topped up by some government funding for postgraduate and research students, plus – and here success depended directly on each institution's individual performance – whatever it could earn through research grants, and the fees paid by self-funded students, including those from overseas.

International student numbers started to rise significantly during the period right across the UK, although some universities found to their cost that reliance on single countries for the pipeline of international student fees could be disastrous if local unrest or changes to government policy suddenly blocked the supply. In 1991–2, the School's first official international undergraduate exchange took place with a group of German graduates from the University of Heidelberg, who studied biochemistry at the School for three months under the Erasmus Scheme. The intake of overseas students at this point was around 20 per year, and the University of London name was invaluable to the School in its growing international recruitment. Today about 25% of the student population, more than 300 each year, comes from outside the UK, and School staff travel the world to attend education fairs, schools and colleges. The School now routinely recruits students from 51 countries. Among these there are European students from Albania, Austria, Germany, Greece, the Netherlands, Poland and Cyprus, while from beyond Europe there are representatives from Kenya, Tanzania, Hong Kong, Malaysia, Singapore, Nigeria, Mauritius, Canada, South Korea, the USA, Jordan, Ghana, India and Egypt.

In 1997, Tony Blair was elected on a commitment to "education, education, education" and, while academe would never admit to a golden age, the late 1990s and early 2000s saw a period of major expansion and investment. The School enjoyed its share of public investment in education, with student numbers rising through the period, significant funding for capital investment coming in periodic and very welcome grants, and its successful research performance earning government grant and charitable funding, as well as industrial sponsorship. The accounts of the period show annual income at £6.7 million in 1991, £8.3 million by 1996, £9.5 million by 2001, £15.6 million by 2006 and over £20 million by 2011. There were some years when expenditure more than matched income, but student numbers rose and investment in research continued apace.

Although the Blair government's ambition for 50% participation in higher education for 18–30-year-olds was not achieved, access to higher education did expand hugely through the late 1990s and 2000s. A series of government funding and policy initiatives and a relatively buoyant economy supported the growth in higher education participation from around 15% of the age group in 1987 to around 44% by 2009–10. This was despite the withdrawal of maintenance grants and their replacement with student loans in 1998, which many expected to halt the expansion. Maintenance grants for students from the lowest income backgrounds were actually reintroduced in 2004.

Much of this growth in numbers came from socioeconomic groups that had not traditionally had access or aspirations to higher education. Thus, the gender, ethnic and economic profile of students through the sector changed very significantly on a national basis. Individual institutions changed in different ways and at their own pace, but one of the most striking phenomena for pharmacy schools throughout the country, and indeed for medical training more generally, was the powerful take-up of places by women, and by very high-achieving first generation British Asian students from state schools. Across the country the feminisation of medical and pharmacy training emerged as a dominant characteristic of the student body, and one which posed long-term issues for the profession. Between 2002 and 2012 the percentage of women undergraduates was typically between 65% and 70%. For the School, and for some others based in large cities, another overwhelming factor was that the undergraduate population was essentially local. There were several years in the early 2000s when over 80% of the School's first year intake was from within the M25.

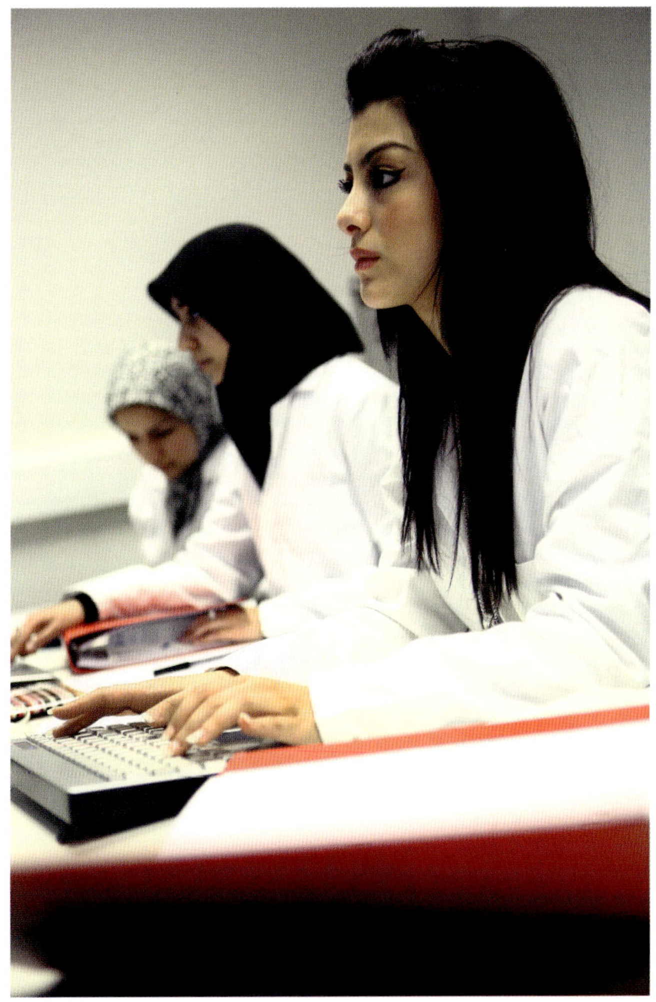

Some of the corporate scandals of the period, as well as the need to account for the huge public investment in university teaching and research, also led to a slow but ultimately transformational governance and accountability regime in the sector. Universities had become charities in law, and successive pieces of legislation and an increasingly articulate national governance structure made ever-clearer statements on the responsibilities of members of governing bodies as charity trustees. By slow degrees through the late twentieth and early twenty-first century, the balance of power within universities shifted from self-governing academic senates to governing bodies, audit functions, professional management and externally facing accountability responsibilities. Academic policy and the monitoring of academic standards remained the proper preserve of the academic community, but responsibility for mission, strategic direction and for resources now lay explicitly with governing bodies, which were almost invariably dominated by external members. By the end

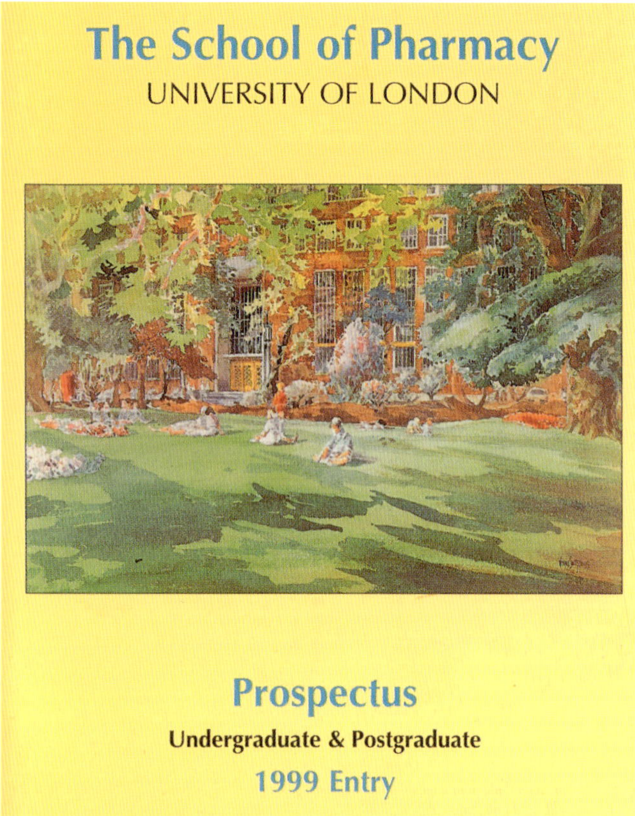

The prospectus design from 1993 to 1999 featured a watercolour of Brunswick Square by John Castle, painted to mark the School's 150th anniversary in 1992.

UCL School of Pharmacy Library

of the 1990s, governing bodies, not senates, were running universities. The School had a long and deep relationship with its professional community, and this served it well through these changing times, with external members of its Council drawn from the Royal Pharmaceutical Society, the NHS, community pharmacists and the pharmaceutical industry.

In higher education as in other areas of public life, the 1990s and 2000s also saw a very strong rise in consumer awareness in its widest sense. For universities, this was partly manifest in the establishment of the Office of the Independent Adjudicator in 2004, which for the first time gave students a route to judgement of their complaints and grievances, independent of their institution. The National Student Satisfaction Survey started in 2005. Whatever the effectiveness of these particular organs, they evidence the mood of regulation and accountability that had surrounded universities by the end of the 2000s, and the growing significance of the student voice.

The great expansionist period had involved not simply numbers of students but also numbers of institutions, a growth in new, usually technology-driven academic disciplines and strategic growth in selective areas, including pharmacy. There were several reasons for pharmacy's growth. Pharmacy was recognised by the Government as a national skills shortage, so funding was available for universities who wanted to train additional MPharm students. It offered full employment to graduates; indeed, junior hospital posts were notoriously difficult to fill, and the profession was propped up by an army of locums. It was anticipated that there would be greater future demand for pharmacists with an expansion and diversification of their roles across the sectors. The British

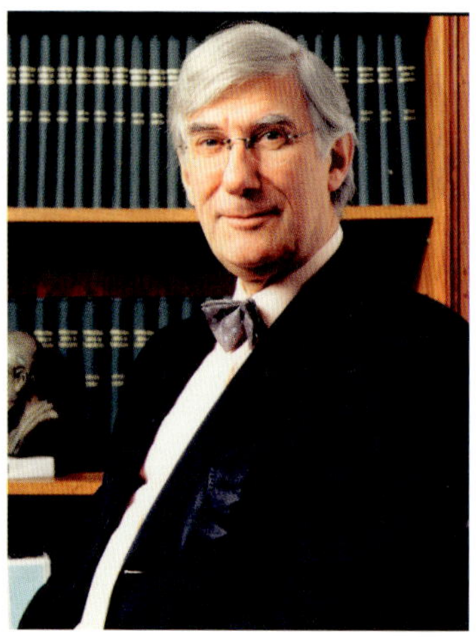

ALEXANDER TAYLOR FLORENCE (1940–)

UCL School of Pharmacy Library

ALEXANDER TAYLOR FLORENCE (1940–)

Sandy Florence graduated in Pharmacy from the University of Glasgow in 1962, and gained his PhD at the University three years later. He spent a year as a junior research fellow at the Medical Research Council, and then joined the staff at the new University of Strathclyde in 1966. Having spent a year as a research associate in the USA at R.J. Reynolds Tobacco Company, he returned to Strathclyde. He was appointed senior lecturer in 1972, J.P. Todd professor of pharmaceutical technology in 1976, and dean of the Strathclyde School of Pharmacy in 1978.

Professor Florence became dean of the School of Pharmacy, University of London in 1988, and continued an active research role alongside his academic post. He retired in 2006. He is editor-in-chief (Europe) of the *International Journal of Pharmaceutics* and was founding co-editor with Professor Vincent Lee of the *Journal of Drug Targeting*. He is the author of more than 250 papers, reviews and chapters in books. He is the co-author, with Professor David Attwood, of *Physicochemical Principles of Pharmacy* and *Surfactant Systems: Their Chemistry, Pharmacy and Biology*. He also co-authored *Solubilization by Surface Active Agents* (1968) with the late Peter H. Elworthy and C.B. Macfarlane.

Professor Florence received the GSK International Achievement award in 2001, the Høst Madsen award from FIP in 1997, the Scheele Prize of the Swedish Academy of Sciences in 1993 and the Harrison memorial medal of the Royal Pharmaceutical Society of Great Britain in 1986. He is a former president of the Controlled Release Society. He was appointed CBE in 1994.

MPharm was recognised internationally as a professional qualification, and Master's degrees were very attractive to an expanding international market. There was also the sheer profitability of the subject in the mix of institutional funding, and in some cases a new pharmacy offering provided a lifeline for long-established chemistry departments which could no longer recruit undergraduates in sustainable numbers. Together, these factors led to the establishment of nine new schools of pharmacy, from 12 to 21, between 2003 and 2009, with another three or four more being planned.

In anticipation of his retirement in March 2006, Professor Florence reflected on the changes that the School had experienced during his time as dean. In 1989, there had been 80 undergraduates in each year and the School had a budget of £5 million. In 2005, this had increased to 192 undergraduates in the first year and a budget of £16 million. Dr Philip Brown, chair of the School's Council, outlined the challenges facing the next dean. With nine new schools of pharmacy approved by the Royal Pharmaceutical Society and others in the pipeline, there was debate about their role. Would the existing schools focus on research while the new ones focused more on the education of much-needed undergraduates? The Square also had to consider its place in the University of London.

Between 2005 and 2007 the School's Council appointed a new dean, Professor Anthony Smith, and a new chair of Council, Lord Tim Clement Jones. In late 2007, in the first reversal of over 10 years of expansionist policy, and with only six months' warning, the Government announced the removal of £100 million from the higher education budget. To find the shortfall, the HEFCE withdrew funding for students studying for qualifications equivalent to or lower than those they already possessed, such as a biochemistry graduate retraining for pharmacy. This new funding policy created acute turbulence across the sector but few institutions were hit as hard as the School, which lost 15% of its undergraduate teaching income.

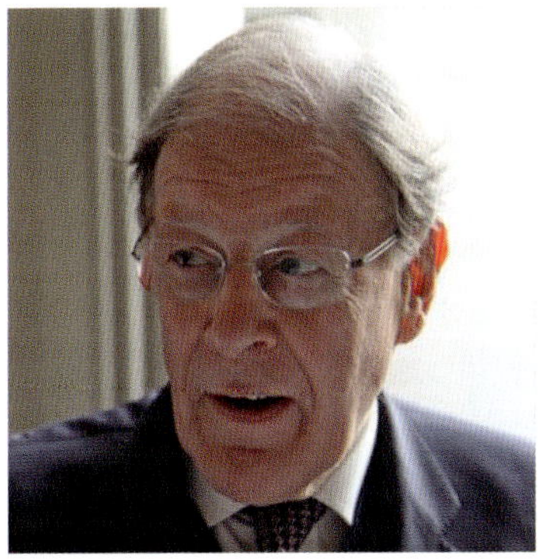

PHILIP J BROWN (1936–)

PHILIP J BROWN (1936–)

In 1954, Philip Brown started a two-year pharmacy apprenticeship at Savory & Moore, New Bond Street, London. He graduated from the School in 1959 with an upper second degree. From then on his career followed a non-pharmacy course. He taught at Guildford Grammar School before going up to Cambridge in 1960 where he studied for his PhD in organic chemistry. In 1963, he joined the Daily Express newspaper as science and medical correspondent, moving onto Sterling Winthrop as Operations Research Manager in 1966. In 1969 he joined the J Walter Thompson advertising agency where he became managing director of the Deltakos subsidiary which specialised in medical advertising. In 1976 Brown set up PJB Publications Ltd which became a leading provider of business and research information for the international healthcare industry. It was sold in 2003. In 1990, he joined the School Council and was Chairman from 2000 to 2007. During this time the degree moved to a four-year course, the staff and student numbers exceeded 1,000, and the lease on the Brunswick Square building was finally secured after 50 years. Brown also served on the management board of the Bloomsbury BioSeed Fund, a joint enterprise with University College set up under the Challenge Fund scheme, and chaired the Board of Pharmovation, a company which developed commercially the School's IP and R&D activities. Philip is now prospective chairman of the School's Foundation which will develop alumni support for the School's academic activities.

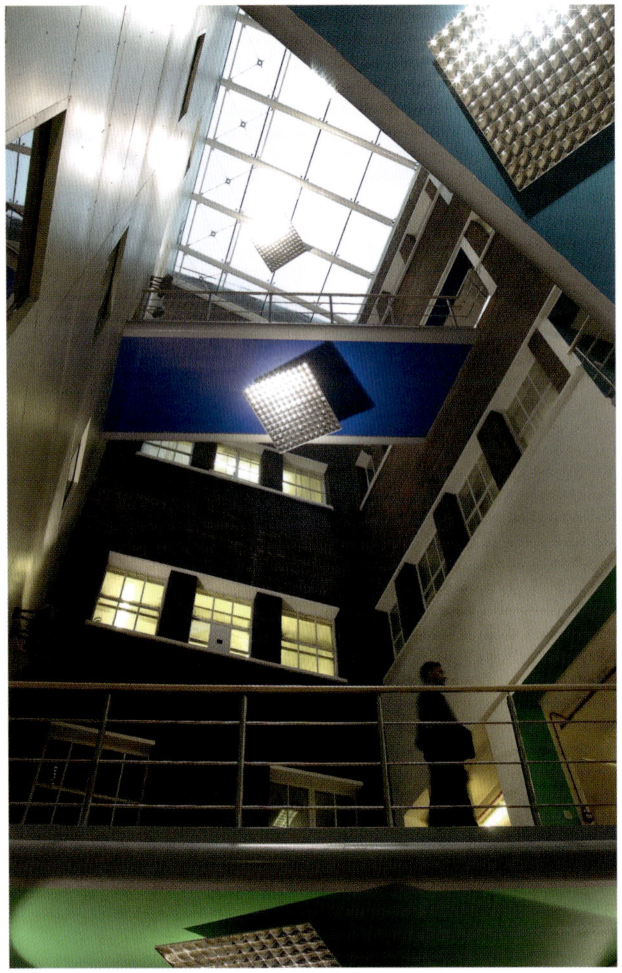

The Molecular Pharmacy Wing was opened by HRH Princess Anne in 2008.

Day and England Stevensen Marsh Architects

THE BUILDING

Unsurprisingly, the Brunswick Square building needed to change to keep up with developments in education and pharmacy. This included keeping up with technology with, for example, the opening of new pharmacy practice laboratories in October 1991, a state-of-the-art development for its time. This was designed to resemble a real-life dispensary, rather than a "wet laboratory" as had previously been the case, together with a fully equipped community pharmacy area in which students could undertake patient counselling and patient history-taking activities. In 1971, the space for the library had been increased by building an extension over what is now the junior common room, to incorporate the senior common room and a corridor. This development, together with a special grant to extend the space in 1996, just about managed to enable the library to support the work of students and staff into the end of the twentieth century. A major refurbishment of the main undergraduate teaching laboratory, funded by the Wolfson Foundation, enabled the School to deliver practical classes to large groups in what was regarded as an enviably well-provided space. The large assembly hall, which had once held degree ceremonies while numbers were still small, was converted into a ground-floor lecture theatre, with a mezzanine floor of offices and small classrooms above.

The biggest construction project of this period was the new seven-storey 980 square metre molecular pharmacy wing, which was completed in 2008. The building infilled the larger of the two light-wells and expanded the basement space. The Princess Royal, as chancellor, officially opened the new wing, which included five floors housing research laboratories, creating a centre for collaborative research into the discovery, design and development of medicines. Each of the new wing's research floors was devoted to a particular discipline: cancer pharmacology, microbiology and infectious diseases, pharmaceutics and nanotechnology, pharmacognosy and phytotherapy, and molecular neuroscience and genetics. The new building also provided a teaching laboratory, seminar and meetings rooms, and a large flexible space on the ground floor as a venue for events. The project was funded by capital grants of £4.1 million, with a further £1 million donation from the Wolfson Foundation to enable the research laboratories to be equipped and furnished to the highest specifications.

"As a University [Pharmaceutical Chemistry] Department this is one of the best equipped in the world for synthetic medicinal, natural product and protein chemistry, for pharmaceutical analysis, and for programmes in drug design based on receptor and enzyme biochemistry."

Annual Report, 1986–7

One of the side-effects of this large project was the relocation of the Department of Practice and Policy (DPP) to rented accommodation in BMA House, Tavistock Square. The move was intended to be temporary while the construction work was underway, but the expansion of Practice and Policy, and its success in attracting research grants, which in turn attracted researchers, meant that it had outgrown itself within two years. The School was forced to recognise that most of the DPP's activity would have to stay outside the main building. A share of a Georgian house in Russell Square, to house the DPP's spin-out activity (the burgeoning continuing professional development work of the Advanced Pharmacy Studies Centre), was also completed at this time. Thus, without actually intending it, the School had permanently become a multisite operation by 2007.

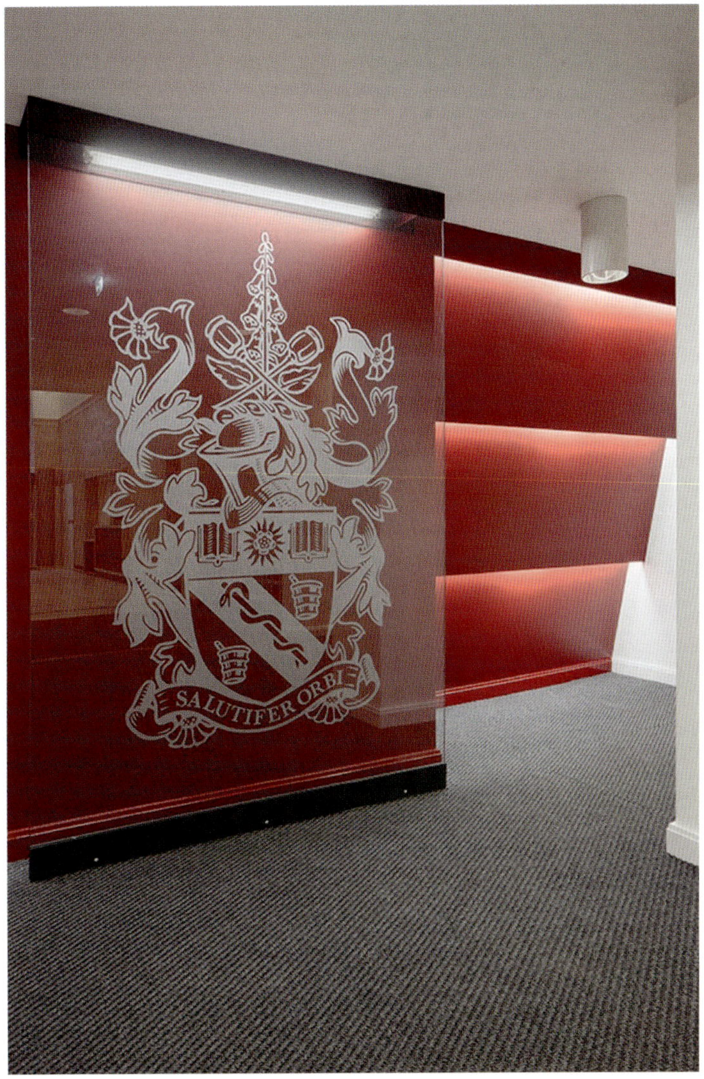

The entrance hall was brought up to date, but with the School's coat of arms as a dominant feature.

The national approach to university capital investment had for some years been supported through periodic grants from the HEFCE, and the School had elected to invest most of its funding in its research infrastructure, with conspicuous success. However, by the middle of the decade, the non-research areas of the School were looking tired. The public areas, classrooms, student facilities and the hidden infrastructure were all suffering from underinvestment. The new National Student Survey revealed that, in the context of increasing student enrolments and the changing nature of the undergraduate course, the library and information technology (IT) provision were in need of major upgrading. Thus, when the next HEFCE capital funding round became available from 2008, the School's leaders decided to invest as much as possible in areas of the building used by the greatest numbers of staff, and in facilities for students.

Over a three-year period, from 2008 to 2011, the School saw the complete refurbishment of the entrance hall (its only previous claim to fame had been as the film location for a magistrates court), the junior common room and bar, one of the two large lecture theatres, several small laboratories and the square lounge (transformed into a Wi-Fi-enabled group study space, exhibition venue, internet café and common room), the provision of bike sheds (which later won the School an environmental awareness award), the creation of individual study spaces for PhD students and, most importantly, the library and IT provision. The library was transformed from a tired and dated facility into a bright, professionally designed space, where the excellent collection again had the surroundings it merited. The newly refurbished library was reopened by the vice-chancellor of the University in December 2010. Students so enjoyed the transformation, however, that usage increased dramatically, bringing new, yet perennial, space challenges.

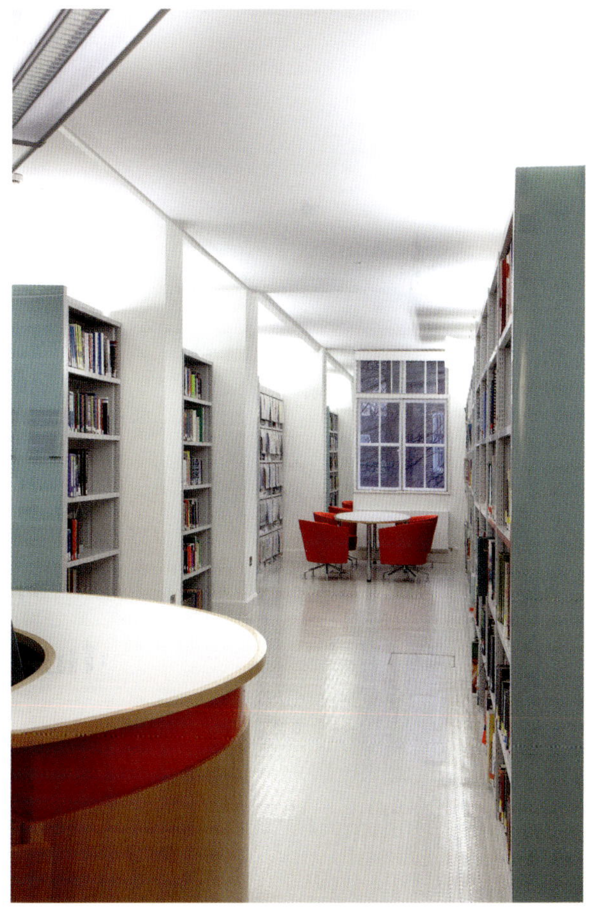

The library was completely refurbished in 2010.

At the same time that the decision was made to refurbish the students' IT provision, the whole of the IT infrastructure was discovered to be at acute risk. The School used the opportunity to recover years of underinvestment with complete replacement of the physical infrastructure and renovation of the

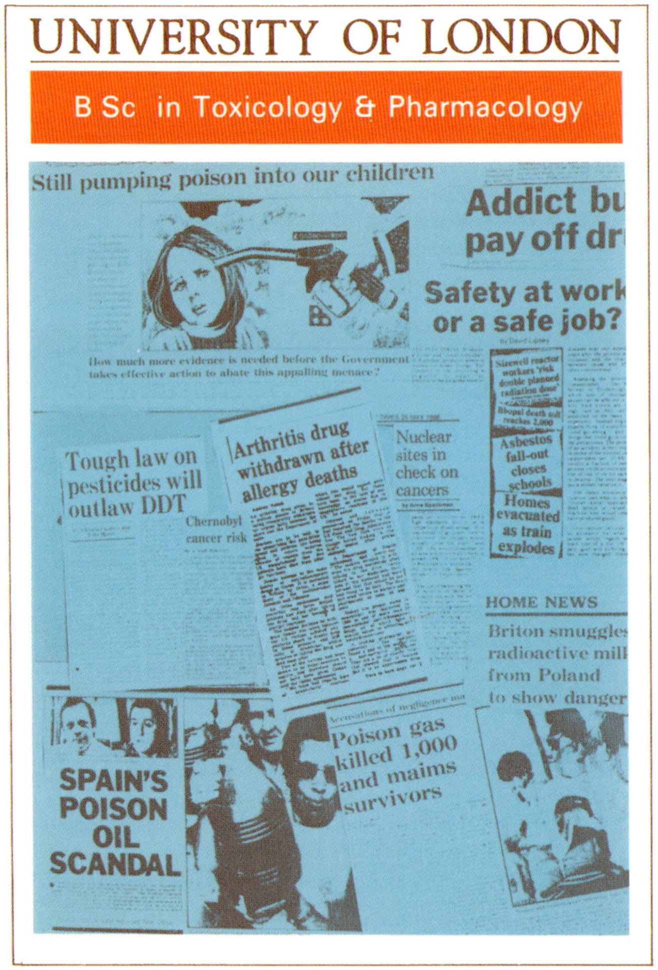
UNIVERSITY OF LONDON
B Sc in Toxicology & Pharmacology
Still pumping poison into our children
Addict bu
pay off dr
Safety at work
or a safe job?
Tough law on pesticides will outlaw DDT
Arthritis drug withdrawn after allergy deaths
Nuclear sites in check on cancers
Chernobyl cancer risk
Asbestos fall-out closes schools
Homes evacuated as train explodes
HOME NEWS
Briton smuggles radioactive mill from Poland to show danger
Poison gas killed 1,000 and maims survivors
SPAIN'S POISON OIL SCANDAL

UCL School of Pharmacy Library

principal IT space. It also exploited the technological developments of recent years to provide Wi-Fi throughout the building, a laptop loan scheme, and to establish little corners of the building where students could work individually or in small groups. Far from simply being a tool for management and research, modern teaching and learning drives a demand for personal computing and adaptive technology that the School successfully prioritised in the last major capital investment of the period.

TEACHING

The original three professors at the School may have managed to grasp the developments in staffing and subject areas that were experienced in the following century, but in recent years the proliferation of posts and specialisms reflect the fact that pharmacy operates in a completely different era. Chairs in botany, chemistry and pharmacy have evolved into more than 50 academic posts including roles devoted to cellular neuroscience, nanomedicine, clinical pharmaceutics, behavioural medicine, public policy and many more.

Events of the past 25 years have continued to act as a catalyst for the School to innovate and develop. In response to the Nuffield Report, changes were made to the teaching staff and style at the Square. In the 1986–7 session, the pharmaceutics department gained approval from the School Council to nominate up to six practising pharmacists as honorary practitioner teachers. Staff introduced lectures on study methods and communication skills into the first year undergraduate course, and created a clinical pharmacy/pharmacy practice working group to focus on these areas across the curriculum. In the late 1980s, the second year dispensing course was completely redesigned to reflect modern practice, and to make use of the new sterile products unit, alongside a new emphasis on powder technology. In the 1987–8 session, a new series of "pharmacy orientation" lectures

" We have done more than merely survive, we have progressed. "

Professor Fish, 1987

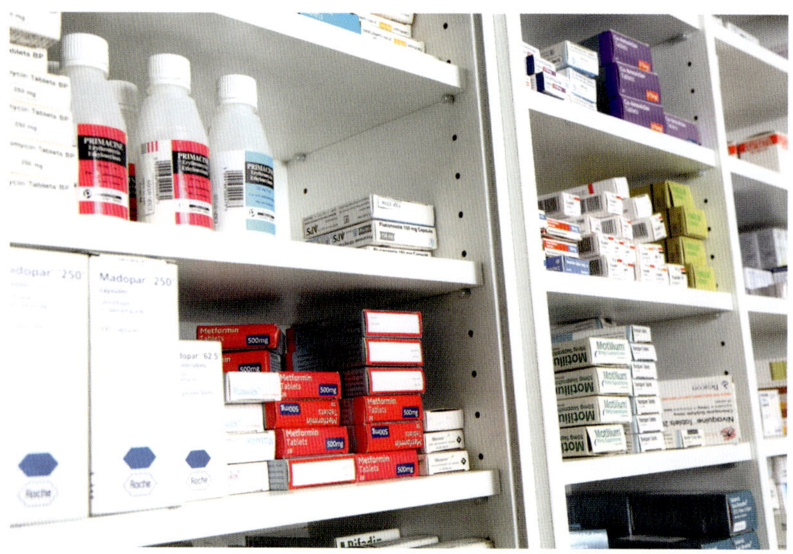

was introduced into the first year course, with more pharmacy practice teaching in the first and second years, and a modified third year core course. All of these elements particularly concentrated on communication and interpersonal skills. In the same year, toxicology was made available as a pharmacology option for third year students. From 1989 onwards, all final year students spent time at the Royal London Hospital for small group teaching, and ward rounds – a first for undergraduate pharmacy students in the UK. In 2012, the School created an innovative partnership with a local community pharmacy to give students hands-on experience of patient interaction, advice services and dispensing.

The School began to develop Master's courses in the 1990s, and they have been characterised by their links both into research and into the profession. In 1992, the pharmacognosy department designed a collaborative MSc in Phytotherapy Research jointly with the School of Hygiene and Tropical Medicine. Although an early and highly innovative programme, it did not attract sufficient numbers to make it viable. However, in 1996, a new MSc in Clinical Pharmacy, International Policy and Practice was launched to extend clinical pharmacy training to overseas pharmacists. The aim of the course was to provide pharmacists with skills to take back to their home countries in order to improve their practice, and develop the pharmacy infrastructure where it may face challenges.

A Master's in Drug Delivery has been offered by the department of pharmaceutics since 2002, followed by Drug Discovery two years later. This MSc in Drug Discovery was set up for those wanting to work in industry, or in government drug licensing and regulatory bodies, and was later expanded as a Master's in Drug Discovery and Pharma Management. An MSc in Pharmacognosy was launched in 2009 by the Centre for Pharmacognosy and Phytotherapy. To support future generations of researchers, the School introduced a Master of Research degree for September 2010. The full 12-month course included taught sessions and research projects in order to prepare students for a PhD or to begin a career in pharmaceutical

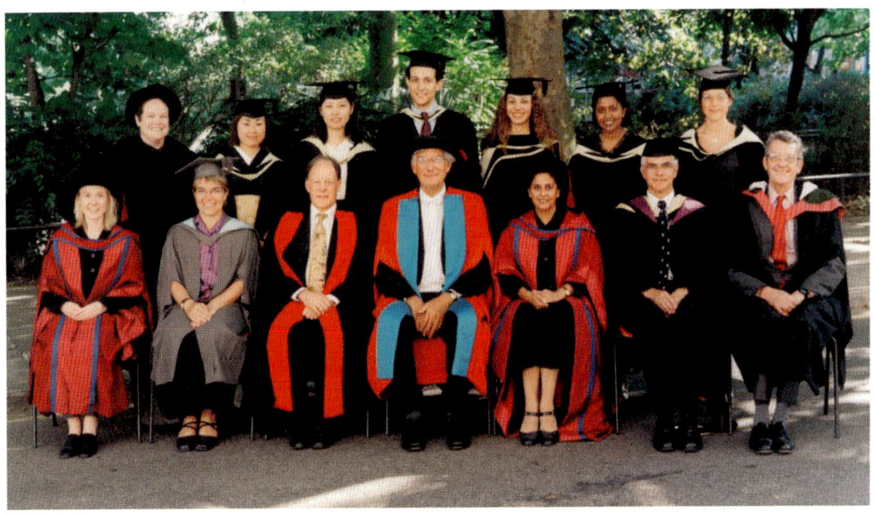

Staff and students at the graduation for MSc in Clinical Pharmacy, International Practice and Policy, 2001.

UCL School of Pharmacy Library

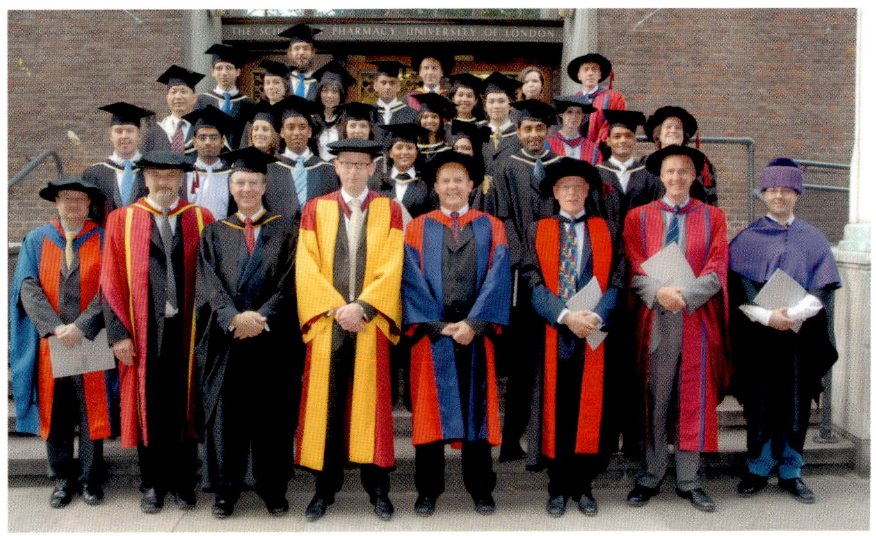

Staff and students at the graduation for MSc in Drug Discovery, 2007.

UCL School of Pharmacy Library

or biotech industries. The potential for new and interdisciplinary Master's teaching with University College London (UCL) is seen as one of the great opportunities for the immediate future.

CONTINUING PROFESSIONAL DEVELOPMENT AND LIFELONG EDUCATIONAL ENGAGEMENT

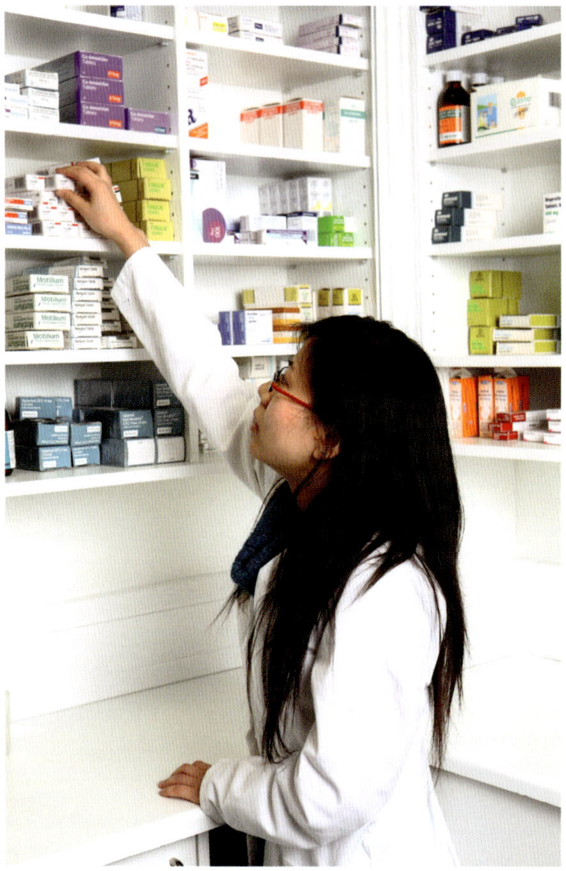

Continuing professional development is now a statutory requirement for pharmacists, and has been encouraged formally for over a decade. However, continuing education, the opportunity for pharmacists to continue to learn throughout their career, has been a key feature of the profession for a long time. It could be traced back to the original founders of the School and the Pharmaceutical Society with the establishment of evening scientific meetings, conversazione, the British Pharmaceutical Conference from 1863, and *The Pharmaceutical Journal* to share research and opinions.

In the late twentieth century, the Square was able to continue this tradition via the Centre for Pharmacy Practice, established in 1990. It had previously established the first full-time post-registration MSc in Clinical Pharmacy in 1989 and the first Chair of Pharmacy Practice in 1992, taken up by Professor Nick Barber, who joined the School in 1990. The MSc in Clinical Pharmacy was developed from the in-service training needs of four regional health authorities and established a culture of collaboration in education. The more accessible, part-time, post-registration Diploma in Clinical Pharmacy, initiated by the School in 1989 in conjunction with local health authorities, was also pioneering. The School further established the very first Chair in Pharmacy Education in 2004 – held by Professor Ian Bates – which led to continued innovations in professional education.

In 2007, a new School-NHS partnership took up residence in the School's advanced pharmacy studies centre in Russell Square, with start-up funds provided by government. The establishment of the Joint Programmes Board (JPB), covering NHS areas across the south of England, meant that all newly qualified NHS Pharmacists, with the support of NHS employers, were enrolled on foundation training which linked the NHS Knowledge and Skills Framework with the competence and capability needs of pharmaceutical care service provision. The aim was to create a standardised postgraduate programme for the post-registration development of pharmacists, which foreshadowed this as a national requirement.

RESEARCH

The School has a long tradition in cutting-edge research, and like every other research institution, the School has been subject to periodic evaluation by an arm of the Funding Council. It achieved an excellent grade 5 rating in every year of the assessment in 1992, 1996 and 2001, and triumphed in 2008 when 25% of its research was recognised as world leading and 90% as internationally significant.

Throughout its history, its research preoccupations have had different professional and social constituencies, as well as tackling different scientific and medical problems. Research leaders have always worked with external grant bodies and governmental departments, sometimes following developments in pharmacy, and sometimes driving the scientific or policy agenda. For example, in the late 1980s the School initiated a major research project, prompted by the Nuffield Report, with support from the Department of Health and Social Security, researching into contributions that health centre pharmacists were making to primary healthcare delivery. In the following decade, the establishment of the National Institute for Clinical Excellence (NICE) in 1999, as a result of increasing government concerns over the cost of medicines, was echoed in the launch of a new research department at the School focused on evidence-based prescribing.

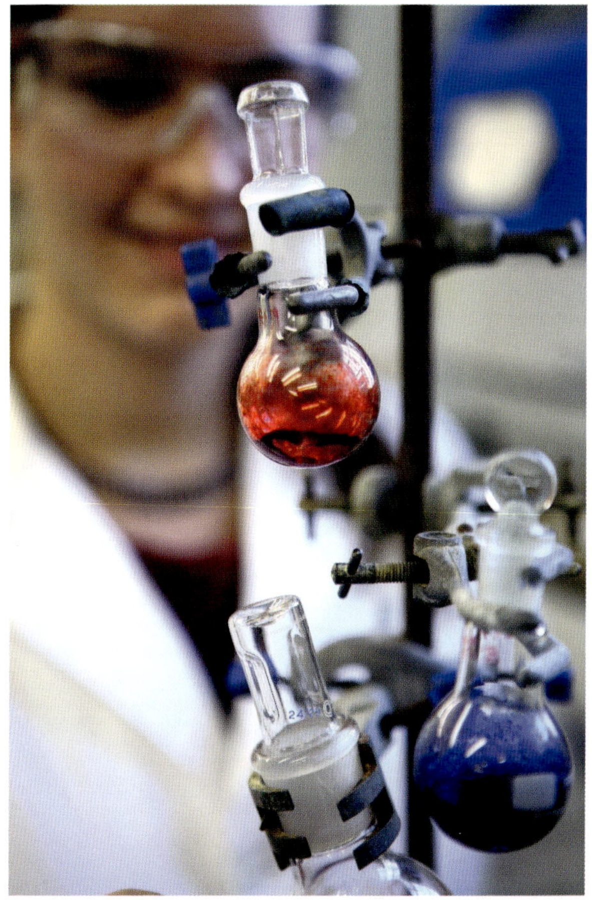

Even very small departments continued to carry out internationally recognised research. In his Annual Report of 1989–90, Professor Florence singled out Professor Phillipson, who with the smallest department of just three academic staff, had been named by the German Körber Foundation as a recipient of the Förderpreis für die Europaische Wissenschaft, in recognition of his achievement in European science. Although land that included the School's medicinal plant garden was sold along with the playing fields at Myddelton House in 2002, researchers in pharmacognosy and phytotherapy were able to develop their work on cannabis and also new areas such as herbal medicines sold in community pharmacies, the development of pharmacovigilance practices, ethnopharmacy, and projects looking at antimicrobial agents from plants in this age of antibiotic resistance.

In 1990, the Centre for Drug Delivery Research was founded to promote interdisciplinary research in drug delivery in the School. Intentionally not attached to any particular department, it was primarily supported by Medical Research Council grants and individual grants awarded to workers and students. As well as research projects, in its early years it was also responsible for the organisation and direction of two NATO Advanced Study Institute series on the "Targeting of Drugs" and on "Vaccines". In the following year, the School set up the University Academic Centre for Pharmaceutical Sciences and the Centre for Material Science, to act similarly as hubs for research in these areas. The Centre for Pharmaceutical Analysis was established in 1994 and developed a worldwide reputation for near-infrared spectroscopy, particularly in the analysis of counterfeit medicines, working in collaboration with the Medicines and Healthcare products Regulatory Agency (MHRA) and the Forensic Science Service. One of its key developments was direct analysis in real time (DART), which gives almost instantaneous results for a test on the composition of a tablet, allowing the potential to identify counterfeit medicines more simply and rapidly than previously possible.

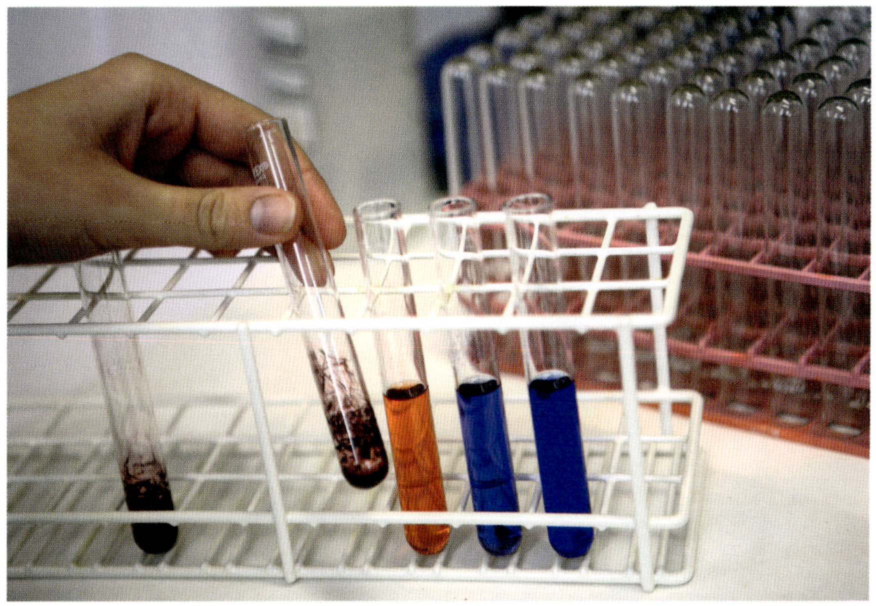

In 2008, the School established the first FIP collaborating centre (FIPCC). Its aim is to work in partnership with the International Pharmaceutical Federation (FIP) to have a global influence on the development of pharmacy and its effect on public health, through links with international health organisations such as the World Health Organization and the Educational, Scientific and Cultural Organization (UNESCO). The FIPCC supports research into pharmacy and public health as well as providing policy analysis and encouraging international collaboration and innovation in pharmacy.

Meanwhile, individual professors and departments continued to carry out projects into topical issues. At the end of the twentieth century, the changing relationship between the pharmacist and the patient was based primarily on the growing availability of information and a sense of patient empowerment. The School took the innovative step of creating the first Chair in Behavioural Medicine in a school of pharmacy anywhere in the world. In 2011, the School embarked on a five-year project, funded by the National Institute for Health Research, to assess adherence to antiretroviral therapy for patients with human immunodeficiency virus (HIV). The Centre for Behavioural Medicine is also exploring issues around adherence for other long-term conditions such as asthma, epilepsy and chronic kidney disease. Staff from the department of practice and policy have also carried out significant work into the use of medicines in care homes, commissioned by the Department of Health, and their research into other areas of medicines use and adherence has underpinned a NHS New Medicine Service, launched in October 2011, to improve patients' use of medicines. Drug delivery systems for children have also formed the focus of work, particularly paediatric formulations, and compliance issues for babies and children. A report exploring these issues in London, published by the School in 2010, revealed a high rate of prescription errors for children being treated in hospital.

The School has carried out a wide range of research into the role that pharmacists can play in improving public health. Recent reports have investigated pain management, the effects of the ageing population, and the value of extended provision of diagnostic tests and healthcare services in community pharmacies. All have concluded that pharmacy has a significant part to play in the twenty-first century, both in the UK and further afield.

Scientists at the Square have played a leading role in the development of cancer medicines and of antimicrobials, especially against methicillin-resistant *Staphylococcus aureus* (MRSA) infection. For example, in 2007, the School was awarded £2.5 million for a five-year programme to discover new cancer drugs that work by blocking proteins within cancer cells to inhibit growth and spread. Its Centre for Cancer Medicines is currently working with Cancer Research UK to develop a treatment that transports genes selectively to cancer cells to destroy tumours.

In the field of neuroscience, the School is leading significant research into the nervous system, synaptic function and the causes of neurological diseases, particularly Parkinson's and Alzheimer's diseases. Cutting-edge developments in nanotechnology are also enabling staff to make exciting discoveries, including the use of carbon nanotubes to deliver short strands of ribonucleic acid (RNA) to treat strokes, and also to treat lung cancer. In both cases, these tiny tubes play their part in silencing genes for specific target areas of the body. The School has also carried out a major project to investigate the use of nanotechnology to detect abnormal blood clots that may lead to a stroke.

COMMERCIAL DEVELOPMENT AND APPLICATION

One of the key areas of development over the past 25 years has been to maximise the opportunities to facilitate commercial exploitation of the School's research. Professor Fish announced the formation of a company to enable the Square to achieve this in 1986. In more recent years, commercial applications of research carried out at the School has been a very exciting area of development. One such initiative, Pharmaterials, a contract drug preformulation and development company, was awarded the Queen's Award for Enterprise for International Trade in 2008. The company was established in 2001 to reap the business potential of the School's excellence in pharmaceutical materials science. Its partnerships with over 80 companies in 16 countries worldwide allowed it to increase its overseas trade by 270% in just three years. In 2010, a new technology platform which enhances delivery of medicines to the colon was developed by researchers at the School and was commercially launched by Tillotts, a Swiss-based pharmaceutical company. In 2011, a company called Therakind, set up by the School, was the first to win a positive opinion for a paediatric-use marketing authorisation from the European Medicines Agency's Committee for Medicinal Products for Human Use (CHMP) under a Directive introduced in 2007 to encourage the development of paediatric medicines. The opinion by CHMP for the use of Buccolam (midazolam) in the treatment of prolonged, acute convulsive seizures in children aged from three months to 18 years is the first step towards the drug being made available as a paediatric medicine across Europe. In 2002, the Centre for Paediatric Pharmacy Research was established jointly with Great Ormond Street Hospital and the Institute of Child Health. By the time it merged with UCL, the School had developed five full spin-out companies and hundreds of patents and licences from its small staff base.

SUPPORT FOR YOUNG RESEARCHERS

In 1986, Professor Fish reported the importance of the recent Maplethorpe Fellowships in replacing lost teaching fellows' posts that were cut by the University Grants Council. Cyril Maplethorpe's will provided funding for postdoctoral fellowships. After his death in 1983, the University of London set up a panel to choose two each year, one each from King's College and the School. The aim of the fellowships was the promotion of pharmaceutical education and research. After an open competition, ideally for two registered pharmacists, the terms of the bequest allowed for each to be funded for a two-year appointment with a strong emphasis on undergraduate teaching alongside the research. These fellowships still continue.

In 1993, the School became a founding member of a consortium to promote pan-European postgraduate research and training in the pharmaceutical sciences. ULLA (named after the founding institutions of Uppsala University; the School of Pharmacy, University of London; Leiden University; and Amsterdam Free University) offers opportunities for collaboration and exchange of staff and students in the pursuit of the highest standards of pharmaceutical research. The expanded consortium holds a summer school every second year at which staff and students get together to attend short courses, exchange research information and hear the views of opinion-formers in the world of pharmaceutical sciences. The first summer school was held at the Square in London in 1993.

THE STUDENT POPULATION

By 2011–12, the School was home to around 1,300 students, including over 200 postgraduates. The student numbers grew steadily through the 1990s and early 2000s to a maximum annual intake of around

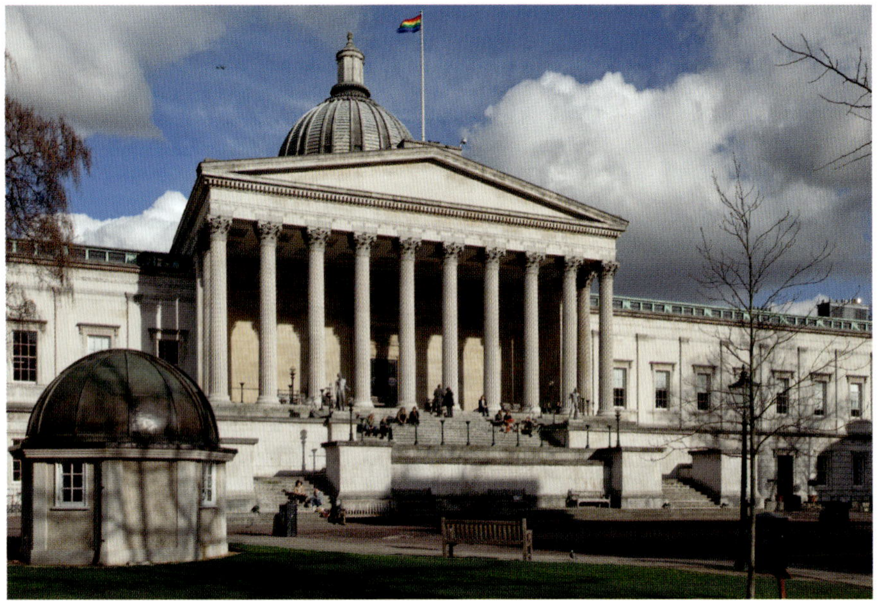

University College London, the Wilkins Portico.

© UCL Creative Media Services

200, somewhat more than the School could comfortably house. As a result, the laboratory classes of the MPharm curriculum had to be delivered more than once in each year in order to reach all students. However, while it continued to recruit strongly, like all pharmacy providers through the past 20 years, by 2000 the School was starting to lose market share to its competitors. Students were increasingly demanding the full student lifestyle experience, in large institutions that could offer up-to-date social and sporting as well as scientific facilities.

Today, around 10,000 students each year enter MPharm programmes across the UK, a figure that would have been unimaginable for John Attfield or C.W. Maplethorpe. Despite the introduction of full-cost tuition fees, there seemed in 2012 to be no shortage nationally of students who saw pharmacy as an excellent academic and career choice, although the profession had started to alert universities to the possibility of overproduction, in contrast to the shortage seen 20 years earlier. Meanwhile, past students continue to support the School, particularly

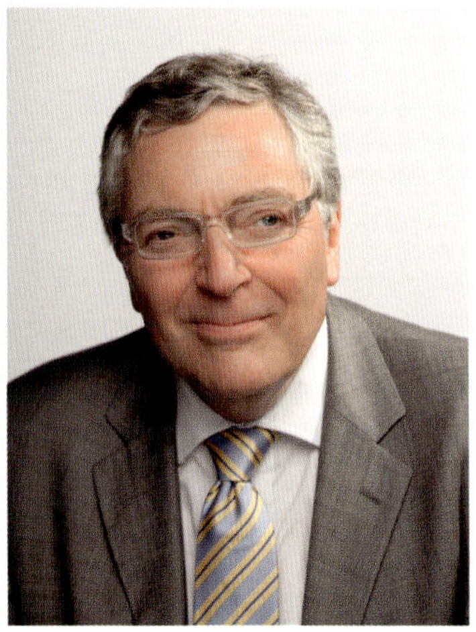

TIM CLEMENT-JONES (1949–)

TIM CLEMENT-JONES (1949–)

Lord Clement-Jones is the London Managing Partner and International Business Relations Partner of DLA Piper, the global law firm.

He was until its merger with University College London, Chairman of the Council of the School of Pharmacy, University of London (2008–2012) and is currently a member of the Council of University College London.

A communications professional and a solicitor, Lord Clement-Jones was Group Company Secretary and Legal Adviser of Kingfisher Plc from 1986 until 1995.

He was Chairman of the Liberal Party from 1986 to 1988 and played a major part in the merger negotiations with the Social Democratic Party to form the Liberal Democrats. He was made CBE for political services in 1988 and was the Chairman of the Liberal Democrats Finance Committee from 1989 to 1998 and Treasurer of the Liberal Democrats from 2005 to 2010.

Lord Clement-Jones was made a life peer in 1998 and until July 2004 was the Liberal Democrat Health Spokesman and thereafter until 2010 Liberal Democrat Spokesman on Culture, Media and Sport, in the House of Lords. He is Deputy Chairman of the All-Party Parliamentary Group on China.

He introduced and sponsored the passage through Parliament of the 2003 Tobacco Advertising and Sponsorship Act and the Live Music Act 2012.

He is President of Ambitious About Autism (formerly Treehouse), an autism education charity and school for children with autism and other communication disorders and was its former Chairman (from 2001–2008). He is a Trustee of the Barbican Centre Trust.

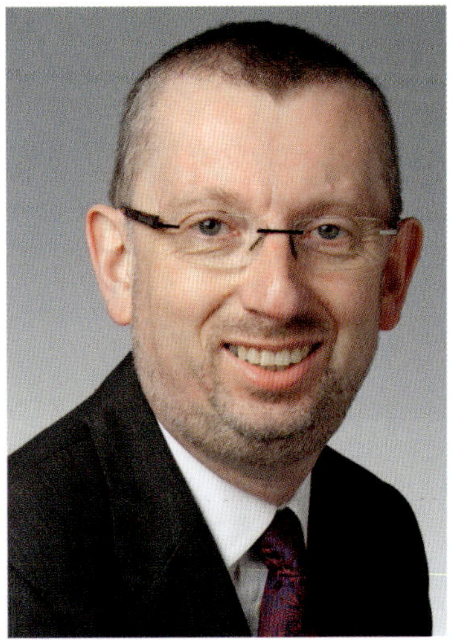

ANTHONY WILLIAM SMITH (1962–)

ANTHONY WILLIAM SMITH (1962–)

Anthony Smith registered as a pharmacist in 1984, completing both his undergraduate degree and a PhD at the University of Bath, before taking a postdoctoral post and his first lectureship at Aston University. He returned to Bath as a lecturer in 1993, became a senior lecturer in 1999 and head of department in 2002. He became dean of the Square in 2006 on Sandy Florence's retirement.

He has served as a member of the Pharmaceutical Society's Adjudicating Committee and its accreditation teams for Overseas Pharmacists Assessment Programme and the MPharm degree. He was also a member of the Transitional Committee for the demerger of RPSGB. He co-led development of the proposals for a new five-year integrated pharmacy degree programme and for four years was chair of Council of University Heads of Pharmacy (now the Pharmacy Schools Council).

Smith left the post of dean when the School merged with University College London, and became UCL's vice-provost (education) on 1st January 2012.

through fund-raising and reunion events. Constant features of reunions seem to be reminiscences about rag week, Friday night discos and the staff pantomimes.

LOOKING TO THE FUTURE

In September 2009 the School's Council held one of its annual planning meetings where it thought very carefully about the economic threats that were then gathering in every area of public funding. "What if," they asked themselves, "the HEFCE grant was reduced by 5 or 10%, the capital investment grant was reduced by maybe 5%, what if undergraduate fees went up to £5,000? What should we do to safeguard the legacy of this important institution?"

The real future was, however, far more serious than anything the Council could have anticipated as the world economy slid into recession in 2009 and 2010. Within 18 months the UK higher education sector was facing a future where £1.9 billion was lost to the higher education budget. Teaching funding had been reduced by 100% for some institutions (pharmacy was one of the lucky subject areas in retaining around 24%), the capital investment grant had been cut by 65% and undergraduate fees had been trebled to £9,000. For the dean and Council the answer was the same: the School was too important to its profession and to the discipline to be put at risk, and as a standalone institution, and the only independent pharmacy school left in Europe, it faced challenges and costs that could sink it, while its small size constrained its ability to grow its way through the recession.

In January 2010, the School's Council started a long and painstaking options review. While staying independent remained an option until the very end, Council also had to consider a "best fit merger partner".

The School's collaborations with UCL were extensive and growing fast. The Council concluded that, if merger were to happen, UCL was the best possible candidate.

“ The opportunities available for pharmacy education and research within UCL are compelling, together with the best possible mitigation of financial risks in what is likely to be an extremely dynamic and unstable system for years to come. ”

Anthony Smith, 2011

The academic collaborations with the School's huge neighbour were already well established, with research synergies that touched on cancer, drug discovery and drug development, behavioural medicine and pharmacology, and the School and UCL formally entered merger discussions in the autumn of 2010. It was a slow process and at times a bitter internal dispute for the School. Many were reluctant to give up the School's independence, fearing it would damage its character forever, whilst others argued that UCL housed one of the greatest medical and biosciences activities in Europe, but lacked a pharmacy presence. The academic “fit” offered incomparable research and teaching opportunities, the students could gain the full university experience that the School had long wanted for them, and both academic and professional support staff would gain access to career opportunities that were impossible to provide in a small institution. On 12th May 2011, after months of debate, the School's Council voted in favour of merger with UCL, and formally started the journey towards the School's future role as part of one of the world's great global universities.

The real and symbolic trappings of the independent School were slowly wound up through late 2011 and 2012 as the assets and liabilities were transferred to UCL. The Council met for the last time in July 2012 to confirm the last set of accounts and to agree the petition to the Privy Council to surrender the Royal Charter. The Privy Council order revoking the Charter was dated 17th October 2012, just over two years after that key Council planning meeting. At the same time, the research collaborations between the two institutions had started to accelerate, students adapted as though membership of this giant neighbour had always been their right, and the first plans for interdisciplinary teaching between medics and pharmacists were tentatively outlined.

“ It is a tremendous honour to be appointed as Director of one of the most internationally respected and iconic pharmacy schools at a time when it has become integrated into one of the world's most prestigious universities. ”

Professor Duncan Craig, 2012

The formal date of merger was 1st January 2012 and the assets (including the staff and students) were transferred and the School formally joined UCL's School of Life and Medical Sciences as the UCL School of Pharmacy. Anthony Smith moved to UCL as vice-provost (education), and the School's transitional management was shared between Maureen Boylan, the chief operating officer, Professor Stephen Neidle, research director, and Dr Brian Pearce as acting director. In July 2012, it was announced that Professor Duncan Craig, an alumnus of the School, was to become the School's new director.

In May 2011, as part of the public debate about the School's future, the dean, Anthony Smith, published an article in *The Pharmaceutical Journal* outlining the rationale for the decision. He confirmed that the School would stay in Brunswick Square, but that students would gradually benefit from increasing contact with UCL's educational, social, welfare and sports facilities. On the research side, the School would be able to

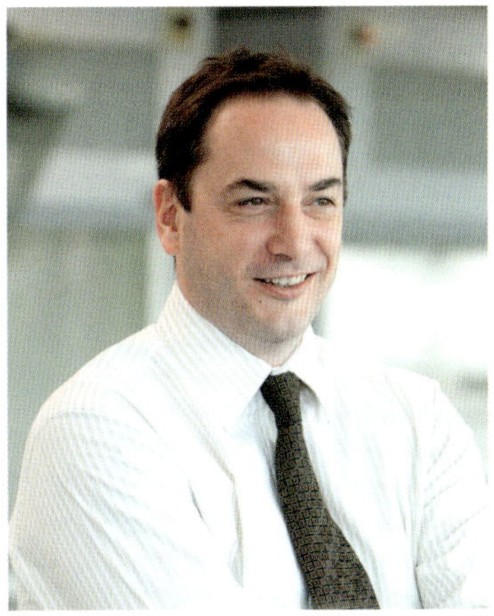

DUNCAN Q.M.CRAIG (1963–)

DUNCAN Q.M.CRAIG (1963–)

Duncan Craig graduated from the University of Bath in 1984 with a first class BPharm and, following pre-registration training at Upjohn Ltd and St Thomas' Hospital, he went on to study for a PhD at the School of Pharmacy, University of London, on the topic of polymeric drug delivery systems. He subsequently joined the staff and rose to the position of Reader in 1999 but left to take up a chair at the Queen's University Belfast, where he stayed for four years before moving to the University of East Anglia to set up the new School of Pharmacy in 2003. The School went on to achieve top ranking in the national student survey for five years in a row and was consistently ranked within the top three UK pharmacy schools in the major league tables under his stewardship. He stepped down as Head of School in 2011 to work for the Vice-Chancellor's Office as Director of Internationalisation, charged with shaping the university's policy on international relations and collaborations. In 2013 he returned to the School of Pharmacy, now part of UCL, to assume the position of Director of the newly merged School. Professor Craig has won numerous prizes including the Glaxo SmithKline International Award, the Controlled Release Society Young Investigator Award and the British Pharmaceutical Conference Science Award.

form part of "Europe's largest grouping of biomedical research", which included the new UK Centre for Medical Research and Innovation, headed by Nobel laureate and current president of the Royal Society, Sir Paul Nurse. Smith described the attraction for research as "compelling": "With UKCMRI's focus on translational biomedical research, taking research from the laboratory all the way through to the patient, pharmacy and the pharmaceutical sciences are ideally placed to make a significant contribution."

Professor Smith concluded the article by writing:

> It is the mission of the School – our teaching and research in pharmacy – which has been foremost in my mind in strongly advocating joining UCL. We have built a precious institution and we all work hard to preserve its values, make it sustainable and allow it to thrive. Those early Victorians who founded the modern profession in Great Britain wanted a school "to elevate the profession of pharmacy by furnishing the proper means of instruction". Within UCL, we have a secure future to do just that – and to retain the special identity and character that staff, students and alumni hold dear.

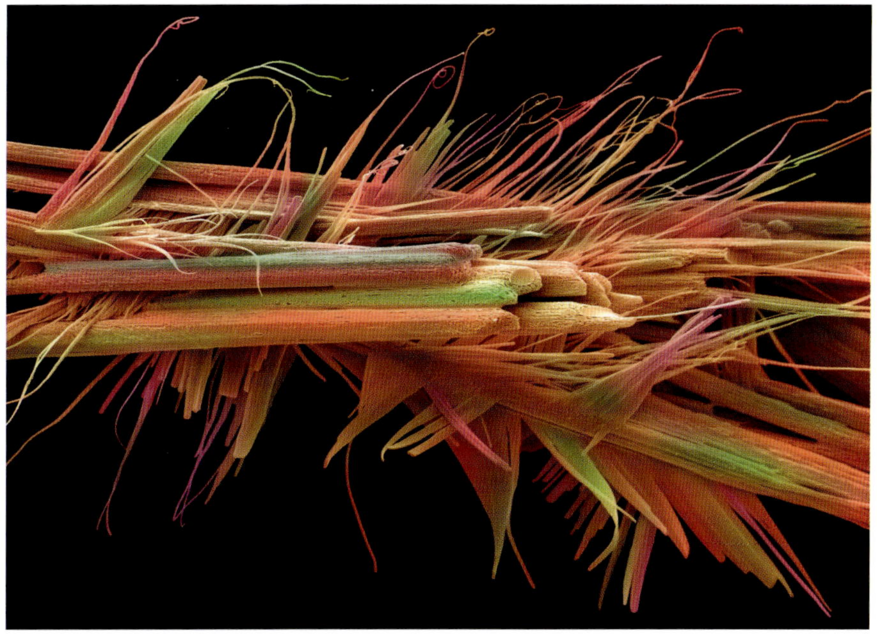

Annie Cavanagh, multimedia unit manager at the School, and David McCarthy, who set up its Electron Microscope Unit in 1977, have won many awards for their images. This false-coloured scanning electron micrograph shows caffeine crystals. It won a Wellcome Image Award in 2012.

Annie Cavanagh and David McCarthy, Wellcome Images

EDUCATION FOR THE FUTURE

The story of the School of Pharmacy started with visionary pharmacists and educators who recognised how important this set of professional skills could be to the scientific development of medicines, to improvements in public health and advances in medical care. The success of this School and the growth of many others has proved them right. The early days included a long struggle to be recognised as a profession alongside medicine and the School's founders saw clearly that a rigorous professional education was the only way to achieve the esteem and influence they felt to be essential.

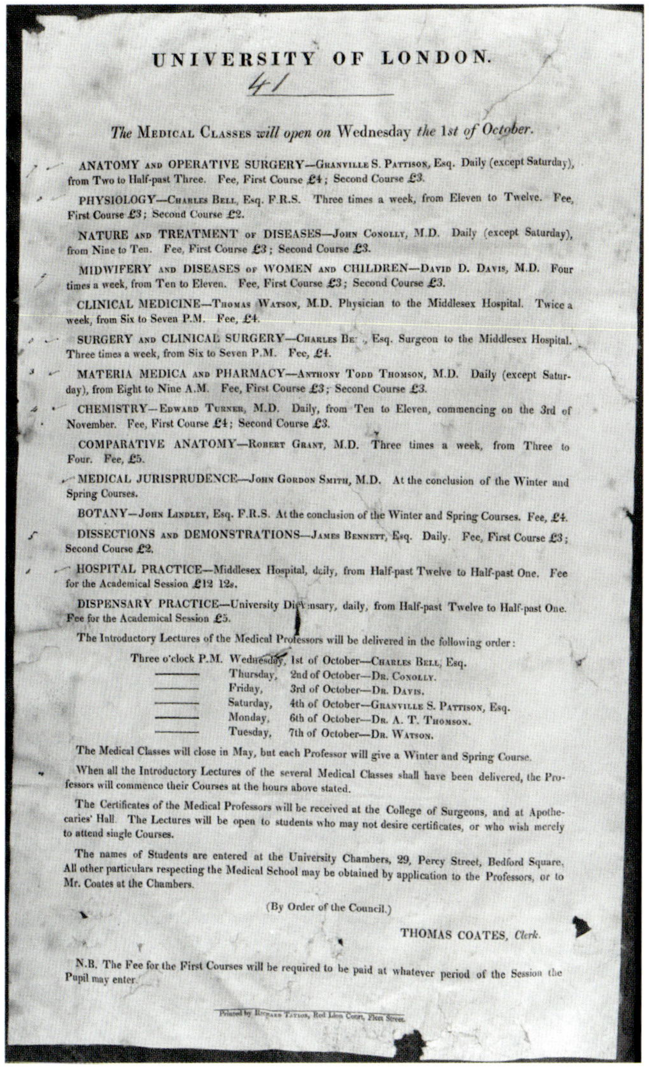

UNIVERSITY OF LONDON.

41

The Medical Classes *will open on* Wednesday *the* 1st *of October.*

ANATOMY and OPERATIVE SURGERY—Granville S. Pattison, Esq. Daily (except Saturday), from Two to Half-past Three. Fee, First Course £4; Second Course £3.

PHYSIOLOGY—Charles Bell, Esq. F.R.S. Three times a week, from Eleven to Twelve. Fee, First Course £3; Second Course £2.

NATURE and TREATMENT of DISEASES—John Conolly, M.D. Daily (except Saturday), from Nine to Ten. Fee, First Course £3; Second Course £3.

MIDWIFERY and DISEASES of WOMEN and CHILDREN—David D. Davis, M.D. Four times a week, from Ten to Eleven. Fee, First Course £3; Second Course £3.

CLINICAL MEDICINE—Thomas Watson, M.D. Physician to the Middlesex Hospital. Twice a week, from Six to Seven P.M. Fee, £4.

SURGERY and CLINICAL SURGERY—Charles Be[illegible], Esq. Surgeon to the Middlesex Hospital. Three times a week, from Six to Seven P.M. Fee, £4.

MATERIA MEDICA and PHARMACY—Anthony Todd Thomson, M.D. Daily (except Saturday), from Eight to Nine A.M. Fee, First Course £3; Second Course £3.

CHEMISTRY—Edward Turner, M.D. Daily, from Ten to Eleven, commencing on the 3rd of November. Fee, First Course £4; Second Course £3.

COMPARATIVE ANATOMY—Robert Grant, M.D. Three times a week, from Three to Four. Fee, £5.

MEDICAL JURISPRUDENCE—John Gordon Smith, M.D. At the conclusion of the Winter and Spring Courses.

BOTANY—John Lindley, Esq. F.R.S. At the conclusion of the Winter and Spring Courses. Fee, £4.

DISSECTIONS and DEMONSTRATIONS—James Bennett, Esq. Daily. Fee, First Course £3; Second Course £2.

HOSPITAL PRACTICE—Middlesex Hospital, daily, from Half-past Twelve to Half-past One. Fee for the Academical Session £12 12*s*.

DISPENSARY PRACTICE—University Dispensary, daily, from Half-past Twelve to Half-past One. Fee for the Academical Session £5.

The Introductory Lectures of the Medical Professors will be delivered in the following order:

Three o'clock P.M.	Wednesday,	1st of October—Charles Bell, Esq.
———	Thursday,	2nd of October—Dr. Conolly.
———	Friday,	3rd of October—Dr. Davis.
———	Saturday,	4th of October—Granville S. Pattison, Esq.
———	Monday,	6th of October—Dr. A. T. Thomson.
———	Tuesday,	7th of October—Dr. Watson.

The Medical Classes will close in May, but each Professor will give a Winter and Spring Course.

When all the Introductory Lectures of the several Medical Classes shall have been delivered, the Professors will commence their Courses at the hours above stated.

The Certificates of the Medical Professors will be received at the College of Surgeons, and at Apothecaries' Hall. The Lectures will be open to students who may not desire certificates, or who wish merely to attend single Courses.

The names of Students are entered at the University Chambers, 29, Percy Street, Bedford Square. All other particulars respecting the Medical School may be obtained by application to the Professors, or to Mr. Coates at the Chambers.

(By Order of the Council.)

THOMAS COATES, *Clerk.*

N.B. The Fee for the First Courses will be required to be paid at whatever period of the Session the Pupil may enter.

Printed by Richard Taylor, Red Lion Court, Fleet Street.

The relationship between the School and the University of London pre-dates the School's foundation in 1842. Anthony Todd Thomson is listed here as the lecturer in materia medica and pharmacy for the University Medical School's first session in 1828. Dr Thomson went on to give the first ever lecture at the School of Pharmacy in 1842 and became its professor of botany and materia medica.

UCL Library Services, Special Collections

The UK's public health planning is faced with major health challenges. Some 15 million people in Britain live with a long-term condition – some linked to public health concerns such as diabetes and heart disease, and others less so such as dementia and arthritis. These account for approximately £7 in every £10 spent on health and care. This figure is set to rise by 25% in the next 25 years. The UK's ageing population and increased public health challenges – obesity, sexual health, alcohol use and smoking-related illness – could add an extra £1 billion to £1.4 billion per year to our health costs. And all of this came before the banking crisis of 2008 and 2009, the deep recession in most developed economies and far-reaching austerity measures to curb levels of debt.

Two watershed events will define how well the profession will respond to these challenges. First, the landmark Pharmacy White Paper, *Pharmacy in England – Building on Strength, Delivering the Future*, was published in April 2008. This not only acknowledged the health challenges of the early to mid-twenty-first century but also set out an ambitious route map about how pharmacy could be part of the solution to these challenges. It is perhaps too much hyperbole for a conservative profession to speak of paradigm shifts in practice resulting from the White Paper, but three initiatives warrant mention. Healthy Living Pharmacies started as a pilot in Portsmouth and the Isle of Wight and demonstrated how the unique accessibility of pharmacies to the public could be used as a new focus for advice and public health interventions. Studies with sexual health, smoking cessation and targeted medicines use reviews, amongst others, demonstrated tangible benefit to patients and the exchequer. The New Medicine Service deserves particular mention as the evidence for it was developed by researchers at the School of Pharmacy: Nick Barber, Rob Horne and Sally-Ann Francis. This service sees pharmacists supporting patients in the early weeks as they take a new medicine for a long-term condition – where evidence indicates that adherence is notoriously poor and non-compliance high. The third area is education, where the White Paper sought far-reaching reform of pharmacy education and training to develop a workforce that would be more ready at registration to support patients to get the best value from their medicines.

The Pharmacy White Paper was published at the same time as the then Health Minister Lord Darzi published his series of Next Stage Reviews for the NHS, including the education and training of health professionals. Darzi took as his starting point the review of medical education chaired by Sir John Tooke (now UCL's Vice-Provost for Health) following the Modernising Medical Careers debacle. The Tooke Report recommended establishing a body that would have oversight of the education of key healthcare professionals. And so Medical Education England (MEE) came into being, which for the first time brought together pharmacy, medical, dental and healthcare scientist education. Also for the first time, pharmacy was properly at "the top table" alongside medicine and dentistry.

Each profession was supported by a Programme Board charged with providing independent advice to MEE and the Secretary of State for Health. Led by the commitment to education reform in the Pharmacy White Paper, the Modernising Pharmacy Careers Board set about to review pharmacy education and training in what was the most wide-ranging review since pharmacy became a graduate-only profession in 1967. The consultation across the profession indicated a genuine appetite for moving on from the crossroads and setting the profession down a path where pharmacists are an even more clinically focused profession, supporting patients in getting the best value from their medicines through optimised therapy and in making healthy living choices by working in partnership with all healthcare practitioners.

Discussions about the future of pharmacy have necessarily precipitated much soul-searching in professionals for whom their whole academic and clinical development has been towards risk aversion. The question of the counterfactual is raised. What future is there for pharmacy if a greater clinical role is not embraced? Lessons from elsewhere in the high street are sobering, where businesses that have failed to adapt with speed to astonishing changes in customers' habits have paid a heavy price. Internet pharmacies remain at the margins and are inadequately regulated but the profession would do well to recognise the impact that companies such as Amazon have had on conventional methods for supplying goods. It continues to be the School's job to train pharmacists to engage with these issues through a curriculum which continues to place the highest value on scientific knowledge.

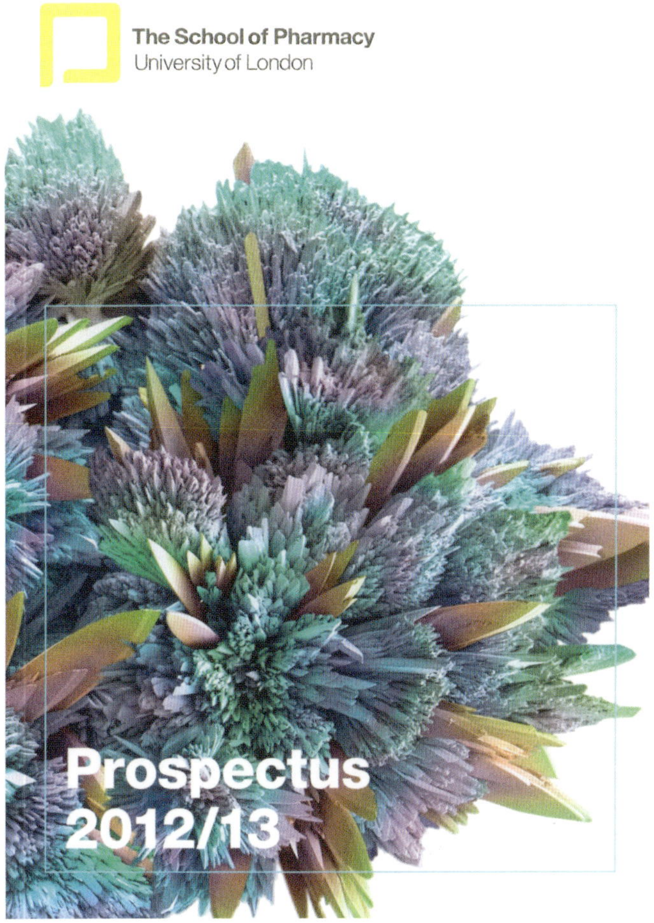

UCL School of Pharmacy Library

So, would those early Victorians who established the modern pharmacy profession in the UK and started the School of Pharmacy recognise what is happening? I believe they would. They had lofty ambitions for the profession based on the highest standard of education. The School of Pharmacy has been doing that for 170 years and as it enters its third age as a part of University College London, it is best placed to continue producing pharmacists who can lead the profession in the twenty-first century, just as it did in the nineteenth and twentieth centuries.

Professor Anthony Smith
Vice-Provost Education, UCL
Dean of the School of Pharmacy 2006–2011

APPENDIX

PHARMACY QUALIFICATIONS AND COURSES AT THE SCHOOL

The founding of the Pharmaceutical Society of Great Britain in 1841 marked the beginning of qualifications relating specifically to pharmacists.

1841

Two exams were established:

- the **Minor examination**, a rudimentary qualification for pharmacists' employed assistants: successful candidates could become Associate Members of the Pharmaceutical Society
- the **Major examination**, intended for established business-owning pharmacists who were, or who aspired to be, members of the Society: successful candidates were called pharmaceutical chemists, and could become Full Members of the Pharmaceutical Society.

Neither exam was compulsory in order to practise as a pharmacist.

1864

The Society created a new **Modified examination**, first held on 26th October 1864. It was intended for established chemists who wanted to codify their educational standing. Candidates had to have been engaged in business for at least five years, or be at least 30 years old.

1868

The Pharmacy Act of 1868 required that *all* individuals dealing in or compounding medicines containing poisons must register with the Society in order to practise. The Act stipulated that the **Minor examination** was to become the legal minimum requirement for new entrants to the profession. Successful candidates were called chemists & druggists. The **Major examination** remained for those wanting to achieve a higher academic level, and successful candidates were still known as pharmaceutical chemists.

For a limited period after the Act, pharmacy assistants who had been working for three years or more prior to 1868 were able to take a special **Modified examination** qualifying them as a chemist & druggist.

1920

The **Minor examination**, now also known as the **Qualifying examination**, was split into two sections: pure science (chemistry, physics and botany) and an applied pharmacy section [materia medica, pharmacy including posology (study of dosages), the translation and dispensing of prescriptions, and poisons laws]. It was possible to take the parts together or separately. The curriculum for the exam was fixed.

Students also had to attend approved courses of instruction in order to enter the exam, and an apprenticeship of 4,000 hours was essential. This could be served either wholly in retail, or half and half in retail and a hospital setting.

1925

The School was formally recognised to teach a two-year **Bachelor of Pharmacy degree course** from 1st January 1925, as a school within the University's Faculty of Medicine. The degree course was approved by the Pharmaceutical Society for registration as a pharmaceutical chemist, subject to a test in forensic pharmacy.

Part I of the Qualifying exam became the **Preliminary Scientific examination**. It included practical exams in physics and botany. This course was no longer taught at the School.

Part II became the **chemist & druggist Qualifying examination**. Students were not allowed to enter for the Preliminary and chemist & druggist exams at the same time.

The Major exam became the **pharmaceutical chemist Qualifying examination**. The pharmaceutical chemist exam now had a compulsory course of study. A student could enter for this exam without passing the chemist & druggist exam if they had attended an approved course over two years after passing the Preliminary exam.

Written exams were instituted in all subjects, and practical exams were required in all subjects apart from forensic pharmacy. Oral exams were discontinued, apart from the pharmacy paper for the chemist & druggist Qualifying exam.

1932

Postgraduate diplomas in Pharmaceutical Analysis and Biochemical Analysis were introduced.

1937

The School stopped teaching for the Major exam. It only ran courses for the chemist & druggist Qualifying exam, the pharmaceutical chemist exam and the final BPharm exams.

1946

The **three-year BPharm honours degree course** was first introduced, with first, second and pass classes.

1950

The three-year degree was the only course on offer at the Square from this date onward.

1953

The Pharmacy Act of 1953 introduced the **pharmaceutical chemist's Diploma** as the new single professional qualification for pharmacists. The last chemist & druggist exam was held in 1954.

Newly qualified pharmacists registering from 1954 having passed the diploma or the BPharm degree were required to complete one year of practical preregistration training after their course, unless they had already served a two-year apprenticeship before they started at the Square.

1957

In 1957, the entrance requirements for the pharmaceutical chemist exam were brought into line with universities, and a three-year course was established to start in 1958.

1967

It became compulsory for all new pharmacists to obtain a Pharmacy degree, followed by a year's practical preregistration experience, in order to register. This marked the end of the pharmaceutical chemist Diploma. At the School, a new undergraduate syllabus was taught for the first time leading to the **First University Examination**, which replaced the School's own exam at the end of the first year.

The **Pharmaceutical Engineering Science Master's** degree by examination was launched.

1981
The **BSc in Toxicology and Pharmacology** was introduced.

1989
The **Diploma in Clinical Pharmacy** was introduced.

The **MSc in Clinical Pharmacy** was established.

1992
The **MSc in Phytotherapy Research** was introduced, organised jointly between the School of Hygiene and Tropical Medicine and the Square.

1997
All British Pharmacy degrees required a four-year course of study for the MPharm from this date.

1998
The **MSc in Clinical Pharmacy, International Policy and Practice** was introduced.

The **Certificate/Diploma in Medicines in Healthcare** was established.

2002
The **MSc in Drug Delivery** was established.

2003
The **MSc in Drug Discovery** was set up.

2005
The first formal education programme for pharmacy technicians was established, the **Certificate in Medicines Management for Pharmacy Technicians** (CMMPT).

The **Foundation Degree in Pharmaceutical Science for Pharmacy Technicians** was set up in partnership with Birkbeck College and Westminster Kingsway College of Further Education.

2006
The first university-NHS partnership model for foundation training for post-registration pharmacists was launched, via the Joint Programmes Board (a partnership between the NHS and five universities). The **Diploma in General Pharmacy Practice** was the first competency-based workplace education model established in GB.

2009
The **MSc in Pharmacognosy** was established.

2010
The **Master of Research** (MRes) degree was introduced.

2012
The **MSc in Drug Discovery and Pharma Management** was launched.

FURTHER READING

The following list is not a comprehensive bibliography, but is intended to enable readers to explore further the topics and sources covered in the book.

KEY RESOURCES

In 1964, the only previous book purely about the history of the School was published. It was written by T.E. Wallis, who had experienced the School as both a student and a staff member, and was illustrated with his own photographs, the originals of which are now held by the Royal Pharmaceutical Society's museum:

Wallis, T.E. (1964). *History of the School of Pharmacy, University of London*. Pharmaceutical Press, London.

The key primary source for events and comment on the history of the Pharmaceutical Society and of the pharmacy profession from 1841 is *The Pharmaceutical Journal*. Its editions since 2005 are available online at www.pjonline.com. Since 1859, an alternative viewpoint has been provided by the *Chemist and Druggist*.

The history of the School is largely told through its *Dean's Reports*, *Annual Reports* and *Prospectuses*. Earlier details are provided in the Pharmaceutical Society's *Calendars* from 1870. A fascinating and entertaining perspective is given in the *Square Chronicle* from 1912 to 1988, produced by alumni and students. Since 2004, *Square Roots* has provided a more recent insight. Since Volume 7, it has been available online at http://www.ucl.ac.uk/pharmacy/alumni/square_roots

The historical collections of the Royal Pharmaceutical Society and of the School of Pharmacy are full of interesting material, not least their photographic archives. Both institutions welcome researchers by prior appointment with the museum and the library, respectively.

MILESTONES AND CONTEXT

Bartlett, S. *A–Z of Medicines Research*. APBI. http://www.abpi.org.uk/our-work/library/medical-disease/Documents/AtoZ.pdf (last accessed 16 October 2012).

Briggs, A. (1990). *Victorian Things*. Penguin Books, London.

UCL Bloomsbury Project: http://www.ucl.ac.uk/bloomsbury-project/streets/bloomsbury_square.htm; http://www.ucl.ac.uk/bloomsbury-project/streets/brunswick_square.htm (last accessed 18 October 2012).

de Vries, L. (1967). *History as Hot News. The World of the Early Victorians through the Eyes of the Illustrated London News, 1842–1865*. John Murray, London.

HISTORY OF THE PHARMACY PROFESSION

150 Years of a Science Based Profession. *Supplement to The Pharmaceutical Journal*, 27 April 1991.

150 Years of The Pharmaceutical Journal. *Supplement to The Pharmaceutical Journal*, 6 July 1991.

Anderson, S. Ed. (2005). *Making Medicines*. Pharmaceutical Press, London. <http://www.pharmpress.com/product/9780857110992/making-medicines>

Bell, J., and Redwood, T. (1880). *Historical Sketch of the Progress of Pharmacy in Great Britain*. Pharmaceutical Society of Great Britain, London.

Court, W.E. (1991). General Practice Pharmacy in the 1840s. *Pharmaceutical Historian* 21 (2), 2–4.

Crellin, J. (1967). Pharmaceutical history and its sources in the Wellcome collections. Part 1: The growth of professionalism in 19th century British pharmacy. *Medical History* 11, 215–227.

Eastoe, J. (2010). *Victorian Pharmacy. Rediscovering Forgotten Remedies and Recipes*. Pavilion, London. <http://store.anovabooks.com/index.php/9781862058903-victorian-pharmacy-remedies-and-recipes.html>

Holloway, S.W.F. (1991). The Royal Pharmaceutical Society 1841–1991: A Political and Social History. Pharmaceutical Press, London. <http://www.rpharms.com/museum-shop/books-and-cards.asp>

Homan, P.G., Hudson, B., and Rowe, R. (2008). *Popular Medicines: An Illustrated History*. Pharmaceutical Press, London. <http://www.pharmpress.com/product/9780853697282/popular-medicines>

Hudson, B., Bridgeman, J. (2009). **Jacob Bell** (1810–59): *A Useful and Honourable Life*. Friends of Woodbury Park Cemetery, Tunbridge Wells. <http://www.fwpc.org.uk/newspublications.html>

Jordan, E. (2001). Admitting … a dozen women into the Society: The first women members of the British Pharmaceutical Society. *Pharmaceutical Historian* 31 (2), 18–26. <http://www.bshp.org/bshpwebsite/index.htm>

Shellard, E.J. (1982). Some early women research workers in British pharmacy, 1886–1912. *Pharmaceutical Historian* 12 (2), 2–3. <http://www.bshp.org/bshpwebsite/index.htm>

Tallis, N., and Arnold-Foster, K. (1991). *Pharmacy History: A Pictorial Record*. Pharmaceutical Press, London. <http://www.rpharms.com/museum-shop/books-and-cards.asp>

HISTORY OF PHARMACY EDUCATION

Attfield, J. (1880). A pamphlet on pharmaceutical education. Personal communication.

Burt, D.G. (1991). A study of the factors contributing to the development of a uniform system of pharmacy education. Unpublished thesis.

Earles, M. (1963). The pharmacy schools of the nineteenth century. In *The Evolution of Pharmacy in Britain* (F.N.L. Poynter, Ed.), pp. 79-95. Pitman Medical Publishing, London.

Earles, M. (1997). *Pharmacy and education* 1841–99. Pharmaceutical Historian 27 (4), 42–45. <http://www.bshp.org/bshpwebsite/index.htm>

Earles, M. (2005). The development of pharmacy education. In *Making Medicines* (S. Anderson, Ed.), pp. 97–113. Pharmaceutical Press, London. <http://www.pharmpress.com/product/9780857110992/making-medicines>

Matthews, L. (1983). The Aldersgate Dispensary and the Aldersgate Medical School. *Pharmaceutical Historian* 13 (3), 7–10. <http://www.bshp.org/bshpwebsite/index.htm>

Nutton, V., and Porter, R. Eds., (1995). *The History of Medical Education in Britain*. Rodopi, Amsterdam/Atlanta.

Poynter, F.N.L. (1966). *The Evolution of Medical Education in Britain*. Pitman Medical Publishing, London.

Whaley, T. (2010). Two tiers of materia medica. *Pharmaceutical Historian* 40 (3), 46–49. <http://www.bshp.org/bshpwebsite/index.htm>

Whaley, T. (2012). From unacceptable to essential: Pharmacology in pharmaceutical education. *Pharmaceutical Historian* 42 (2), 40–43. <http://www.bshp.org/bshpwebsite/index.htm>

HISTORY OF THE SCHOOL

150 Years of "The Square". *Supplement to The Pharmaceutical Journal*, 21 March 1992. <http://www.pjonline.com>

Bellot, A. (1929). *University College London (1828–1926)*. University of London Press, London.

Callingham, B.A., Simmonds, M.A., and Straughan, D.W. (1976). *Frontiers of Pharmacy. A Collection of Papers to mark the Fiftieth Anniversary of the Founding of the Pharmacological Laboratories of the Pharmaceutical Society of Great Britain*. Supplement to the *Journal of Pharmacy and Pharmacology* 28, 333–405. PSBG, London. <http://www.pharmpress.com/product/00223573/jpp>.

Harte, N., and North, J. (1991). *The World of University College London 1828–1978*, 2nd edn. University Press, London.

Holloway, S.W.F. (1991). *The Royal Pharmaceutical Society 1841–1991: A Political and Social History*. Pharmaceutical Press, London. <http://www.rpharms.com/museum-shop/books-and-cards.asp>

Holloway, S.W.F. (1995). Producing experts, constructing expertise: The School of Pharmacy of the Pharmaceutical Society of Great Britain, 1842–1896. In *The History of Medical Education in Britain* (Nutton, V., Porter, R. Eds.), pp. 116–140. Rodopi, Amsterdam/Atlanta.

Morson, A. (1990). T.N.R. Morson and his scientific friends. *Pharmaceutical Historian* 20 (4), 6–7. <http://www.bshp.org/bshpwebsite/index.htm>

Tallis, N., and Arnold-Foster, K. (1991). *Pharmacy History: A Pictorial Record*. Pharmaceutical Press, London. <http://www.rpharms.com/museum-shop/books-and-cards.asp>

Wallis, T.E. (1964). *History of the School of Pharmacy, University of London*. Pharmaceutical Press, London.

INDEX

Note: Page numbers followed by "*f*" and "*b*" refer to figures and boxes, respectively.